NATURAL PRODUCTS AND THERAPEUTICS

GINGER'S ANTIMICROBIAL, ANTI-NAUSEA AND ANTI-OSTEOARTHRITIC ACTIVITIES

Natural Products and Therapeutics

Additional books and e-books in this series can be found on Nova's website under the Series tab.

NATURAL PRODUCTS AND THERAPEUTICS

GINGER'S ANTIMICROBIAL, ANTI-NAUSEA AND ANTI-OSTEOARTHRITIC ACTIVITIES

DIANA R. CUNDELL
EDITOR

nova
Medicine & Health
New York

https://doi.org/10.52305/HHIR2325

NOTICE TO THE READER

The Publisher has taken reasonable care in the preparation of this book, but makes no expressed or implied warranty of any kind and assumes no responsibility for any errors or omissions. No liability is assumed for incidental or consequential damages in connection with or arising out of information contained in this book. The Publisher shall not be liable for any special, consequential, or exemplary damages resulting, in whole or in part, from the readers' use of, or reliance upon, this material. Any parts of this book based on government reports are so indicated and copyright is claimed for those parts to the extent applicable to compilations of such works.

Independent verification should be sought for any data, advice or recommendations contained in this book. In addition, no responsibility is assumed by the Publisher for any injury and/or damage to persons or property arising from any methods, products, instructions, ideas or otherwise contained in this publication.

This publication is designed to provide accurate and authoritative information with regard to the subject matter covered herein. It is sold with the clear understanding that the Publisher is not engaged in rendering legal or any other professional services. If legal or any other expert assistance is required, the services of a competent person should be sought. FROM A DECLARATION OF PARTICIPANTS JOINTLY ADOPTED BY A COMMITTEE OF THE AMERICAN BAR ASSOCIATION AND A COMMITTEE OF PUBLISHERS.

Additional color graphics may be available in the e-book version of this book.

Library of Congress Cataloging-in-Publication Data

ISBN: 978-1-68507-117-2

Published by Nova Science Publishers, Inc. † New York

Contents

PREFACE

Ginger has a strong reputation as an anti-nausea agent but our understanding of the roles played by its important biological constituents (gingerols and shogaols) as antimicrobial and anti-inflammatory agents has not been examined in detail. This series of monographs seeks to look first at how and why ginger was used as an ethnomedicine and how this expanded into general antimicrobial studies. One cardinal use for ginger and its constituents may be in the topical management of osteoarthritis. Given the widespread nature of this condition and ginger's ability to block pain receptors it may join other molecules such as capsaicin in this mode of treatment.

Chapter 1 - Ayurvedic and traditional Chinese medicines have used ginger root in their formulations for the treatment of infection, and arthritic syndromes as well as nausea and indigestion for at least 5,000 years. Ancient Rome and Greece placed ginger firmly in the role of stomach settler and anti-emetic and that has been its primary use ever since. Chemical analysis of the ginger root in the 20th century revealed that the active components of gingerols and their metabolites, the shogaols, are non-competitive inhibitors of the serotonin and cholinergic receptors of the gastrointestinal tract. Gingerols and shogaols are also potent anti-inflammatory agents, able to block a variety of enzymes including cyclooxygenase (COX) enzymes. Indeed, this latter property along with other anti-inflammatory activities may allow ginger to leave its typecast role as anti-nausea agent and allow its development for a wide range of chronic conditions. This chapter will discuss the history of the use of ginger, the bioavailability of its components, evaluate clinical trials of its anti-nausea and anti-emesis effects and explore the development of novel delivery technologies. Finally, given our understanding of the molecular mechanisms of actions of ginger an overview of potential new roles in the treatment of chronic gastrointestinal conditions will be made.

Chapter 2 - Bacterial infections represent one of the leading causes of death worldwide. With the drastic rise in bacterial-related infections, it has become shockingly apparent that the once effective sources of treatment have begun to lose its potency. The use of antibiotics has been the primary therapy against bacterial infections for years. Unfortunately, many bacteria are developing resistance resulting in the inefficacy of many antibiotics. The race to find a solution to antibiotic resistance has focused in on the potential of plants and their active constituents as novel antimicrobials. Phytochemicals have been used for centuries in alternative medicine in remedies against different malaises. *Zingiber officinale* (ginger) rhizome has been used as a spice and as a health supplement due to its numerous properties. Over the recent years the interest in ginger and its compounds has increase, so scientific research which has generated a great amount of data on the efficacy of these chemicals against different diseases. In this review the authors present an overview of studies conducted on the antibacterial efficacy of ginger against the causative agents of infections in 4 major body systems; skin and joints, respiratory, digestive, and the oral cavity.

Chapter 3 - Fungal infections are on the rise globally with an increase in immunocompromised populations and a corresponding decrease in effectiveness of selective pharmaceuticals for treatment due to cost, availability and resistance. Ginger *(Zingiber officinale* Roscoe) has been used for centuries in both the Traditional Chinese Medicine (TCM) and Ayurvedic traditional systems for a wide range of uses including as an antifungal agent and as an immunomodulator. This review explores ginger's production of antifungal enzymes and chemicals in the soil environment, the physiological and biochemical mechanism of how ginger changes cell membranes and inhibits hyphal growth in comparison to other antifungal plant species. The antifungal effectiveness of ginger essential oils to other plant species are systematically reviewed based on chemical constituents, geographic range, and mechanism of action. The cumulative scientific evidence establishes the potential of ginger as an adjuvant treatment in an integrative medicine system to address the two leading fungal pathogens *Candida* and *Aspergillus*.

Chapter 4 - Ginger is on a growing list of natural sources under consideration in development of new antiviral compounds. This chapter is a comprehensive review of research investigating the use of ginger as an antiviral agent. Compounds and mixtures isolated from ginger and tested for antiviral activity include 6-gingerols, 6-shogaol, sesquiterpenes, mixed polysaccharides, essential oils, and aqueous or solvent extracts. These compounds appear to exert several activities such as disruption of the viral life cycle, destabilization of the virion, and host immunity support. In some cases, viral proteins were predicted or found to bind to individual ginger compounds resulting in disruption of viral protein activity. To evaluate these compounds or extracts, a variety of methods were employed including molecular docking, viral plaque assays, viral titer, gene expression, histopathological score, symptom scoring markers of host immunity, and animal mortality. Viruses that infect a variety of human tissues, animals, and plant species were used as model systems for testing of the ginger compounds. A unifying conclusion from these studies is that ginger exhibits several antiviral activities that can be utilized in further development of new antiviral compounds for therapeutic use.

Chapter 5 - Ginger is a traditional medicine used by many cultures as a poultice or compress to alleviate pain and inflammation associated with swollen joints and rheumatic disorders. The primary activity of ginger involves phenolic gingerols, that are unstable and rapidly undergo decomposition to spicy shogaols. Studies have appeared in the literature that reported excellent anti-inflammatory activity for both gingerols and shogaols against isolated cells, as well as in animal models of osteoarthritis. Several meta-analyses of double-blind randomized placebo-controlled clinical trials (DBRPCT) of ginger have also suggested its potential use for human osteoarthritis patients. Osteoarthritis is a major cause of significant morbidity worldwide and current pharmaceutical interventions demonstrate both a lack of efficacy combined with significant side effects associated with long-term use. No current strategies exist to halt or reverse the condition. Patients with osteoarthritis and their health providers are therefore seeking newer, safer alternatives to manage this chronic condition. For many, the answer lies in the incorporation of phytomedicines as complementary therapies. To evaluate whether ginger and its bioactive phenols are potential candidates in managing osteoarthritis, this paper will discuss the history of the use of ginger for this condition and evaluate the scientific evidence from *in vitro* studies and animal models to DBRPCT of the condition. Finally, currently available effective delivery systems for gingerols and shogaols will be discussed as well as potential future strategies.

ACKNOWLEDGMENTS

Many individuals are involved in the creation of a book, providing a support system that allows it to grow and develop as an entity. First, my thanks go to my daughter Olivia and husband Michael who have been my sounding boards and supports throughout. My fellow authors approached the unsung abilities of ginger with various strategies and used their own styles to create a blend of approaches that makes for an excellent story. Our reviewers added and molded these chapters to become the final product you see now. We all learned a great deal from their supportive critique. Finally, thank you reader for your interest in the field of herbal medicine and particularly ginger. It is only through the spread of information about this field that it has the chance to continue to develop to its full potential.

In: Ginger's Antimicrobial ... ISBN: 978-1-68507-117-2
Editor: Diana R. Cundell

Chapter 1

GINGER AND THE GASTROINTESTINAL TRACT: BIOACTIVE EFFECTOR MOLECULES AND POSSIBLE FUTURE USES

Diana R. Cundell*, PhD
College of Life Sciences, Jefferson University,
Philadelphia, PA, USA

ABSTRACT

Ayurvedic and traditional Chinese medicines have used ginger root in their formulations for the treatment of infection, and arthritic syndromes as well as nausea and indigestion for at least 5,000 years. Ancient Rome and Greece placed ginger firmly in the role of stomach settler and anti-emetic and that has been its primary use ever since. Chemical analysis of the ginger root in the 20th century revealed that the active components of gingerols and their metabolites, the shogaols, are non-competitive inhibitors of the serotonin and cholinergic receptors of the gastrointestinal tract. Gingerols and shogaols are also potent anti-inflammatory agents, able to block a variety of enzymes including cyclooxygenase (COX) enzymes. Indeed, this latter property along with other anti-inflammatory

* Corresponding Author's E-mail: Diana.Cundell@jefferson.edu.

activities may allow ginger to leave its typecast role as anti-nausea agent and allow its development for a wide range of chronic conditions. This chapter will discuss the history of the use of ginger, the bioavailability of its components, evaluate clinical trials of its anti-nausea and anti-emesis effects and explore the development of novel delivery technologies. Finally, given our understanding of the molecular mechanisms of actions of ginger an overview of potential new roles in the treatment of chronic gastrointestinal conditions will be made.

Keywords: herbal medicine, phytochemical, shogaol, gingerol, gastrointestinal

INTRODUCTION

When most people think of ginger they think primarily of ginger ale for an upset stomach but this spice has been used for over 5000 years to treat not only gastrointestinal discomfort [1-3] but also infections, arthritis and hypertension [1,2]. The ginger plant (*Zingiber officinalis*), thrives in tropical and semi-tropical climates and was originally locally sourced in India and China, where it was incorporated into Ayurvedic and traditional Chinese medicines (TCM) [2, 3]. Medicinal use of ginger spread throughout south East Asia [4], with the Japanese using it to improve blood circulation and Indonesian people to prevent rheumatism [5]. During the 1st Century A.D., ginger rhizomes were traded from China and India along the major spice routes to Europe, where they rapidly gained medicinal and nutritional popularity [3, 5]. At this point ginger was used medicinally as a stomach settler and anti-emetic [3, 4], possibly reflecting the original Ayurvedic customs [6]. Leading ancient physicians who endorsed this use of ginger included the Greek physician Discorides who stated that "*it gently stimulates the gut and is profitable for the stomach*" [7]. Indeed, after one particularly indulgent Greek orgy ancient scholars report that nausea was combatted by consumption of whole ginger wrapped in bread [5].

Given that the teachings of Greek and Roman physicians were followed in many European nations, this may well be where ginger's usage became focused on gastrointestinal treatments [5-7]. From Europe ginger use spread to the Middle East and Africa, and later to the New World where the use of the spice was more diverse [8]. For example, in the Congo, ginger paste was used for headaches and in mixtures with mango juice for respiratory infections [8]. In the New World Latin American countries, the ginger plant thrived and began its commercial cultivation that has continued to this day [5]. Although still a central component of many folk remedies, ginger is now primarily advocated for gastrointestinal discomfort due to motion sickness, morning sickness and other emetic syndromes [5].

Ginger, like any other plant, consists of multiple components and an understanding of its efficacy must first identify which of these can individually or in concert with others produce physiological activities [1]. The part of ginger that is used are its rhizomes, which consist of starch (40-60%), proteins (up to 20%), lipids (up to 15%) and fibers (up to 7%) [3]. When ginger rhizomes are processed by steam distillation (currently, the major method used to produce medicinal ginger) the resultant oil contains over one hundred bioactive compounds [9]. Phenolic gingerols and their metabolites the shogaols are both the most abundant in ginger oil [10] and are now widely accepted as responsible for ginger's diverse biological activities [4].

Given that ginger's bioactivity is primarily tied to the phenolic gingerols and shogaols it contains, this editorial will focus on these moieties in evaluating the evidence supporting the potential use of ginger in the clinical setting. It will review our current understanding of the bioavailability of gingerols and shogaols, as well as their mechanism of action against nausea and emesis seen in pregnancy, chemotherapy treatment and post-surgical procedures. Finally, the modes of action of gingerols and shogaols will be discussed as to their future potential uses to prevent other inflammatory conditions. A more extensive evaluation of the antimicrobial and anti-inflammatory activities of gingerols and shogaols are the topics of future chapters in this book.

Gingerol and Shogaol Chemistry and Availability

Gingerols are chemically defined as a series of aromatic polyphenols with an α, β-unsaturated ketone structure with a varied unbranched alkyl chain [11]. They were discovered in 1879 when 6-gingerol ((S)-5-hydroxy-1-(4-hydroxy-3-methoxy)-3-decanone) was isolated as a yellow, pungent oil from the fresh, crushed ginger rhizome [12]. The ginger rhizome is now known to contain over thirty different members of this phenolic family [13], with 4-, 6-, 8- and 10-gingerols being isolated in lesser amounts [3, 5]. When exposed to heat gingerols undergo a dehydration reaction that converts them to the corresponding shogaol e.g., 6-gingerol becomes 6-shogaol ((E)-1-(4-hydroxy-3-methoxyphenyl) dec-4-en-3-one) [5]. Shogaols are spicier, more aromatic and have a higher stability than their corresponding gingerols [11, 14]. Comparison studies of shogaols and their gingerol parent molecules have reported a two to three-fold increase in the potency of antibacterial [15], antifungal [15], antioxidant [15, 16] and inflammatory [17] activity. Structures of the three common gingerols and shogaols appear in Figure 1.

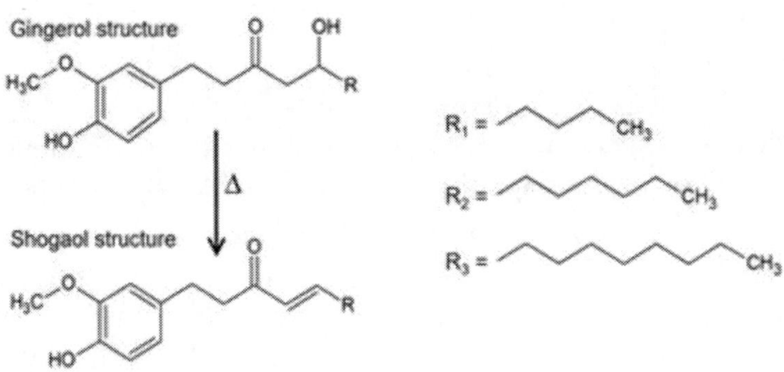

Figure 1. Figure illustrating comparative structures of the common gingerols and shogaols isolated from ginger. R represents differential chain structures for 6-, 8- and 10 forms of gingerol or shogaol. Figure modified from reference [5].

Metabolism and Bioavailability of Gingerols and Shogaols

Mammalian metabolism of 6-gingerol appears to primarily occur in the liver where uridine diphosphate glucuronosyltransferase enzymes add a glucuronide conjugate [18, 19]. Modified gingerols and shogaols, but not the free forms, are able to enter the circulation where they show different kinetics of absorption [11, 20-22]. Studies by Mukkavilli et al. [20], reported that ten minutes after mice were gavaged with ginger extract (250 mg/kg), 6-shogaol conjugates reached peak plasma levels, whereas 6-gingerol took two hours but reached peak levels nearly ten-fold higher. A second animal study by Jiang et al. [21] gavaged rats with a ginger extract containing 53% 6-gingerol (240 mg/kg). These authors only assayed 6-gingerol metabolites but reported that a peak plasma level occurred within ten minutes and reached maximal concentrations in the liver, kidney and especially the gastrointestinal tract by thirty minutes [21]. A more recent rodent study reported that 6-gingerol and 6-shogaol reached maximal plasma levels approximately fifty-four and forty minutes after the animals were gavaged with ginger extract (400 mg/kg) [11]. Maximal absorption of the 8-gingerols and shogaols occurred, approximately one hour after gavage and 10-gingerol and 10-shogaol required nearly ninety minutes to reach maximal levels [11]. Li et al. [11] reported that in each case the shogaol metabolite was absorbed more rapidly than the gingerol. In addition, both 6- and 8-gingerols and shogaols showed a second absorption spike approximately three hours following initial gavage [11]. These authors also determined a similar tissue distribution for the gingerol and shogaol metabolites into the rodent tissues as Jiang et al. [31], noting that it appeared they could easily cross the blood brain barrier [11].

Only one human study has appeared in the literature that explores the absorption of gingerols and shogaols in human subjects. Zick et al. [22] evaluated the oral absorption of ginger extract (0.1-2 g) into the plasma of twenty-seven healthy volunteers. They reported similar kinetics for 6-, 8- and 10-gingerol and 6-shogaol-conjugate appearance into the plasma within one hour of ingestion and full elimination two hours after ginger ingestion [22]. These studies strongly suggest that more data is needed to elucidate the pharmacokinetics of gingerols and shogaols, especially if animal models are used.

Ginger, Nausea and Emesis: Reviewing the Evidence

Nausea is a common problem and results from a multifactorial set of causes that commonly include infection, medication, hormonal changes during pregnancy and during chemotherapy [23]. Along with emesis, nausea is the most commonly reported gastrointestinal problem in population studies [24]. The uncomfortable and distressing symptoms of nausea with or without vomiting also account in a loss of at least $4 billion to the United States economy alone [23]. Nausea and vomiting are a common issue during the first trimester of pregnancy where symptoms can affect as many as 90% of all women [25]. Also termed nausea and vomiting of pregnancy (NVP), the loss of fluids to the mother and nutrients to the developing fetus can become a life-threatening condition in up to 2% of pregnancy when it is termed *hyperemesis gravitarum* (HG) [25]. Classic pharmacological interventions for NVP and HG are complicated by the physiological changes that occur during pregnancy coupled with the fact that most emetics are unsafe for the fetus [25]. As a result, ginger, acupressure and dietary changes are considered the three most acceptable and safe methodologies to control these conditions [25].

Around 60% of patients undergoing aggressive chemotherapy also commonly suffer with nausea and emesis, despite the availability of conventional anti-emetics that include $5HT_3$ antagonists and neurokinin (NK_1) inhibitors [26]. Termed chemotherapy-induced nausea and vomiting, or CINV, the adverse effects of chemotherapy can be so severe that patients cease eating or fail to maintain a balanced diet [26]. Some patients can also not afford the financial burden of these anti-emetics, which may be as much as $2,000 per cycle even with health insurance [26, 27]. This combination of adverse effects and monetary cost of anti-emetics has led many oncologists and their patients to seek reliable, safe and affordable alternatives [26, 27].

Another major cause of nausea and vomiting in a patient population are the sedation and opioid medications prescribed for patients undergoing surgery [28]. Termed postoperative nausea and vomiting (PONV), in serious cases this can result in dehydration and aspiration pneumonia, and extends the time patients take to heal and increases medical costs [28]. Similar medications as those utilized for CINV are prescribed for PONV together with dopamine D_2 antagonists [28]. As with CINV, the cost and side effects of these medications may be prohibitive for many patients [27, 28]. Adverse effects of $5HT_3$ antagonists, for example, include constipation and headache [26].

For CINV and PONV patients, one size does not fit all in terms of prescribing and this has led oncologists and surgeons to look for safer, less expensive alternatives that might be used more routinely [26, 28]. Ginger's reputation as a safe, anti-emetic and anti-nausea agent in pregnancy [25, 29, 30, 32-39] has led to it also being extensively studied for the alleviation of CINV [26, 39-54] and PONV [28, 39, 55-66]. The data from both recent meta analyses [25, 26, 28-30, 39, 40], together with reputable, without bias human double-blind, randomized, placebo-controlled clinical trials (DBRPCT) [32-38, 41-66] of patients in these three categories is evaluated in the section below.

Ginger and Nausea: Evidence from Human Double-Blind, Randomized, Placebo-Controlled Clinical Trials

Enough human clinical trials have been performed on the effects of whole or extracts of ginger on both nausea and emesis to allow seven major meta-analyses to appear in the literature [25, 26, 28-30, 39, 40]. Combining articles identified from the meta-analyses with additional literature publications identified thirty-four DBRPCT of ginger or its constituents [25, 26, 28-30, 32-67].

Three groups of patients were investigated namely, women with morning sickness (NVP) or *hyperemesis gravidarum* [32-38], patients with chemotherapy-induced vomiting (CINV) [41-54] and patients with post-operative nausea and vomiting (PONV) [55-67]. The study designs and results of these studies are shown in Tables 1-3 below.

Data from the seven studies of NVP or HG were highly consistent in reporting a significant decrease in the incidence of nausea and emesis compared to placebo ($p < 0.01$) using dosages of between 1,000 mg and 2,500 mg per day [32-38].

Table 1. Human clinical trials of the efficacy of ginger products in preventing nausea and vomiting in pregnancy or *hyperemesis gravidarum**

Study design	Results#	Reference
27 women with HG, 4 days of capsules with or without 1 g (4 x 250 mg) ginger powder, two-day washout and then 4 days of capsules.	Significant ↓ (p<0.002) in nausea and emesis in ginger treated group.	[32]
75 women with NVP, 4 days of capsules with or without ginger powder (1 g).	Significant ↓ (p<0.014) in nausea and emesis in ginger treated group.	[33]
26 women with NVP, syrup with or without 1g ginger, q.i.d. for 9 days.	Significant ↓ (p<0.01) in nausea and emesis in ginger treated group.	[34]
120 women with NVP, 125 mg ginger extract (equivalent to 1.5 g dried ginger) or placebo q.i.d. 4 days.	Significant ↓ (p<0.01) in nausea but not emesis in ginger treated group.	[35]
65 women with NVP, 5 cookies (biscuits) with or without 0.5 g of ginger powder (2.5 g)/day 4 days.	Significant ↓ (p<0.002) in nausea but not emesis in ginger treated group.	[36]
56 women with NVP, 200 mg ginger essence or 10 mg metoclopramide or placebo t.i.d. for 5 days.	Significant ↓ (p<0.001) in nausea and emesis in ginger treated group. Similar in efficacy to metoclopramide.	[37]
120 women, 250 mg ginger powder or placebo t.i.d. for 4 days.	Significant ↓ (p<0.001) in nausea and emesis in ginger treated group.	[38]

* Only double-blind randomized placebo-controlled data are presented in this table.
#Patients self-reported symptoms, q.i.d. = four times daily, t.i.d. = three times daily,

Table 2. Human clinical trials of the efficacy of ginger products in preventing chemotherapy-induced vomiting (CINV) nausea and vomiting*

Study design	Results#	Reference
Cross over trial 50 cancer (various) patients, received either 2 g total of ginger (4 x 500 mg capsules) or placebo for 3 days. 21-day washout period.	No significant difference in efficacy of ginger compared with metoclopramide.	[41]
Cross over trial 43 ovarian/cervical cancer patients, received either 1 g ginger for 5 days after chemotherapy or 1 g placebo and immediately the anti-emetic metoclopramide.	No significant difference seen in efficacy of ginger versus placebo.	[42]
129 cancer (various) patients, received capsules containing either 1g or 2 g of ginger or placebo for 3 days. Patients were also receiving standard anti-emetics (5-HT3 antagonist or aprepitant).	No significant difference seen in efficacy of ginger versus placebo. Patients taking aprepitant and ginger described an increase in symptoms.	[43]
Cross over trial of 36 cancer (various) patients, received 4 commercial ginger capsules (1 g total; Zintoma®, Gol Daru) or placebo one hour before and three days after chemotherapy. Three-week washout period and then a further three days with the alternative regimen of capsules.	No significant difference seen in efficacy of ginger versus placebo.	[44]
58 child cancer patients, received either 1 g ginger (6 × 167 mg) or 2 g (5 × 400 mg) based on patients' weight, or placebo for 3 days then observed for a further 10 days.	Significantly ↓ moderate and severe emesis ($p < 0.003$), severe delayed nausea ($p < 0.001$) and emesis ($p < 0.01$).	[45]
576 cancer (various) mostly female patients, received either 0.5, 1.0, 1.5 of ginger or placebo in 6 capsules for two six-day periods.	All doses reduced acute, but not delayed, nausea ($p = 0.003$). 0.5 and 1.0 g doses were optimal.	[46]
80 breast cancer patients received either 250 mg powdered ginger or placebo q.i.d.	Significant ↓in nausea, early and delayed emesis in ginger treated group ($p < 0.05$).	[47]
65 breast cancer patients received either 500 mg powdered ginger or placebo b.i.d. 5 days before and 5 days after chemotherapy.	Significant ↓in nausea and emesis in ginger treated group ($p < 0.05$).	[48]

Table 2. (Continued)

Study design	Results#	Reference
150 breast cancer patients received either 250 mg powdered ginger (5% gingerols) or placebo b.i.d for 3 days of 3 cycles.	Ginger ↓in nausea and vomiting but not significantly compared to placebo group.	[49]
Cross over trial of 34 breast cancer patients, received either 1 g ginger or placebo for 5 days, then washout period for 5 days.	No significant difference seen in efficacy of ginger versus placebo.	[50]
244 cancer (various) patients received either 160 mg of ginger capsules (shogaol and gingerol concentrations similar to fresh rhizome) or placebo for two treatment periods (42-56 days).	Significant ↓in nausea was identified for females and head and neck tumor patients ($p < 0.05$).	[51]
88 cancer (various) patients received either 10 mg 6-gingerol or placebo for 84 days.	Significant ↓in nausea, fatigue and ↑ in appetite was identified for patients receiving 6-gingerol ($p < 0.05$).	[52]
51 cancer (various) patients received either 300 mg (containing 60 mg of 5% standardized gingerols) or placebo for three cycles of chemotherapy. Outcomes assessed over 7 days of each cycle.	Significant ↓in nausea, fatigue and emesis identified for patients receiving ginger ($p < 0.05$) compared with placebo group over all three cycles of chemotherapy.	[53]
140 lung cancer patients received either 250 mg powdered ginger (5% gingerols) or placebo b.i.d for 5 days.	No significant difference seen in efficacy of ginger versus placebo.	[54]

* Only double-blind randomized placebo-controlled data are presented in this table.
#Patients self-reported symptoms, q.i.d. = four times daily, t.i.d. = three times daily.

The fourteen CINV studies showed more variability in ginger efficacy even when similar patients were considered [41-54]. Nine studies (64%) reported a significantly ($p < 0.05$) positive outcome for ginger's use in the suppression of nausea only [46, 51] or both nausea and vomiting [41, 45, 47, 48, 52, 53]. A tenth study reported a decrease in nausea incidence in the ginger group but this did not reach statistical significance [49]. The remaining five CINV studies recorded that ginger was not superior to placebo [42-44, 50, 54].

Table 3. Human clinical trials of the efficacy of ginger products in preventing post-operative nausea and vomiting (PONV)*

Study design	Results#	Reference
60 female laproscopic patients received 1 g ginger powder capsules, IV metoclopramide (10 mg) or placebo 1 h prior to the operation and assessed 4, 12 and 24 h post-surgery.	Significant ↓ in nausea and vomiting at in ginger group ($p<0.05$) but not at 24 h compared with placebo. Similar in efficacy to metoclopramide.	[55]
120 female laproscopic patients received 1 g ginger powder capsules, metoclopramide capsules (10 mg) or placebo 1 h prior to the operation and assessed 24 h post-surgery.	Significant ↓ in nausea and vomiting at in ginger group ($p<0.05$) at 24 h compared with placebo. Similar in efficacy to metoclopramide.	[56]
108 female laparoscopic patients received either 500 mg or 1 g powdered ginger or placebo, single dose, 1 h prior to operation.	No significant difference seen in efficacy of ginger versus placebo.	[57]
180 female laparoscopic patients received 300 mg capsule (ginger extract) or placebo 1 h before and 100 mg ginger or placebo 3 and 6 h after surgery.	No significant difference seen in efficacy of ginger versus placebo.	[58]
80 female laparoscopic patients received 1.5 g ginger powder capsules or placebo 1 h prior to the operation and assessed 2, 6 h and 24 h post-surgery.	Significant ↓ in nausea but not vomiting at 2 and 6h in ginger group ($p<0.05$) but not at 24 h compared with placebo.	[59]
60 female laparoscopic patients received 1.5 g ginger powder capsules or placebo 1 h prior to the operation and assessed 2 and 6 h post-surgery.	Significant ↓ in nausea and vomiting in ginger group at 6 h compared with placebo following procedure ($p < 0.05$).	[60]
120 gynecology patients received either ginger powder (1 g) or placebo 1 h prior to surgery and were assessed between 1 and 24 h post procedure.	Significant ($p < 0.05$) ↓ in PONV in ginger group seen 2 h and 6 h post operation.	[61]
120 patients (103♀ and 17♂) received either fresh ginger (250 mg), metoclopramide (10 mg), prochlorperazine (5 mg), promethazine (20 mg), ondansetron (4 mg) or placebo 1 h prior to and at 8 h intervals for 24 h post-surgery.	No patients in ginger group had nausea (15% vomited) 6 h after surgery. This was significantly ↓ compared with the classic anti-emetic medications (25-40% vomiting).	[62]

Table 3. (Continued)

Study design	Results#	Reference
160 ambulatory surgical patients received capsules of either ginger powder (1 g) or placebo 1 h after surgery.	Significant ($p<0.05$) ↓ in PONV in ginger group seen 2 h post operation.	[63]
100 ambulatory surgical patients (20 ♀ and 80♂) (received IV ondansetron (4 mg) with capsules of either ginger powder (1 g) or placebo 1 h after surgery.	No significant difference seen in efficacy of ginger versus placebo.	[64]
100 patients (71♀ and 29♂) undergoing cholecystectomy laparoscopic surgery received ginger powder capsules (1 g) or placebo with IV ondansetron (4 mg) 1 h prior to surgery and evaluated up to 24 h after surgery.	Significant ($p < 0.05$) ↓ in nausea in ginger group seen at all times post operation but no difference in vomiting compared with placebo.	[65]
150 female patients undergoing cholecystectomy laparoscopic surgery received either ginger powder capsules (0.5 g) or placebo 1 h prior to surgery and evaluated up to 12 h after surgery.	Nausea severity but not vomiting incidence was significantly ↓ in ginger group 2 hours after surgery ($p < 0.05$).	[66]
120 eye surgery patients (~ 60:40 ratio of males: females in ginger group) received capsules of ginger powder (1 g) or placebo 1 h prior to surgery and evaluated at up to 2 h post procedure.	Nausea severity and vomiting incidence was significantly ↓ in ginger group, 2 hours and up to 12 hours after surgery ($p < 0.05$).	[67]

* Only double-blind randomized placebo-controlled data are presented in this table.
# patients self-reported symptoms, h = hour, IV = intravenous.

One of these trials was a cross over design and did not employ a wash out period between ginger and placebo administration [50]. This is a poor study design as it means any benefits from one treatment may superimpose on the other. It may explain why ginger and placebo were not found to be significantly different in efficacy in preventing nausea and vomiting in these CINV patients [50]. Powdered ginger capsules were used in all but one of the studies [52] and only five studies utilized any standardization of ginger for gingerols or shagoals [49, 51, 53, 54] or purified 6-gingerol itself [52].

It is encouraging that the single trial in which 6-gingerol was employed utilized both a low dose to produce efficacy (10 mg) and was shown to significantly reduce nausea and increase patient appetite $p < 0.05$ [52].

Identifying which CINV patients might respond best to ginger using the data from these DBRPCT has proven difficult, although one study did report that female patients showed enhanced responsiveness to the spice [51]. Of the six studies that involved solely female patients or identified female patients' responsiveness, ginger was reported as without effect in two studies [42, 50], approached significance in a third [49] and was significantly better at controlling emesis and vomiting in the remaining four [46-49].

Ten of the thirteen DBRPCT investigated PONV either only in female patients [55-61, 66] or primarily female patients [62,65]. Interestingly, eight of the ten DBRPCT (80%) reported that ginger significantly decreased PONV symptoms ($p<0.05$) [55-59, 62, 65, 66]. In contrast, the single study of primarily male surgical patients reported no efficacy for ginger [64]. Seven of the DBRPCT evaluated the effect of ginger at preventing PONV in female patients undergoing various gynecological procedures [55-61]. Five studies reported a significant ($p<0.05$) decrease in PONV symptoms post-surgery [55-59], while the remaining two [60, 61] did not. This observation that female nausea and vomiting maybe more responsive to ginger was also suggested by Anh et al. in a recent meta-analysis [39]. There is also evidence that female patients are more likely to experience more emesis and nausea following chemotherapy than males [68]. Given that male patients experience, or describe, fewer symptoms it would therefore be more difficult to achieve significance in those clinical trials of ginger products in which males predominate or are a significant component.

Clearly gender is not the only correlate, given that two large studies demonstrated no efficacy for ginger [60, 61], and other issues such as inconsistency of ginger preparations, dosages, times of administration and study design have been raised in several meta-analyses [25, 26, 28-30, 39, 40] also make interpretation difficult.

Most investigators used ginger powder, which can contain anywhere from 0.036–13.8 mg/g of gingerols and 0.2-6.62 mg/g of shogaols [69-71]. Studies by Marx et al. [70] and Shwertner et al. [71], reported the presence of all three major gingerols, namely 6-, 8- and 10-gingerol, 6-shogaol and 10-shogaol in ginger powder (spice) and commercial ginger supplements. Both studies reported a wide variation in gingerol levels of between 0 and 82.2 mg/g, with 6-gingerol being the most predominant component at between 0 and 66.5 mg/g [70, 71]. 6-shogaol levels in the supplements examined ranged 0 and 16.6 mg/g.

This large variation in gingerol and shogaol content may go some way to explain why 1 g or even 2.5 g of ginger powders or supplements might be without significant effect. So, when a dose of 2.0 g of ginger was reported as "without adverse effects" [72], it may also be because it lacks biological activity. Even in studies that stated they used "5% gingerols", (see Table 1) the ginger powder was not directly tested prior to the trial and so may not have actually contained sufficient active ingredient.

Although none of the DBRPCT was performed in Germany, this is one of few countries where spices are nationally regulated and approved as non-prescription medications [73]. The German Commission E on nutraceuticals recommends 1 g per day of ginger [73] to prevent nausea and emesis, which may be where the DBRPCT obtained their dosages. Although 1 g of well-prepared ginger powder could, in practice, contain anywhere up to 13.8 mg of gingerols, the actual minimum effective human dosage of these agents has not yet been determined.

Biochemically, it may also be that gingerols display optimal kinetics only at lower concentrations [46]. For example, studies by Ryan et al. [46] suggested that once ginger's bioactive components saturate receptors higher doses would be ineffective. It is to be hoped that future studies will employ purified gingerols and shogaols, and with a single ginger component and dosage then producing data to confirm or refute the existing DBRPCT. Identifying optimal uses for ginger and its constituents to prevent nausea and emesis also requires an understanding of how they impact the mechanisms involved in these reflexes at the molecular level.

MOLECULAR MECHANISMSOF NAUSEA AND EMESIS

Nausea results from stimulation of the *nucleus tractus solitarius* (NTS) in the medulla oblongata of the brain [74-76]. Four separate pathways of NTS activation have been identified [74-76] and their mode of action is summarized in Figure 2.

Nausea and Vomiting in Pregnancy: Pathophysiology and Management

Predisposition to NVP and HG appears to involve a variety of factors [78] but researchers have suggested roles for gastrointestinal inflammation, through elevated inflammatory factors such as prostaglandin E_2 (PGE_2) and interleukin 1 (IL-1) [79]. Several researchers have also correlated HG with an increased frequency of infection with the bacterium *Helicobacter pylori* [80-82]. *H. pylori* appears able to colonize pregnant women more successfully due to changes in the stomach pH [83] and possibly local immunosuppression [84]. Management of NVP and HG has to proceed with caution to avoid harming the fetus [78]. Primarily, for pregnant women management of NVP and HG involves prevention of nausea through ingestion of lighter and more frequent meals and a focus on hydration [78]. Ginger is an advocated complementary medicine for both NVP and HG and has generally been successful for this treatment group [78].

Chemotherapy-Induced Nausea and Vomiting: Pathophysiology and Treatment

CINV appears to be initiated by damage to the enterochromaffin cells in the gastrointestinal tract and their consequent inflammation and release of free radicals [85, 86].

Elevations in free radical levels induce the enterochromaffin cells to secrete serotonin (5-HT) and this can activate or sensitize the vagal nerve by binding to local serotonin (5-HT3) receptors [85, 86]. Acute CINV (appears within 24 hours and is maximal at 6 hours) is believed to be mediated directly through a direct 5-HT3 receptor-initiated pathway involving the NTS [85, 87]. In contrast, delayed CINV (appears after 24 hours and lasts up to 6 days) is associated with sensitization of the vagus nerve to other neurotransmitters such as substance P and NK-1 [85, 87]. As previously stated, substance P acts as an intermediary in transferring signals from activated 5-HT3 receptors to the *area postrema* and NTS using the NK-1 receptors (Figure 2). Cross talk between 5-HT3 and NK-1 receptors may also potentiate these effects, according to animal studies [85-89]. To underline the differences between CINV and NVP/HG, serotonin levels in the latter conditions have been shown to show no correlation with either nausea or emesis [90, 91]. Although the gender component of CINV is poorly understood, women do seem more likely to report more severe symptoms [68]. This observation means that any studies of CINV remediation need to identify males and females in the study groups to identify efficacy.

Treatment of CINV is optimally achieved through a combination of three medications [92, 93]. Use of the 5-HT3 antagonist ondansetron together with the anti-inflammatory steroid dexamethasone and the NK-1 inhibitor aprepitant was shown to prevent vomiting in up to 78% of patients receiving cisplatin chemotherapy [93]. For delayed CINV, 5-HT3 medications alone are ineffective, with dexamethasone and NK-1 inhibitors instead preventing nausea and emesis in these patients [92]. Dopamine antagonists such as metoclopramide are typically reserved as rescue medications for CINV patients [92, 94]. These agents bind to D2 and D3 receptors in the *area postrema*, thereby directly preventing emesis [95]. Metoclopramide is particularly useful in that its structure allows it to antagonize not only D2 but also 5-HT3 and histamine (H1) receptors [95].

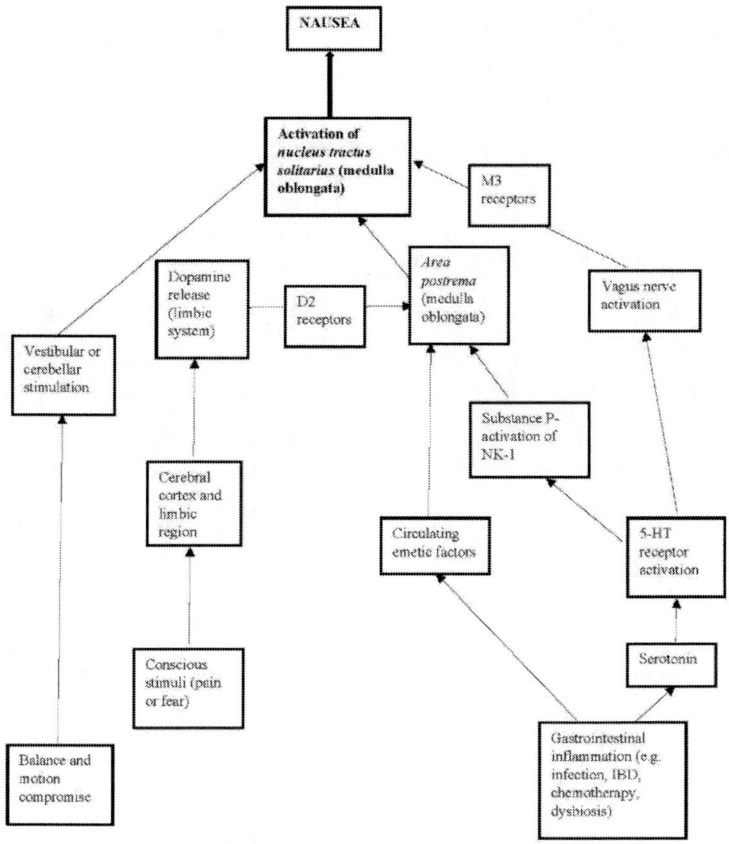

Figure 2. Central to nausea is activation of the *nucleus tractus solitarius* (NTS) in the medulla oblongata of the brain. This can occur by one of four separate pathways. Balance anomalies such as dizziness or motion can activate vestibular and cerebellar stimulation of the NTS [75]. Conscious stimuli of nausea e.g., smell, fear can affect the cerebral cortex and limbic system also stimulating NTS-induced nausea [74]. Chemical messengers including blood toxins (possibly from gastrointestinal infection) or other emesis-inducing factors can stimulate the *area postrema* of the medulla oblongata and in turn the NTS [75]. Abdominal vagal afferent nerves that detect gastric tone and contents can directly stimulate the NTS during gastrointestinal anomalies through muscarinic receptors [75]. This latter effect may result from serotonin (5-hydroxytryptamine; 5-HT) release during gastrointestinal inflammation and its stimulation of 5-HT3 receptors on vagal and spinal nerves [77]. Substance P picks up the signals from 5-HT3 receptors and then transfers them, via the neurokinin-1 (NK-1) receptors, to the *area postrema* and then the NTS [74-77]. Limbic system activation releases dopamine, which interacts with D2 receptors in the *area postrema* [74]. Activation of NTS through all these mechanisms can then induce nausea [74-77].

Post-Operative Nausea and Vomiting: Pathophysiology and Treatment

PONV appears to be directly connected with the duration of anesthesia the patient experiences with volatile agents such as nitrous oxide more likely to produce PONV than intravenous variants [96]. Administration of IV opioids, both during and after surgery, can also directly activate emesis via direct interaction with the brainstem but may also affect gut motility and thereby sensitize the vagal nerve to communicate with the NTS [96, 97]. Inhaled anesthetics can also potentiate 5-HT3 signals to induce emesis [98]. Opioids may also cause emesis by binding directly to mu receptors in the *area postrema* [97]. Both anesthetics and opioids are believed to affect gastric motility through their ability to increase levels of circulating vasopressin in a similar manner to the physiology of motion sickness [96, 99] i.e., vestibular or cerebellar stimulation of the NTS [75]. A combination of endogenously released gastrointestinal opioids due to surgical stress and exogenous opioids can result in a condition termed postoperative ileum in which peristalsis is impaired and passage of stool is inhibited [100].

Most of the current understanding of how PONV works has derived from studies in which various anti-emetic agents were effective when administered to patients either individually or as combination therapy [96]. Similar medications are used as those for CINV [85, 87], but for PONV antagonism of 5-HT3-mediated pathways by medications such as ondansetron has been the most effective [96], followed by dopamine antagonists [93, 95] and NK-1 receptor antagonists [101]. PONV is also prevented by dexamethasone when combined with 5-HT3 antagonists [102]. Dexamethasone's mechanism of action in preventing PONV is unclear but believed to stem from its prevention of nerve sensitization by preventing inflammatory mediator release [103]. Glucocorticoids, like dexamethasone, may also directly interact with steroid receptors in the NTS [104] and inhibit 5-HT3 receptors [105].

Mechanisms of Anti-Emetic and Anti-Nausea Action of Gingerols and Shogaols: Implications for NVP, CINV and PONV

Patients with NVP, CINV and PONV clearly have divergent mechanisms involved in their nausea and emesis [78, 80-86, 95-100]. The fact that these symptoms still is an issue, despite pharmaceutical interventions, means that it is important to identify for any new therapy how and where it might fill in the gaps or substitute for an existing medication. Much of the understanding of how ginger and its components reduce emesis and vomiting has been gained from studies using isolated animal small intestine [106-108] or vagal nodose ganglia [109]. Ginger components 6-gingerol and 6-shogaol inhibited acetylcholine-, serotonin- and carbachol-induced contractions of the guinea pig ileum [106-108]. Several studies also suggest potent anti-inflammatory effects for 6-, 8- and 10-gingerols or 6-shogaols, using various systems including isolated mouse macrophages [110], human neutrophils [110], lipopolysaccharide (LPS)-activated human macrophages (U937 cells) [111], human hepatic cancer cells (HuH7) [112] and human colorectal cells [113]. Gingerols have been found to be antimicrobial both against gastrointestinal pathogens [114, 115] as well as those producing antibiotic-resistant biofilms [116, 117].

Most importantly, gingerols and shogaols may have direct effects on several nausea and emesis-inducing pathways by interacting with muscarinic (M3), 5-HT3 and dopamine (D2) receptors. Molecular binding studies by Abdel-Aziz et al. [106] concluded that 6-, 8- and 10-gingerol together with 6-shogaol may be able to directly inhibit emesis by binding to ileal 5-HT3 receptors. These findings were confirmed by Pertz et al. [107], who also described the antagonism of guinea pig ileal muscarinic M3 receptors by 6-, 8- and 10-gingerol. Further, *in vitro* studies of dispersed visceral afferent neurons rat nodose ganglia reported that 6-gingerol and 6-shogaol could directly inhibit 5-HT3 responses [109].

Interestingly in this latter study, the two ginger phenols were able to behave as non-competitive inhibitors of the 5-HT3 receptor, making them different from current classic 5-HT3 inhibitors which are competitive antagonists [109]. Several animal models of emesis reported a significant decrease ($p < 0.05$) in retching and vomiting symptoms when gingerol was administered prior to cisplatin [118-121]. At the molecular level, this correlated with a significant decrease ($p < 0.05$) in expression of substance P [118, 119, 121], 5-HT3 [118, 121], NK-1 receptors [119, 121] and dopamine (D2) receptors [118, 120, 121] in both the ileal mucosa and *area postrema* of these animals.

Gingerols and Shogaols Anti-Nausea and Emesis Mechanisms in Pregnancy-Induced Vomiting

Gastrointestinal inflammation, in particular that mediated by cyclooxygenase-2 (COX-2)-induced prostaglandin E_2 (PGE_2), is believed to play a major role in the pathophysiology of NVP [79]. Several reports have appeared in the literature that demonstrate gingerols and or shogaols down-regulate COX-2 expression in resting [110] or activated [111-113] cells. Shogaols, in particular 6-shogaol, were reported to be superior to 6-gingerol in reducing COX-2 expression in resting human cells [110]. Expression of COX-2 was decreased by 6-, 8- and 10-gingerol in LPS-activated murine macrophages [111] and 6-gingerol in interleukin-1beta (IL-1β)-stimulated human hepatocytes [113]. Interestingly, no effect was seen in on LPS-stimulated murine macrophage COX-2 expression when 6-shogaol was used; data which may suggest a species difference [111].

Lantz et al. also reported that the release of nitric oxide (NO) and PGE_2 from N-formyl-l-methionyl-leucyl-methionyl-phenylalanine (FMLP)-stimulated human neutrophils was inhibited by both gingerols and shogaols [111]. Finally, studies by Breemen et al. [122] further demonstrated that both gingerols and shogaols (8- and 10-series) were able to directly bind to and inhibit the enzyme COX-2 but not its analog "housekeeping" enzyme COX-1 using *in vitro* biochemical studies.

Given that the major product of COX-2 is PGE_2, these data together suggest that gingerols and or shogaols may be acting to impair NVP in part by preventing the generation of this prostaglandin. In the DBRPCT of the effect of ginger on NVP, several preparations of ginger were used namely ginger powder [33, 34, 36, 38], ginger essence [37] and ginger extract [35]. Optimization of gingerol content has been described using ginger oil from steam distillation [123] and a microwave-ethanol extraction [124], methods which potentially correlate with at least two of the DBRPCT [35, 37]. Ginger powders may have various preparative processes but are likely to contain a relatively equivalent mixture of both gingerol and shogaol constituents [70, 71]. This may explain why the DBRPCT were effective as the various ginger sources would all be expected to contain some variant of anti-inflammatory gingerols and shogaols.

A second component to NVP, and particularly its HG variant is infection of the pregnant patient with *H. pylori* [80-84]. Studies by Mahady et al. [114] have reported that 6-, 8-, and 10-gingerols together with 6-shogaol were able to kill nineteen clinical isolates of *H. pylori in vitro*. Interestingly, five of the nineteen clinical strains investigated possessed the *Cag+* gene i.e., were linked to the development of severe gastritis and adenocarcinoma [114]. Minimum inhibitory concentrations (MIC) for the gingerols for these five *Cag+ H. pylori* strains was between 1.56 and 6.25 μg/ml and demonstrated increasing antibacterial activity with increasing gingerol chain length [114]. 6-shogoal was not as active as the gingerols against the five *Cag+ H. pylori* strains with an MIC of 12.25-25 μg/ml [114].

So, how do gingerols compare with conventional antibiotics at killing *H. pylori*? The two most commonly used antibiotics for *H. pylori* are metronidazole and ciprofloxacin [125]. Most *H pylori* clinical isolates display MIC of >8 μg/ml for metronidazole and >1 μg/ml for ciprofloxacin [125], so clearly gingerols are at least as effective. Both metronidazole [126] and ciprofloxacin [127] act by diffusing into the bacterial cell and disrupting DNA synthesis. In contrast, gingerols appear to bind to the bacterial cell membrane and allow nucleic acids and other proteins to leak out of the bacterial cells [128]. Certainly, the DBRPCT involving subjects with NVP or HG all used dosages of ginger powder/ supplement of between 1 and 2.5 g [32-38]. Given that 1 g of ginger powder has been reported to contain at least 36 μg of gingerols [70, 71], all these studies would have used a sufficient dosage to kill *H. pylori* in these subjects.

Gingerols and Shogaols Anti-Nausea and Emesis Mechanisms in Chemotherapy-Induced Vomiting

CINV is the only one of the three syndromes that ginger has been tested on to be investigated using animal models of the condition [118-121, 129]. Five studies have, to date, appeared in the literature that report the ability of gingerols to significantly decrease ($p < 0.05$) decrease pica (non-food ingestion) in cisplatin-induced vomiting models of mink [118, 119, 121] or rats [120, 121, 129]. Performed by two research groups, these studies all administered gingerol or the vehicle (saline) by gavage to either Wistar rats (10-40 mg/kg) or mink (50-200 mg/ kg) thirty minutes before intraperitoneal administration of cisplatin (rats 3 or 6 mg/kg and mink 6 mg/kg) [118-121, 129].

The most recent of these, by Tian et al. [121], demonstrated that gingerol treatment had decreased the number of abnormal neurons in the *area postrema* of these animals as well as protecting the normal ileal structure over a period of three days [121]. The study by Tian et al. [121] is the only one to date in which gingerol was directly compared with metoclopramide, in terms of both efficacy and dosage. In terms of dosages, metoclopramide at 2.5 mg/kg for rats and 4.0 mg/kg for mink was significantly less effective ($p < 0.05$) than 40 mg/kg of gingerol and 200 mg/kg at preventing emesis and retching in rats and mink, respectively [121]. No actual dosage equivalents were identified in this study between gingerol and metoclopramide in preventing animal CINV [121]. Feng et al. [129], reported that similar significant effects ($p < 0.05$) on rat retching and vomiting were seen with 25 mg/kg of 6-gingerol and 1.3 mg/kg of the 5-HT3 antagonist ondansetron.

Although the above studies are encouraging and provide an explanation of the mechanism of action of gingerols in preventing nausea and emesis they have to be interpreted with caution. The animal models used contain similar receptor and neurological pathways involved in initiating nausea [118-121, 129]. It is important to note that rats and mink do not actually vomit but retch and exhibit pica (eat non-food items to settle their stomachs) [118-121, 129]. Animals in these models of CINV received similar levels of cisplatin, weight-wise (3 or 6 mg/kg) [118-121, 129] as human oncology patients (60 mg/ mm^2) [130]. In contrast, the amount of anti-emetic/ anti-nausea agents is much higher for animals in terms of a weight: agent ratio [118-121, 129]. Metoclopramide and ondansetron were given to rats at dosages of 2.5 mg/kg [121] and 1.3 mg/kg [129], respectively whereas the human dosages of both medications is only10 mg total [131, 132].

These limitations mean that translating the efficacy of gingerols in rats and mink to human subjects is challenging. Evidence that supports further research in this field has, however, come from the recent human DBRPCT that investigated the efficacy of purified 6-gingerol rather than ginger powder on CINV [52]. Over a period of 84 days, oral 6-gingerol at an identical dose to that of either intravenous metoclopramide or ondansetron, namely 10 mg [131, 132], significantly prevented nausea and encouraged eating in chemotherapy patients [52]. At this point new DBRPCT, which add gingerol to existing combination therapies, may also determine which medications the phenol may either substitute for or provided additive or complementary activities.

Gingerols and Shogaols Anti-Nausea and Emesis Mechanisms in Post-Operative Vomiting

Although no selective animal models are currently available for studies of PONV, given that the symptoms are treated using similar antagonists as CINV [93, 102-105] it may be anticipated that any benefits of gingerols involve similar targets. One difference for PONV pathophysiology is its being triggered by post-operative administration of opioids [96, 97]. Opioids block pain by binding to mu receptors but cause nausea as an adverse effect when those receptors are in the *area postrema* [97]. Gingerols and shogaols have also been reported to be analgesic (antinociceptive) in several rat models of pain induced by carrageenan [133, 134], formalin [134] or applied heat [135].

Antinociceptive activity of gingerols and shogaols appears unrelated to their antagonism of 5-HT3, dopamine and substance P pathways [136, 137]. Instead, like other plant-based phenols such as vanillin and capsaicin, gingerols and shogaols are agonists of the transient receptor potential cation channel subfamily V member 1 (TRPV1) or vanillin (VR1) receptor [136, 137]. Studies by Dedov et al. [137] first reported that 6- and 8-gingerol were able to directly bind to TRPV1/VR1 receptors in isolated rat dorsal root ganglion neurons with a sensitivity similar to capsaicin. Later docking studies, using an immobilized silica model, confirmed this finding and also reported that 10-gingerol as well as 6-8 and 10-shogaol analogs were also able to bind to TRPV1/VR1 receptors with high affinity [137].

The TRPV1/VR1 receptor is found in tissues throughout the human central and peripheral nervous system, but most strongly concentrated in the brainstem [138, 139]. To take this one level further, TRPV1/VR1 pathways are also involved with the induction of emesis and nausea [139, 140]. Early studies, by Andrews and Bhandari [139] of the capsaicin analog and TRPV1/VR1-inhibitor resinferatoxin (RTX), observed that this agent blocked the emesis in ferrets exposed to radiation (200 rads) or who were gavaged with copper sulfate (40 mg/ml). Similar anti-emetic results have been found using capsaicin (0.033-33 mM) or RTX (16-160 μM) pre-treatment of vagally-stimulated paralyzed dogs [141].

While the mechanism underpinning how agents interacting with TRPV1/VR1 receptors block emesis is currently unclear, Rudd et al. [140], suggest that they act to reduce intracellular substance P and internalize NK-1 receptors on neurons in the NTS. As previously stated, several authors reported a 6-gingerol-induced inhibition in emesis in animal models of CINV that correlated with a significant decrease ($p < 0.05$) in expression of substance P [118, 119], and NK-1 receptors [119, 121] in the *area postrema* of these animals. Clearly, if gingerols and shogaols can interact with these receptors their development as a mainstream pharmaceutical might well provide an alternative therapy that might combine analgesia with nausea prevention. Time of administration prior to surgery to prevent PONV is also important given that the TRPV1/VR1 inhibitor RFX required administration at least twenty minutes in ferrets [139] and forty minutes in dogs [141] to be effective.

Probiotic Effects of Gingerols and Shogaols: Important in Managing NVP and CINV

During pregnancy the gut microbiome population changes and shows an increased risk for the development of abnormal shifts in species distribution coupled with a decrease in microbial diversity (dysbiosis) [142]. Patients undergoing chemotherapy display inflammatory changes in their intestinal lining (mucositis) and a narrowing in the diversity of their intestinal flora, which play a role in delayed CINV symptoms [130]. Recent studies by Elmrassy et al. [143] described a shift of bacterial flora towards beneficial bacteria in rodents fed gingerols and shogaols for up to thirty days. Feng et al. [129] further reported that 6-gingerol, but not ondansetron, could reverse the gastrointestinal dysbiosis induced by cisplatin in rats. Taken together these results suggestive of a probiotic amplifying role for ginger and its components, which, if it translates to human patients, would add another potential role to the use of ginger components in NVP and CINV management.

Strategies to Standardize and Deliver Gingerols and Shogaols

Currently the only way to potentially obtain gingerols and shogaols at levels that might provide potential physiological effects is to purchase them as ginger supplements termed nutraceuticals, but even this is a variable proposition [70, 71, 144]. Nutraceuticals receive no standardization in most countries, excepting those in Europe [1, 73] and so can contain any amount of bioactivity or even none at all; a factor which plays a major role in perpetuating a distrust of their usage [70, 71, 144].

To put this in perspective, three studies of more than twenty commercial ginger supplements or powders reported that gingerol and shogaol levels ranged from between 0 to 66 mg/kg and 0 to 16 mg/kg, respectively [70, 71 and 144]. One reason for this may also be due to there being no stated shelf life or storage conditions for nutraceuticals as they are considered "food items" [1, 145]. Studies by Ghasamzedeh et al. [145] reported that, even in fresh rhizomes, levels of 6-gingerol and 6-shagoal fell by more than seventy percent after eight months of storage. No stability studies even exist in the literature for ginger supplements.

Some researchers have addressed the problem of gingerols and shogaol lability through the development of various semi-synthetic forms of the phenols [146-150]. At least nine studies have also recently appeared in the literature where gingerols and or shogaols have been immobilized inside nanoparticles, or micelles or bound to inert surfaces [151-159]. Each of these methods would allow standardized doses to be tested for efficacy in preventing nausea and emesis in a variety of gastrointestinal syndromes.

Current State of the Art of Semi-Synthetic Forms of Gingerols and Shogaols

Seven synthetic variants of 6-gingerol and related phenylalkanol analogs were first created by Koo et al. [146], who used them to impair human platelet aggregation. Koo et al. [146] determined that at least two of the analogs were at least twice as effective on a mol for mol basis as aspirin at impairing platelet aggregation and COX-2 *in vitro*. These authors did not, however, identify the structural components of gingerols needed to be most effective [146]. Morera et al. [147], created twenty analogs of 6-gingerol and used these to investigate their bioactivity against TRPV1 pain receptors. These authors identified that optimal activity of synthetic 6-gingerol analogs required the presence of a phenolic hydroxyl group and increasing lipophilic activity of the side chain with variants in the ketone region providing only minimal effects on bioactivity [147]. Seven of the twenty analogs were highly active, stable and selective: three against TRPV1 receptors and four TRPA1 antagonists [147].

Two *in vitro* studies investigated the ability of semi-synthetic derivatives of 6-gingerol [148, 149] or 6-shogaol [148] to be tumoricidal. Kumboonma et al. [148], generated a total of thirteen analogs of 6-gingerol and 6-gingerol and evaluated their activity as antioxidants and inhibitors of histone deacetylase (HDAC) activity in human kidney tumor cells (HeLa). Demethylated 6-shogaol demonstrated optimal stability and inhibition of both these activities with a half maximal inhibitory concentration (IC_{50}) of 45 μM against the HeLa cells [148]. Recently the semi-synthetic analogue SSi6, generated by chemical modification of [6]-gingerol, was shown to be both more effective than the parent molecule in killing breast cancer cells *in vitro* [148]. Further, Luna-Dulcey et al. [148] reported that SSi6 killed tumor cells through initiating autophagy followed by caspase-independent apoptosis whereas for 6- cell death did not involve the autophagy precursor.

At least a dozen HDAC inhibitors are either going through clinical trials or currently approved for use [160]. Of the approved HDAC, the most potent is considered to be vorinostat (SAHA), with an *in vitro* IC_{50} ranging from 0.5 μM in some lymphoma and leukemia cells to as much as 83 μM for B-cell follicular lymphomas [161]. Clearly, the IC_{50} of the demethylated 6-shogaol is comparable to HDAC under development and future studies using different cell lines are also warranted. No commercial chemotherapeutic agents are able to stimulate tumor cell autophagy. Synthetic gingerols are clearly in their infancy but the findings of increased stability, bioavailability and even separate mechanisms of action suggest this line of research is worthy of further investigation in the potential development of future anti-inflammatory agents.

Zhu et al. [150] are the only group to date that have reported the creation of semi-synthetic versions of 6-shogaol with Kelch-like ECH-associated protein 1 (Keap1)–nuclear factor erythroid 2 p45-related factor 2 (Nrf2) activity. The authors reported that optimal activity was associated with the inclusion of both an *α, β*-unsaturated carbonyl and catechol groups [150]. Zhu et al. [150] hypothesized that the carbonyl and catechol groups were able to bind to reactive sulfur-containing cysteine amino acids in Keap1, preventing its downregulation of Nrf2. Nrf2 dysregulation is common in many chronic inflammatory conditions [162].

Current State of the Art in the Development of Stabilized Gingerols and Shogaols

Nine reports of effective stabilized/immobilized forms of gingerols or shogaols have recently appeared in the literature [151-159]. Five of these involve the use of edible nanoparticle carriers (ENP) of ginger (GDNP) [151-154, 157]. Two involves micelles composed of either soy lecithin [159] or polyethylene glycolate-linoleic acid (mPEG$_{2k}$-LA) [159]. Individual compositions were a γ-cyclodextrin-modified gingerol microcrystal nanoparticle [155] and a solid gingerol-alginate-coupled nanoparticle carrier [156]. Seven of these studies either determined levels of gingerol and shogaol [151, 152] or utilized pure gingerols [155, 158], or shogaols [156-158] and will be focused on in this chapter. Gingerols and shogaols are being evaluated for many properties, particularly as tumoricidal agents, and therefore many of these studies report the biological activity of these phenols in *in vitro* cell lines [148, 149, 151, 152, 156, 158] and animal models [158, 159]. These data are valid since they support the preservation of the biological activity of these molecules and are therefore included here.

Gingerol and Shogaol Nanoparticles as Potential Tumoricidal Agents and to Remediate Intestinal Inflammation

Zhang et al. [151, 152] created GDNP containing 6-gingerol and 6-shogaol at levels of 0.56-5.68 μg/ml and 1 0.22-2.95 μg/ml, respectively. These authors confirmed that the created GDNP were easily taken up by murine macrophages (RAW 264.7) [151, 152], murine colon cancer cells (Colon-26) [151, 152] and human adenocarcinoma cells (Caco-2BBE) [152]. In their second study, Zhang et al. [152] added small interfering RNA for CD98 (siRNA-CD98) to their GDNP and demonstrated that these could silence the gene for CD98 in both RAW 264.7 and Colon-26 cell lines. Mice gavaged with these GDNP demonstrated selective binding of the nanoparticles to the ileum and colon and no toxicity elsewhere to the animal in both studies as evidenced by normal bloodwork [151,152]. Interestingly CD98 is a gene that has been shown to play a major role in the pathophysiology of both intestinal inflammation, colitis and their progression into colon cancer [163] so this strategy may be well worth revisiting.

Stabilized Shogaol Micelles as Tumoricidal Agents

Micelles offer a method of preserving non-polar agents inside a hydrophobic shell, which both improves their bioavailability and stability [158, 159]. Two separate approaches have been taken to stabilize 6-shogaol using this strategy [158, 159]. Kemkar et al. [158], utilized a soy lecithin carrier and reported the resulting 6-shogaol micelles able to induce cytotoxicity *in vitro* against human breast cancer (MCF-7) cells as well as *in vivo* in a murine model of Dalton's ascitic leukemia. No toxicity effects were reported for the 6-shogaol micelles [158]. The lifespan of the leukemic mice was reported to be nearly doubled (84% compared with 48% in control group) after 14 days of treatment with 400 mg/kg of the 6-shogaol micelles [158]. By comparison, 94% of the animals that received the standard chemotherapeutic drug 5-fluorouracil (5-FU; 20 mg/kg) were alive after 14 days [158]. No combination therapy i.e., 5-FU plus 6-shogaol was assessed. Zhang et al. [159] constructed $mPEG_{2k}$-LA, which they reported were both non-toxic and demonstrated good blood and tissue bioavailability in healthy Sprague Dawley rats and Kunming mice. In contrast, the $mPEG_{2k}$-LA were tumoricidal and prevented the cell proliferation of human liver tumor (HepG2) cells *in vitro* [158]. Finally, these authors also observed that gavage of Kunming mice (100 mg/kg) with the $mPEG_{2k}$-LA for seven days could significantly reduce carbon tetrachloride (CCL_4)-induced hepatic damage compared with controls [158]. This latter effect was suggested to involve decrease of hepatic ROS levels and an increase in superoxide dismutase (SOD) levels [158].

Other Methodologies for Stabilizing Gingerol as an Antioxidant and Tumoricidal Agent

Studies by Pais et al. [155] are the only group, to date, that have immobilized purified mixtures of gingerols (6-, 8- and 10-gingerol) by conversion to a γ-cyclodextrin form and attachment to an alginate carrier. The γ-cyclodextrin gingerols (approximately 54% 6-gingerol, 19.5% 8-gingerol and 26.5% 10-gingerol) bound in a 1:1 ratio with the alginate carrier and possessed similar anti-inflammatory and antioxidant activities as the parent gingerols [155]. Most interestingly, Pais et al. [155] reported that the γ-cyclodextrin-alginate mixed well into yogurt and created a fortified food that displayed a five-fold increase in antioxidant activity as well as improved shelf life.

Finally, Manatunga et al. [156], recently designed a magnetic apatite alginate nanocarrier in which they incorporated both doxorubicin (0.06 mg/ml) and 6-gingerol (23 mg/ml) (6-gin + Dox-M-HAP), which they used *in vitro* as anti-proliferative agents against human breast (MCF-7) and liver (HepG2) tumor cell lines. Exposure of the MCF-7 to various concentrations of the 6-gin + Dox-M-HAP nanoparticles (0-150 μg/ml) for up to 72 hours, demonstrated that these were superior to doxorubicin alone and nanoparticle-bound doxorubicin throughout the time period. Indeed, IC_{50} for the 6-gin + Dox-M-HAP nanoparticles was relatively unchanged between 24 hours (0.58 μg/ml) and 72 hours (0.45 μg/ml).

In contrast, apatite alginate nanoparticles with doxorubicin alone or 6-gingerol alone displayed closely similar, much higher IC_{50} at 24 hours (2.25 and 2.96 μg/ml, respectively) and each required at least 48 hours to demonstrate efficacy [156]. Manatunga et al. [156], observed that HepG2 tumor cell lines were relatively insensitive to the effects of doxorubicin alone or doxorubicin nanoparticles after 24 hours (IC_{50} of 53 and 7.7 μg/ml, respectively) when compared with 6-gin + Dox-M-HAP (0.55 μg/ml) [156]. By 72 hours, the IC_{50} of doxorubicin and 6-gin + Dox-M-HAP had become more similar (0.58 and 0.19 μg/ml, respectively), with the 6-gin + Dox-M-HAP still remaining superior [156]. No concentrations of the 6-gin + Dox-M-HAP nanoparticles had any *in vitro* effects on a healthy human epithelial

(Vero) cell line [156]. Given that direct doxorubicin administration is associated with significant adverse effects, nanoparticle forms of the drug are already under investigation [164]. Any substance, such as 6-gingerol, that enhances doxorubicin's antitumor clearly warrant further testing.

Nanoparticles and micelles in all these studies were small with sizes of around 23 nm [156], 77 nm [158], 200 nm [151, 152, 155-157] or 300-400 nm [159]. All could easily be incorporated into either a dissolvable capsule, eaten or delivered by injection to the target. At this point having a reproducible and standardized form of gingerol and shogaol would allow their realistic evaluation in both pre-clinical (animal) and human subjects.

CONCLUSION AND POTENTIAL FUTURE DIRECTIONS

Ginger has a long and successful history of a safe medicinal anti-nausea and anti-emesis agent in pregnancy that has been supported by unbiased DBRPCT human clinical trials. Because it helped NVP, ginger was explored as a treatment for nausea and emesis in CINV and PONV, despite the fact that these involve different physiological pathways. Conflicting results from a number of DBRPCT resulted in a loss of support for ginger use in these conditions and no real development of the phytochemical for mainstream use. In fact, until recently the instability of gingerol and shogaol meant that the diverse anti-inflammatory, anti-microbial, and antinociceptive activities they demonstrated in animal models did not have any hope of being used as even complementary therapies in clinical trials. As researchers have developed an understanding of how to optimize these phenolic ginger moieties, as well as stabilize them, semi-synthetic and nanoparticle forms now offer the hope of providing future safe and therapies for emesis and vomiting in CINV and PONV. Apart from these two conditions, how might gingerols and shogaols be next developed? In searching the literature, two main fields are currently in the spotlight for gingerols and shogaols: chemotherapy [112, 113, 152, 156-159, 165-179] and chronic inflammatory bowel disease IBD [151, 152, 180-182].

Potential for Gingerol and Shogaol in the Management of Neoplastic Disease

Focusing in on just the CINV potential for gingerol, if all it did was prevent emesis it could potentially be used for the over one in five chemotherapy patients for whom conventional medicines is ineffective [93]. If the 6-gingerol-doxyrubicin nanoparticles recently created by Manatunga et al. [156] could be successfully used in human patients, these would allow direct targeting of tumors with a known chemotherapeutic agent and its potentiation by gingerol. Studies have reported in vitro tumoricidal activity for 6-gingerol against human breast (MDA-MB-231) [165]. cervical (HeLa) [166], colorectal [113, 152, 167], liver (HuH7) [112], lung (H1299) [167] and oral (SCC4 KB) [166] tumor cells. 6-shogaol demonstrated direct in vitro tumoricidal activity against human breast (MDA-MB-231) [168, 169], cervical (HeLa) [170], colorectal [171], primary leukemia [172], liver (HepG2) [158], non-small cell lung cancer (NCI-H1650, NCI-H520, NCI-H1975, HEK 293T) [173] and prostate cancer [174] cells. Animal studies demonstrated that 6-gingerol significantly ($p < 0.05$) inhibited angiogenesis (new tumor blood vessel growth) and the metastasis of breast [165, 175], liver [175], melanoma [176], colon [177] and prostate [178] cancer cells. Similar data were also reported for 6-shogaol in models of prostate [174] and skin cancer [179]. One animal study reported that 6-shogaol was superior to 6-gingerol in preventing 2-O-tetradecanoylphorbol 13-acetate (TPA)-induced murine skin tumors [179]. Taken together these data gingerols and shogaols have the potential to provide more than the alleviation of emesis and vomiting in tumor patients and may instead offer a complementary therapy that improves overall outcomes and quality of life.

Potential for Gingerol and Shogaol in the Management of Inflammatory Bowel Disease

Inflammatory bowel disease (IBD), most commonly manifested as either ulcerative colitis (UC) or Crohn's disease (CD), are currently managed by an individualized combination of corticosteroids, antibiotics and aminosalicylates [183]. However, in spite of these treatments many patients with IBD, particularly UC, often require surgical removal of their colon (colectomy) in the later stages of the condition and are at increased risk for the development of colon cancer [183]. The underlying pathophysiology of IBD revolves around cycles of involving a combination of gastrointestinal dysbiosis and faulty immune cell-mediated inflammation [183, 184].

Animal studies of UC and CD pathophysiology have typically employed either knockout animals, that spontaneously develop disease, or chemically-induced conditions including dextran sulfate injection [185]. Four studies have appeared in the literature to suggest that native gingerols are able to significantly decrease ($p < 0.05$) colonic damage in rodent models of dextran sulfate-induced IBD [151, 180-182]. Several mechanisms of action for purified 6-gingerol were proposed by these authors including impairment of reactive oxygen species (ROS), inflammatory cytokines [180], COX-2 activity [181] and Th17 cell levels [182]. Stabilized gingerol as GDNP (administered by gavage 3 mg/mouse for 1-19 weeks depending on the model) were able to reduce inflammatory colitis changes in models of C57BL/6 dextran sulfate-induced ulcerative colitis, IL10 spontaneous colitis and FVB/NJ azoxymethane-induced colon cancer [152]. A murine model of IBD reported that 6-gingerol (100 mg/kg by gavage) was comparable with the pharmacological IBD agent mesalazine (20 mg/kg) in reducing colonic inflammation and preventing weight loss [182]. Increases in cytokines, Th17 cells and COX2-2 activation together with decreased Treg function are well documented as playing a central role in the pathophysiology of IBD [183, 184, 186, 187].

Finally, although untested in these animal models of IBD, at least two studies have reported a strong probiotic function for both gingerols and shogaols [129, 143]. Probiotic use was found to significantly reduce patient symptoms ($p < 0.05$) in DBRPCT of IBD [188, 189]. Even if gingerols and shogaols only acted as effective probiotics by helping to reverse gut dysbiosis this would translate into more symptom-free days for IBD patients. Probiotic bacteria secrete short chain fatty acids (SCFA), which regulate the local inflammatory response and prevent bacterial binding to and damage of colonic epithelium [190]. As the numbers of probiotic bacteria decrease, SCFA manufacture is replaced by that of trimethylamine *N*-oxide (TMAO) metabolites of phosphatidylcholine [190, 191]. By interfering with cholesterol sequestration and platelet activation, TMAO are now recognized to be a major contributors to the generation of systemic atherosclerosis and cardiovascular disease [190, 191]. In spite of current interventions, patients with UC and CD remain at an increased risk of developing both colorectal cancer [183] and coronary artery disease [192]. Given the positive findings in animal models of these conditions further exploration of the potential of gingerols and shogaols in managing human IBD is also clearly warranted.

References

[1] Cundell, Diana R. 2014. "Herbal phytochemicals as immunomodulators." *Current Immunology Reviews* 10(2): 64-81. Accessed April 6, 2021. http://benthamscience.com/journal/index.hp?journalID=cir.

[2] Bode, Anne M., and Zigang Dong. "Chapter 7: The amazing and mighty ginger." In *Herbal Medicine: Biomolecular and Clinical Aspects*. Eds. Benzie IFF, Wachtel-Galor S 2011. 2nd edition. Boca Raton (FL): CRC Press/Taylor & Francis.

[3] Santos Braga, Susanna 2019. "Ginger: Panacea or Consumer's Hype? *Appl. Sci.,* 9: 1570. Accessed April 6, 2021. https://doi.org/10.3390/app9081570.

[4] Whiman, Liisa 2016. *The story of ginger. Metropolis*. Posted on December 30, 2016. Accessed April 6, 2021. https://metropolisjapan.com/the-story-of-ginger/

[5] Semwal, Ruchi B, Deepak K Semwal, Sandra Combrinck, and Alvaro M. Viljoen 2015. "Gingerols and shogaols: Important nutraceutical principles from ginger." *Phytochemistry,* 117:554-568. Accessed April 6, 2021 doi: 10.1016/j.phytochem.2015.07.012

[6] Tapsell, Lindsey C, Ian Hemphill, Lynne Cobiac, David R. Sulliva, Michael Fenech, Craig S. Patch CS, Stephen Roodenry, Jennifer B. Keogh, Peter M. Clifton, Peter G. Williams, Virginia A. Fazio, and Karen E. Inge 2006. "Health benefits of herbs and spices: The past, the present, the future." *Med. J. Aust.,* 185: S4–S24. Accessed on April 6, 2021 https://ro.uow.edu.au/hbspapers/1397/

[7] Khodaie, Laleh, and Omid Sadeghpoor 2015 "Ginger from ancient times to the new outlook." *Jundishapur Journal of Natural Pharmaceutical Products,* 10(1): e18402. Accessed on April 6, 2021. doi:10.17795/jjnpp-18402.

[8] Khaki, Arash, and Fatimezeh Fathiazad 2012. "Diabetic nephropathy – using herbals in diabetic nephropathy prevention and treatment – the role of ginger (*Zingiber officinale*) and onion (*Allium cepa*) in diabetics' nephropathy." A. Bhattacharya (Ed.), In: *A Compendium of Essays on Alternative Therapy*, InTech Publisher, Rijeka, Croatia, pp. 207-232. Accessed on April 6, 2021. https://citeseerx.ist.psu.edu/viewdoc/download?doi=10.1.1.463.8546&rep=rep1&type=pdf.

[9] Pratap, Singh R., H.V. Gandadharappa, and K. Mruthunjaya 2017. "Ginger: a potent nutraceutical, an updated review." *Int. J. Pharmacogn. Phytochem. Res.*, 9:1227-1238.

[10] Schulick, Paul 2012. "Ginger; common spice and wonder drug." 3rd Ed, Hohm Press, Prescott, AZ, USA ISBN: 978-1935826224.

[11] Li, Ling L., Ying Cui, Xing-Han Guo, Kai Ma, Ping Tian, Jing Feng, and Jun-Ming Wang 2019. "Pharmacokinetics and Tissue Distribution of Gingerols and Shogaols from Ginger (*Zingiber officinale* Rosc.) in Rats by UPLC⁻Q-Exactive⁻HRMS." *Molecules*, 2019 24(3):512. Accessed on April 7, 2021. doi: 10.3390 /molecules24030512.

[12] Thresh, J.C. 1879. Proximate analysis of the rhizome of *Zingiber officinale* and comparative examination of typical specimens of commercial gingers. *Pharm. J.*, 10: 171.

[13] Jiang Hongliang, Anikó M. Solyom, Barbara N. Timmerman, and David R. Gang 2005. "Characterization of gingerol-related compounds in ginger rhizome (*Zingiber oficinale* Rosc.) by high-

performance liquid chromatography/electrospray ionization mass spectrometry." *Rapid Commun. Mass Spectrom.,* 19; 2957-2964. Accessed on April 7, 2021 doi: 10.1002/rcm.2140.

[14] Bak, Min-Ji, Seon Ok, Mira Jun, and Woo-Sik Jeong 2012. "6-shogaol-rich extract from ginger up-regulates the antioxidant defense systems in cells and mice." *Molecules,* 17(7):8037-55. Accessed on April 7, 2021 doi: 10.3390/molecules17078037.

[15] Ghasemzadeh, Ali, Hawa Z.E. Jaafar, Ali Baghdadi, and Amin Tayebi-Meigooni A 2018. "Formation of 6-, 8- and 10-Shogaol in Ginger through Application of Different Drying Methods: Altered Antioxidant and Antimicrobial Activity." *Molecules,* 5;23(7):1646. Accessed on April 7, 2021 doi: 10.3390/molecules23071646.

[16] Dugasani, Swarnalatha, Mallikarjuna R. Pichika, Visha N. Devi, Madhu K. Balijepall, Satyanarayana Tandra, and Jayaveera N. Korlakunta 2010. "Comparative antioxidant and anti-inflammatory effects of [6]-gingerol, [8]-gingerol, [10]-gingerol and [6]-shogaol." *Journal of Ethnopharmacology,* 127(2): 515-520. Accessed on April 7, 2021. https://doi.org/10.1016/j.jep.2009.10.004.

[17] Ho, Su-Chen, and Yi-Huang Chang 2018. "Comparison of Inhibitory Capacities of 6-, 8- and 10-Gingerols/Shogaols on the Canonical NLRP3 Inflammasome-Mediated IL-1β Secretion." *Molecules,* 21;23(2):466. Accessed on April 7, 2021. doi: 10.3390/ molecules23020466.

[18] Nakazawa, Takaharo, and Keisuke Ohsawa 2002. "Metabolism of [6]-gingerol in rats." *Life Sci.,* 70:2165-2175. Accessed on April 7, 2021 doi: 10.1016/s0024-3205(01)01551-x.

[19] Hoehle, Simone I., Erica Pfeiffer and Manfred Metzler 2007. "Glucuronidation of curcuminoids by human microsomal and recombinant UDP-glucuronosyltransferases." *Mol. Nutr. Food Res.,* 51:932-938. Accessed on April 7, 2021. doi 10.1002/mnfr. 200600283.

[20] Mukkavalli, Rao, Chinhua Yang, Reenu S. Tanwar, Ahmed Ghareeb, Lateeka Luthra, and Ritu Aneja 2008. "Absorption, metabolic stability, and pharmacokinetics of 6-gingerol, 8-gingerol, 10-

gingerol, and 6-shogaol and conjugate metabolites in healthy human subjects." *Cancer Epidemiol. Biomark Prev.,* 17:1930-1936. Accessed on April 7, 2021. doi: 10.3390/molecules22040553.

[21] Jiang Su-zhen, Wang Ning-sheng, and Sui-qing Mi2008. "Plasma pharmacokinetics and tissue distribution of [6]-gingerol in rats." *Biopharm. Drug Dispos.,* 29:529-537. Accessed on April 7, 2021. Doi:10.1002/bdd.638.

[22] Zick, Suzanna M., Zora Djuric, Mack T. Ruffin, Amie J. Litzinger, Daniel P. Normolle, Sara Alrawi, Meihua R. Feng, and Dean E. Brenner 2017. "Pharmacokinetics of ginger phytochemicals." *Molecules*, 17:1930-1936. Accessed on April 7, 2021. doi: 10.1158/1055-9965.EPI-07-2934.

[23] Hasler William L., and William D. Chey. 2003. "Nausea and vomiting." *Clinical Management,* 125(6): 1860-1867. Accessed on April 7, 2021. doi: https//doi.org/10.1053/j.gastro.2003.09.40.

[24] Frese, Thomas, Steffi Klauss, Kristen Herrmann, and Hagen Sandholzer 2011. "Nausea and vomiting as the reasons for encounter in general practice." *J. Clin. Med. Res.*, 3(1):23-29. Accessed on April 7, 2021. doi:10.4021/jocmr410w.

[25] Viljoen, Estelle, Janicke Visser, Nelene Koen, and Alfred Musekiwa 2014. "A systematic review and meta-analysis of the effect and safety of ginger in the treatment of pregnancy-associated nausea and vomiting." *Nutr. J.*, 19; 13:20. Accessed on April 7, 2021. doi: 10.1186/1475-2891-13-20.

[26] Marx, Wolfgang M., Laisa Teleni, Alexandra L. McCarthy, Luis Vitetta, Dan McKavanagh, Damien Thomson, and Elisabeth Isenring 2013. "Ginger (*Zingiber officinale*) and chemotherapy-induced nausea and vomiting: a systematic literature review." *Nutrition Reviews*, 71(4): 245–254. Accessed on April 7, 2021. doi: 10.1111/nure.12016.

[27] Encinosa, William, and Amy J. Davidoff 2017. "Changes in Antiemetic Overuse in Response to Choosing Wisely Recommendations." *JAMA Oncol.*, 3(3):320–326. Accessed on April 7, 2021. doi:10.1001/jamaoncol.2016.2530.

[28] Tóth, Barbara, Tomás Lantos, Péter Hegyi, Réka Viola, Andrea Vasas, Riya Benkő, Zoltán Gyöngi, Áron Vincze, Péter Csécsei, Alexandra Mika, Dávid Hegyi, Andrea Szentesi, Mária Matusz, and Dezső Csupor 2018. "Ginger (Zingiber officinale): An alternative for the prevention of postoperative nausea and vomiting. A meta-analysis." *Phytomedicine: International Journal of Phytotherapy and Phytopharmacology,* 50:8-18. doi: 10.1016/j.phymed.2018.09.007.

[29] Thompson, Maggie, Renee Corbin, and Lawrence Leung 2014. "The effects of ginger for nausea and vomiting in early pregnancy: A meta-analysis." *J. Am. Board Fam. Med.,* 27(1):115-122. Accessed on April 7, 2021. Doi:10.3122/jabfm.2014.01.130167.

[30] AlHajiri, Lamia, Moaza Alfasi, Munira Abdelrahim, and Rawdha AlKaabi R 2017. "The efficacy of ginger for pregnancy-induced nausea and vomiting: a systematic review." *Journal of Natural Remedies,* 17(2). Accessed on April 8, 2021. https://doi.org /10.18311/jnr/2017/18012.

[31] Hu, Youchun, Adwoa N. Amoah, Han Zhang, Rong Fu, Yanfang Qiu, Yuan Cao, Yafei Sun, Huanan Chen, Yanhua Liu, and Quanjun Lyu 2020. "Effect of ginger in the treatment of nausea and vomiting compared with vitamin B6 and placebo during pregnancy: a meta-analysis." *The Journal of Maternal-Fetal & Neonatal Medicine,* 14:1-10. Accessed on April 8, 2021. doi: 10.1080/14767058. 2020.1712714.

[32] Fischer-Rasmussen, Wiggo, Susanne K. Kjaer, Claus Dahl, and Ulla Asping 1991. "Ginger treatment of hyperemesis gravidarum." *Eur. J. Obstet. Gynecol. Reprod. Biol.*, 38:19–24. Accessed on April 8, 2021.

[33] Vutyavanich, T, T. Kraisarin, and R. Ruangsri 2001. "Ginger for nausea and vomiting in pregnancy: randomized, double-masked, placebo-controlled trial." *Obstet. Gynecol.,* 97:577–82. Accessed on April 8, 2021. doi: 10.1016/s0029-7844(00)01228-x.

[34] Keating, Angela, and Ronald A. Chez 2002. "Ginger syrup as an antiemetic in early pregnancy." *Altern. Ther. Health Med.,* 8:89–91. Accessed on April 8, 2021. PMID: 12233808.

[35] Willetts, Karen E., Abie Ekangaki, and John A. Eden 2003. "Effect of a ginger extract on pregnancy-induced nausea: A randomised controlled trial." *Aust. N. Z. J. Obstet. Gynaecol.*, 43:139–144. Accessed on April 8, 2021. doi: 10.1046/j.0004-8666.2003.00039.x.

[36] Basirat, Zahra, Ali Moghadamnia, Mehrdad Kashifard, and Atena Sarifi-Razavi 2009. "The effect of ginger biscuit on nausea and vomiting in early pregnancy." *Acta Medica Iranica*, 47:51–56. Accessed on April 8, 2021. https://acta.tums.ac.ir/index.php/acta/article/view/3543

[37] Mohammadbeigi, Robababeh, Shaleah Shahgeibi, Nazrin Soufizadeh, Masoumeh Rezaiie, and Fariba Farhadifar 2011. "Comparing the effects of ginger and metoclopramide on the treatment of pregnancy nausea." *Pak. J. Biol. Sci.*, 14:817–820. Accessed on April 8, 2021. doi: 10.3923/pjbs.2011.817.820.

[38] Firouzbakht, Mozhgan., Maryam Nikpour, Bita Jamali, and Shabnam Omidvar 2014. "Comparison of ginger with vitamin B6 in relieving nausea and vomiting during pregnancy." *Ayu.,* 35:289–293. Accessed on April 8, 2021. doi: 10.4103/0974-8520.153746.

[39] Anh, Nguyen H., Sun J. Kim, Nguyen P. Long, Jung E. Min, Young C. Yoon, Eun G. Lee, Mina Kim, Tae J. Kim, Yoon Y. Yang, Eui Y. Son, Sang J. Yoon, Nguyen C. Diem, Hyung M. Kim, and Sung W. Kwon 2020. "Ginger on Human Health: A Comprehensive Systematic Review of 109 Randomized Controlled Trials." *Nutrients,* 12(1):157. Accessed on April 8, 2021. doi:10.3390/nu12010157.

[40] Lee, Jiyeon, and Heeyoung Oh 2013. "Ginger as an antiemetic modality for chemotherapy-induced nausea and vomiting: a systematic review and meta-analysis." *Oncol. Nurs. Forum,* 40(2):163-170. Accessed on April 8, 2021. doi:10.1188/13.ONF.163-170.

[41] Sontakke, S, V. Thawani, and S.M. Naik 2003. "Ginger as an antiemetic in nausea and vomiting induced by chemotherapy: A randomized, cross-over, double blind study." *Ind. J. Pharmacol.,* 35:32–36.

[42] Manusirivathaya, S, M. Sripramote, S. Tangjitgamol, C. Sheanukul, S. Leelahakorn, T. Thavaramara, and K. Tangcharoenpnich 2004. "Antiemetic effect of ginger in gynecologic oncology patients receiving cisplatin." *International Journal of Gynecologic Cancer,* 14:1063-1069. Accessed on April 8, 2021. doi: 10.1111/j.1048-891X.2004.14603.x.

[43] Zick, Suzanna M., Mack T. Ruffin, Julia Lee, Daniel P. Normolle, Rivka Siden, Sara Alrawi, and Dean E, Brenner 2009. "Phase II trial of encapsulated ginger as a treatment for chemotherapy-induced nausea and vomiting." *Support Care Cancer*, 17(5):563-72. Accessed on April 8, 2021. doi: 10.1007/s00520-008-0528-8.

[44] Fahimi, Fanack, Kian Khodadad, Somayeh Amini, Farzaneh Naghibi, Jamshid Salamzadeh, and Shadi Baniasadi 2011. "Evaluating the effect of zingiber officinalis on nausea and vomiting in patients receiving Cisplatin based regimens." *Iran J. Pharm. Res.*, 10(2):379-84. Accessed on April 8, 2021. PMID: 24250368.

[45] Pillai, Anu K., Kamlesh K. Sharma, Yogendra K. Gupta, and Sameer Bakhshi 2011. Anti-emetic effect of ginger powder versus placebo as an add-on therapy in children and young adults receiving high emetogenic chemotherapy. *Pediatr. Blood Cancer,* 56: 234-238. Accessed on April 8, 2021. doi:10.1002/pbc.22778.

[46] Ryan, Julie L., Charles E. Heckler, Joseph A. Roscoe, Shaker R. Dakhil, Jeffrey Kirshner, Patrick J. Flynn, Jane T. Hickok, and Gary R. Morrow 2012. "Ginger (*Zingiber officinale*) reduces acute chemotherapy-induced nausea: a URCC CCOP study of 576 patients." *Support Care Cancer,* 2012 20(7):1479-89. Accessed on April 8, 2021. doi: 10.1007/s00520-011-1236-3.

[47] Yekta, Zohreh P., Seyyed M. Ebrahimi, Mostafa Hosseini, Alireza N. Nasrabadi, Sanambar Sedighi, Mohammad-Hosein Surmaghi, and Hossein Madani 2012. "Ginger as a miracle against chemotherapy-induced vomiting." *Iran. J. Nurs. Midwifery Res.*, 17:325–329. Accessed on April 8, 2021. PMID: 23853643.

[48] Sanaati, Fateme, Safa Najafi, Zhara Kashaninia, and Masoud Sadeghi 2016. "Effect of ginger and chamomile on nausea and vomiting

caused by chemotherapy in Iranian women with breast cancer." *Asian Pac. J. Cancer Prev.,* 17:4125–4129. Accessed on April 8, 2021. PMID: 27644672.

[49] Ansari, Mansour, Pezhman Porouhan, Mohammad Mohammadianpanah, Shapour Omidvari, Ahmad Mosalaei, Niloofar Ahmadloo, Hamid Nasrollahi, and Seyed H. Hamedi 2016. "Efficacy of ginger in control of chemotherapy induced nausea and vomiting in breast cancer patients receiving doxorubicin-based chemotherapy." *Asian Pac. J. Cancer Prev.*, 17:3877–3880. Accessed on April 8, 2021. PMID: 27644633.

[50] Thamlikitkul, Lucksamon, Vichien Srimuninnimit, Charowan Akewanlop, Suthinee Ithimakin, Sirisopa Techawathanawanna, Krittya Korphaisarn, Jomjit Chantharamassee, Pongwut Danchaivijtr, and Nopadol Soparattanapaisarn 2017. "Efficacy of ginger for prophylaxis of chemotherapy-induced nausea and vomiting in breast cancer patients receiving adriamycin-cyclophosphamide regimen: a randomized, double-blind, placebo-controlled, crossover study." *Support Care Cancer,* 25(2):459-464. Accessed on April 8, 2021. doi:10.1007/s00520-016-3423-8.

[51] Bossi, P., D. Cortinovis, S. Fatigoni, M. Cossu Rocca, A. Fabi, P. Seminara, C. Ripamonti, S. Alfieri, R. Granata, C. Bergamini, F. Agustoni, P. Bidoli, F. Nolé, M. A. Pessi, F. Macchi, L. Michellini, F. Montanaro, and F. Roila 2017. "A randomized, double-blind, placebo-controlled, multicenter study of a ginger extract in the management of chemotherapy-induced nausea-induced vomiting (CINV) in patients receiving high dose cisplatin." *Annals Oncol.,* 124(10): P2547-P2551. Accessed on April 8, 2021. doi: https://doi.org/10.1093/annonc/mdx315.

[52] Konmun, J., K. Danwilai, N. Ngamphaiboon, B. Sripanidkulchai, A. Sookprasert, and S. Subongkot 2017. "A phase II randomized double-blind placebo-controlled study of 6-gingerol as an anti-emetic in solid tumor patients receiving moderately to highly emetogenic chemotherapy." *Med Oncol.,* 34(4):69. Accessed on April 8, 2021. doi:10.1007/s12032-017-0931-4.

[53] Marx, Wolfgang, Alexandra L. McCarthy, Karin Ried, Dan McKavanagh, Luis Vitetta, Avni Sali, Anna Lohning, and Elisabeth Isenring 2017. "The Effect of a Standardized Ginger Extract on Chemotherapy-Induced Nausea-Rclated Quality of Life in Patients Undergoing Moderately or Highly Emetogenic Chemotherapy: A Double Blind, Randomized, Placebo Controlled Trial." *Nutrients,* 9(8):867. Accessed on April 8, 2021. doi:10.3390/nu9080867.

[54] Li, Xiangfeng, Ying Qin, Wei Liu W, Xiao-Yu Zhou, Ya-Nan Li, and Li-Ying Wang 2018. "Efficacy of ginger in ameliorating acute and delayed chemotherapy-induced nausea and vomiting among patients with lung cancer receiving cisplatin-based regimens: A randomized controlled trial." *Integr. Cancer,* 17:747–754. Accessed on April 8, 2021. doi: 10.1177/1534735417753541.

[55] Bone, M. E., D. J. Wilkinson, J. R. Young, J. McNeil, and S. Charlton 1990. "Ginger root—a new antiemetic. The effect of ginger root on postoperative nausea and vomiting after major gynaecological surgery." *Anaesthesia,* 45: 669-671. Accessed on April 8, 2021. doi:10.1111/j.1365-2044.1990.tb14395.x.

[56] Phillips, S., R. Ruggier, and S.E. Hutchinson 1993. "*Zingiber officinale* (Ginger)–an antiemetic for day case surgery." *Anaesthesia*, 48: 715-717. Accessed on April 8, 2021. doi:10.1111/j.1365-2044.1993.tb07188.x

[57] Arfeen, Z., H. Owen, J. L. Plummer, A. H. Ilsley, R. A. Sorby-Adams, and C. J. Doecke 1995. "A double-blind randomized controlled trial of ginger for the prevention of postoperative nausea and vomiting." *Anaesth. Intensive Care*, 23:449–452. Accessed on April 8, 2021. doi: 10.1177/0310057X9502300406.

[58] Eberhart, Leopold H., Roswitha Mayer, Oliver Betz, Stergios Tsolakidis, Wolfgang Hilpert, Astrid M. Morin, Gőtz Geldner, Hinnerk Wulf, and Seeling Wulf 2003. "Ginger does not prevent postoperative nausea and vomiting after laparoscopic surgery." *Anesth. Analg.*, 96:995–998. Accessed on April 8, 2021. doi: 10.1213/01.ANE.0000055818.64084.41.

[59] Pongrojpaw, Densak, and Charoenchai Chiamchanya 2003. "The Efficacy of Ginger in Prevention of Post-operative nausea and vomiting after outpatient gynecological laparoscopy." *J. Med. Assoc. Thai.* 86:244. Accessed on April 8, 2021. PMID: 12757064.

[60] Apariman, Sirirat, Sawinee Ratchanon, and Budsaba Wiriyasirivej B 2006. "Effectiveness of ginger for prevention of nausea and vomiting after gynecological laparoscopy." *J. Med. Assoc. Thai.,* 89(12):2003-2009. Accessed on April 8, 2021. PMID: 17214049.

[61] Nanthakomon, Tonkta, and Densak Pongrojpaw 2006. "The efficacy of ginger in prevention of postoperative nausea and vomiting after major gynecologic surgery." *J. Med. Assoc. Thai.,* 89 Suppl 4: S130-S136. Accessed on April 8, 2021. PMID: 17725149.

[62] Nale, Ravikiran, Sachin Bhave, and D. S. Divekar 2007. "A comparative study of ginger and other routinely used antiemetics for prevention of postoperative nausea and vomiting." *J. Anesth. Clin. Pharmacolology*, 23(4)454-410. Accessed on April 8, 2021.

[63] Montazeri, Akram S., Azam Hamidzadeh, Medhi Raei, Malihe Mohammadium, Azam S. Montazeri, Reza Mirshahi, and Hosein Roshani 2014. "Evaluation of Oral Ginger Efficacy against Postoperative Nausea and Vomiting: A Randomized, Double - Blinded Clinical Trial." *Iran Red Crescent Med J.*, 15(12):e12268. Accessed on April 8, 2021. doi: 10.5812/ircmj.12268.

[64] Mandal, Pragnadyuti, Anjan Das, Saikat Majumdar, Tapas Bhattacharyya, Tapobrata Mitra, and Ratul Kundul 2014. "The efficacy of ginger added to ondansetron for preventing postoperative nausea and vomiting in ambulatory surgery." *Pharmacogn. Res.,* 6:52–57. Accessed on April 8, 2021. doi: 10.4103/0974-8490.122918.

[65] Soltani, E., A. Jangjoo, M. Afzal Aghaei, and A. Dalili 2018." Effects of preoperative administration of ginger (*Zingiber officinale* Roscoe) on postoperative nausea and vomiting after laparoscopic cholecystectomy." *Journal of Traditional and Complementary Medicine,* 8(3): 387-390. Accessed on April 8, 2021. https://doi.org/10.1016/j.jtcme.2017.06.008.

[66] Bameshki, Alireza, Mohammad N. Namaiee, Ali Jangjoo, Maliheh Dadgarmoghaddam, Mohammad H.E. Ghalibaf, Atefeh Ghorbanzadeh, and Shima Sheybani 2018. "Effect of oral ginger on prevention of nausea and vomiting after laparoscopic cholecystectomy: a double-blind, randomized, placebo-controlled trial." *Electron Physician*, 10(2):6354-6362. Accessed on April 8, 2021. doi:10.19082/6354.

[67] Sedigh Maroufi, Shahnam, Parisa Moradimajd, Seyed A.A. Moosavi, Farnad Imani, Hamidreza Samaee, and Mehmet Oguz 2019. "Dose Ginger Have Preventative Effects on PONV-Related Eye Surgery? A Clinical Trial." *Anesth. Pain Med.,* 9(5):e92072. Accessed on April 8, 2021. doi:10.5812/aapm.92072.

[68] Marx, Wolfgang M., Laisa Teleni, Alexandra L. McCarthy, Luis Vittetta, Dan McKavanagh, Damien Thomson, and Elisabeth Isenring 2012. "Is ginger supplementation effective in ameliorating chemotherapy-induced nausea and vomiting?" *Cosa 39Th Annual Scientific Meeting and IPOS 14Th World Congress of Psycho-Oncology. Asia Pac. J. Clin. Oncol.,* 8(Suppl-3):323. Accessed on April 8, 2021. https://doi.org/10.1111/ajco.12030.

[69] Park, Ji S, and Mun Y. Jung 2012. "Development of high-performance liquid chromatography-time-of-flight mass spectrometry for the simultaneous characterization and quantitative analysis of gingerol-related compounds in ginger products." *J. Agric. Food Chem.,* 60: 10015-10026. Accessed on April 8, 2021. https://doi.org/10.1021/jf302944p.

[70] Marx, Wolfgang, Elisabeth A. Isenring, and Anna E. Lohning 2017. "Determination of the concentration of major anti-emetic constituents within commercial ginger food products and dietary supplements." *Eur J. Integ. Med.*, 10:19-24. Accessed on April 9, 2021. doi: 10.1016/j.eujim.2017.02.001.

[71] Schwertner, Harvey A., Deborah C. Rios, and Joshua E. Pascoe 2006. "Variation in concentration and labeling of ginger root supplements." *Obstet. Gynecol.,* 107:1337-1443. Accessed on April 9, 2021. doi: 10.1097/01.AOG.0000217697.33787.8c.

[72] Zick, Suzanna M, Zora Djuric, Mack T. Ruffin, Amie J. Litzinger, Daniel P. Normolle, Sara Alrawi, Meihua R. Feng, and Dean E. Brenner 2008. "Pharmacokinetics of 6-Gingerol, 8-Gingerol, 10-Gingerol, and 6-Shogaol and Conjugate Metabolites in Healthy Human Subjects." *Cancer Epidemiol. Biomarkers Prev.*, 17 (8): 1930- 1936. Accessed on April 9, 2021. doi: 10.1158/1055-9965.EPI-07-2934.

[73] Blumenthal, Mark 1998. 1998. "The complete German Commission E Monographs: therapeutic guide to herbal medicines." W.R. Busse, A. Goldberg, J. Gruenwald, T. Hall, W. Riggins, and R.S. Rister, editors American Botanical Council, Austin Texas. *Boston (MA): Integrative Medicine Communications* 135-136. Accessed on April 9, 2021. http://www.gbv.de/dms/bs/toc/302401350.pdf.

[74] Singh, Prashant, Sonia S. Yoon, and Braden Kuo 2006. "Nausea: a review of pathophysiology and therapeutics." *Therap. Adv. Gastroenterol.,* 9(1):98-112. Accessed on April 9, 2021. doi: 10.1177/1756283X15618131.

[75] Hornby, Pamela J. 2001. "Central neurocircuitry associated with emesis." *Am. J. Med.*, 111:106S–112S. Accessed on April 9, 2021. doi: 10.1016/s0002-9343(01)00849-x.

[76] Napadow, Vitaly, James D. Sheehan, Jieun Kim, Lauren T. Lacount, Kyungmo Park, Ted D. Kaptchuk, Bruce R. Rosen, and Braden Kuo 2013. "The brain circuitry underlying the temporal evolution of nausea in humans." *Cereb. Cortex,* 23: 806–813. Accessed on April 9, 2021. doi: 10.1093/cercor/bhs073.

[77] Camilleri, Michael 2009. "Serotonin in the gastrointestinal tract." *Curr. Opin. Endocrinol. Diabetes Obes.,* 16(1):53-9. Accessed on April 9, 2021. doi: 10.1097/med.0b013e32831e9c8e.

[78] Lee, Noel M., and Sumona Saha 2011. "Nausea and vomiting of pregnancy." *Gastroenterol. Clin. North Am.*, 40(2):309-vii. Accessed on April 9, 2021. doi:10.1016/j.gtc.2011.03.009.

[79] North, R .A., R. Whitehead, and R. G. Larkins 1991. Stimulation by human chorionic gonadotropin of prostaglandin synthesis by early

human placental tissue. *J. Clin. Endocrinol. Metab.*, 73:60–70. Accessed on April 9, 2021. doi: 10.1210/jcem-73-1-60.

[80] Golberg, Deborah, Andrew Szilagyi, and Lisa Graves 2007. Hyperemesis gravidarum and *Helicobacter pylori* infection: a systemic review. *Obstet. Gynecol.*, 110:695–703. Accessed on April 9, 2021. doi: 10.1097/01.AOG.0000278571.93861.26.

[81] Sandven, Irene, Michael Abdelnoor, Britt I. Nesheim, and Kjetl K. Melby 2009. "*Helicobacter pylori* infection and hyperemesis gravidarum: a systematic review and meta-analysis of case-control studies. *Acta Obstet. Gynecol. Scand.*, 88:1190–1200. Accessed on April 9, 2021. doi: 10.3109/00016340903284927.

[82] Bagis, T., Y. Gumurdulu, F. Kayaselcuk, E. S. Yilmaz, E. Killicadag, and E. Tarim 2002. "Endoscopy in hyperemesis gravidarum and *Helicobacter pylori* infection." *Int. J. Gynaecol. Obstet.*, 79:105–109. Accessed on April 9, 2021. doi: 10.1016/s0020-7292(02)00230-8.

[83] Kocak, I., Y. Akcan, C. Ustun, C. Demirel, F. Cengiz, and F. Yanik 1999. "*Helicobacter pylori* seropositivity in patients with hyperemesis gravidarum." *Int. J. Gynaecol. Obstet.*, 66:251–254. Accessed on April 9, 2021. https://doi.org/10.1016/S0020-7292(99)00091-0.

[84] Lanciers, S., B. Despinasse, D.I. Mehta, and U. Blecker 1999. Increased susceptibility to *Helicobacter pylori* infection in pregnancy. *Infect. Dis. Obstet. Gynecol.,* 7:195–198. Accessed on April 9, 2021. doi: 10.1002/(SICI)1098-0997(1999)7:4<195::AID-IDOG6>3.0.CO;2-R.

[85] Janelsins, Michelle C., Mohamedtaki A. Tejani, Charles Kamen, Anita R. Peoples, Karen M. Mustian, and Gary R. Morrow 2013. "Current pharmacotherapy for chemotherapy-induced nausea and vomiting in cancer patients." *Expert Opin. Pharmacother.,* 14(6):757-766. Accessed on April 9, 2021. doi:10.1517/14656566.2013.776541.

[86] Blackshaw, L.A., S.J. Brookes, D. Grundy, and M. Schemann 2007. "Sensory transmission in the gastrointestinal tract."

Neurogastroenterol. Motil., 19:1–19. Accessed on April 9, 2021. doi: 10.1111/j.1365-2982.2006.00871.x.

[87] Gershon, M.D. 2004. "Review article: serotonin receptors and transporters-roles in normal and abnormal gastrointestinal motility." *Aliment Pharmacol. Ther.*, 20:3–14. Accessed on April 9, 2021. doi: 10.1111/j.1365-2036.2004.02180.x.

[88] Darmani, Nissar A., Seetha Chebolu, Barry Amos, and Tursun Alkam 2011. "Synergistic antiemetic interactions between serotonergic 5-HT(3) and tachykininergic NK(1)-receptor antagonists in the least shrew (*Cryptotis parva*)." *Pharmacol. Biochem. Behav.,* 99:573–579. Accessed on April 9, 2021. doi: 10.1016/j.pbb.2011.05.025.

[89] Rojas, Camilo, Ying Li, Jie Zhang, Marigo Stathis, Jesse Alt, Agit G. Thomas, Sergio Santoreggi, Silvia Sebastiani, Claudia Pietra, and Barbara S. Slusher 2010. "The antiemetic 5-HT3 receptor antagonist palonosetron inhibits substance P-mediated responses *in vitro* and *in vivo*." *J. Pharmacol. Exp. Ther.,* 335:362–368. Accessed on April 9, 2021. doi: 10.1124/jpet.110.166181.

[90] Borgeat, Alain, Marc Fathi, and Antonella Valiton 1997. "Hyperemesis gravidarum: is serotonin implicated?" *Am. J. Obstet. Gynecol.,* 176:476–477. Accessed on April 9, 2021. doi: 10.1016/s0002-9378(97)70518-0.

[91] Sullivan, Christopher A., Cheryl A. Johnson, Holli Roach, Rick W. Martin, Deanna K. Stewart, and John C. Morrison 1996. "A pilot study of intravenous ondansteron for hyperemesis gravidarum." *Am. J. Obstet. Gynecol.,* 174:1565–1568. Accessed on April 9, 2021. doi: 10.1016/s0002-9378(96)70607-5.

[92] Ryan, Julie L. 2010. "Treatment of Chemotherapy-Induced Nausea in Cancer Patients." *Eur. Oncol.,* 6(2):14-16. Accessed on April 9, 2021. doi:10.17925/eoh.2010.06.02.14.

[93] Hickok, Jane T., Joseph A. Roscoe, Gary R. Morrow, David K. King, James N. Atkins, and Tom R. Fitch 2003. "Nausea and emesis remain significant problems of chemotherapy despite prophylaxis with 5-Hydroxytryptamine-3 antiemetics." *Cancer,* 97(11):2880–2886. Accessed on April 9, 2021. https://doi.org/10.1002/cncr.11408

[94] Herrstedt, Jørn 2008. "Antiemetics: an update and the MASCC guidelines applied in clinical practice." *Nature Clinical Practice Oncology*, 5(1):32–43. Accessed on April 9, 2021. doi: 10.1038/ncponc1021.

[95] Sanger, Gareth J., and Paul L.R. Andrews 2006. "Treatment of nausea and vomiting: gaps in our knowledge." *Auton. Neurosci.,* 129:3–16. Accessed on April 9, 2021. doi: 10.3389/fphar.2018.00913.

[96] Horn, Charles C., William J. Wallisch, Gregg E. Homanics, and John P. Williams 2014. "Pathophysiological and neurochemical mechanisms of postoperative nausea and vomiting." *Eur. J. Pharmacol.,* 722:55-66. Accessed on April 9, 2021. doi:10.1016/ j.ejphar.2013.10.037.

[97] Barnes, N. M., K. T. Bunce, R. J. Naylor, and J. A. Rudd 1991. "The actions of fentanyl to inhibit drug-induced emesis." *Neuropharmacology,* 30:1073–1083. Accessed on April 9, 2021. doi: 10.1016/0028-3908(91)90136-y.

[98] Parker, Rachel M.C., Kim R. Bentley, and Nicholas M. Barnes 1996. "Allosteric modulation of 5-HT3 receptors: focus on alcohols and anaesthetic agents." *Trends Pharmacol. Sci.,* 17:95–99. Accessed on April 9, 2021.

[99] Kim, M.S., W.D. Chey, C. Owyang, and W.L. Hasler 1997. "Role of plasma vasopressin as a mediator of nausea and gastric slow wave dysrhythmias in motion sickness." *Am. J. Physiol.,* 272(4 Pt 1):G853-G862. Accessed on April 9, 2021. doi:10.1152/ajpgi.1997. 272.4.G853.

[100] Viscusi, Eugene R., Tong Gan, John Leslie, Joseph Foss, Mark Talon, Wei Du, and Gay Owens 2009. "Peripherally Acting Mu-Opioid Receptor Antagonists and Postoperative Ileus: Mechanisms of Action and Clinical Applicability." *Anesthesia & Analgesia,* 108(6); 1811-1822. Accessed on April 9, 2021. doi: 10.1213/ane. 0b013e31819e0d3a.

[101] Jung, Wol S., Yong B., Hee Y. Park, Woo J. Choi, and Hong S. Yang 2013. "Oral administration of aprepitant to prevent postoperative nausea in highly susceptible patients after gynecological

laparoscopy." *J Anesth.,* 27(3):396-401. Accessed on April 9, 2021. doi:10.1007/s00540-012-1529-9.

[102] Ormel, G., L. Romundstad, P. Lambert-Jensen, and A. Stubhaug 2011. "Dexamethasone has additive effect when combined with ondansetron and droperidol for treatment of established PONV." *Acta Anaesthesiologica Scandinavica*, 55:1196–1205. Accessed on April 9, 2021. doi: 10.1111/j.1399-6576.2011.02536.x.

[103] Grundy, David 2004. "What activates visceral afferents?" *Gut,* 53(Suppl 2): ii5–8. Accessed on April 9, 2021. doi: 10.1136/gut.2003.033415.

[104] Ho, Chiu-Ming, Shung-Tai Ho, Jhi-Joung Wang, Shen-Kou Tsai, and Chok-Yung Chai 2004. "Dexamethasone has a central antiemetic mechanism in decerebrated cats." *Anesthesia and Analgesia,* 99:734–739. Accessed on April 9, 2021. doi: 10.1213/01.ANE.0000130003.68288.C7.

[105] Suzuki, Takahiro, Masahiro Sugimoto, Hideki Koyama, Takashi Mashimo, and Ichiro Uchida 2004. "Inhibitory effect of glucocorticoids on human-cloned 5-hydroxytryptamine3A receptor expressed in xenopus oocytes." *Anesthesiology,* 101:660–665. Accessed on April 9, 2021. doi: 10.1097/00000542-200409000-00014.

[106] Abdel-Aziz, Heba, Tibo Windeck, Michael Ploch, and Eugen J. Verspohl 2006. "Mode of action of gingerols and shogaols on 5-HT 3 receptors: binding studies, cation uptake by the receptor channel and contraction of isolated guinea-pig ileum." *Eur. J. Pharmacol.,* 530:136–143. Accessed on April 9, 2021. doi: 10.1016/j.ejphar.2005.10.049.

[107] Pertz, Heinz H., Jochen Lehmann, Rene Roth-Ehrang, and Sigurd Elz 2011. "Effects of ginger constituents on the gastrointestinal tract: role of cholinergic M3 and serotonergic 5-HT3 and 5-HT4 receptors." *Planta Med.*, 77:973–978. Accessed on April 9, 2021. doi: 10.1055/s-0030-1270747.

[108] Chatturong, Usana, Tanwarat Kajsonkram, Sakanara Tunsophon, Rachanee Chanasong, and Krongkarn Chootip 2018. "Ginger extract

and [6]-gingerol inhibit contraction of entire rat small intestine." *Journal of Evidence Based Integrative Medicine,* 23: 1-9. Accessed on April 9, 2021. https://doi.org/10.1177/2515690X18774273.

[109] Jin, Zhenhua, Goeun Lee, Sojin Kim, Cheung-Seog Park, Yong S. Park, and Young-Ho Jin 2014. "Ginger and its pungent constituents non-competitively inhibit serotonin currents on visceral afferent neurons." *Korean J. Physiol. Pharmacol.*, 18:149–153. Accessed on April 9, 2021. doi: 10.4196/kjpp.2014.18.2.149.

[110] Dugasani, Swarnalatha, Mallikarjuna R. Pichika, Vishna D. Nadarajah, Madhu K. Ballijepalli, Satyanarayana Tandra, and Jayaveera N. Korlakunta 2010. "Comparative antioxidant and anti-inflammatory effects of [6]-gingerol, [8]-gingerol, [10]-gingerol and [6]-shogaol." *Journal of Ethnopharmacology*, 127(2):515-520. Accessed on April 9, 2021. doi: 10.1016/j.jep.2009.10.004.

[111] Lantz, R. C., G. J. Chen, M. Sarihan, A. M. Sólyom, S. D. Jolad, and B. N. Timmermann 2007. "The effect of extracts from ginger rhizome on inflammatory mediator production." *Phytomedicine*, 14:123–8. Accessed on April 9, 2021. doi: 10.1016/j.phymed.2006.03.003.

[112] Li, Xiao-Hong, Kristine C. Y. McGrath, Van H. Tran, Yi-Ming Li, Colin C. Duke, Basil D. Roufogalis, and Alison D. Heather 2013. "Attenuation of proinflammatory responses by S-[6]-gingerol via inhibition of ROS/NF-kappa B/COX2 activation of HuH7 cells." *Evidence-Based Complementary and Alternative Medicine*, 13:14612. Accessed on April 10, 2021. doi: 10.1155/2013/146142

[113] Pan, Min-Hsiung, Min-Chi Hsieh, Jin-Min Kuo, Ching-Shu Lai, Hou Wu, Shengming Sang, and Chi-Tang Ho 2008. "[6]-Shogaol induces apoptosis in human colorectal carcinoma cells via ROS production, caspase activation, and GADD 153 expression." *Mol. Nutr. Food Res.*, 52:527–37. Accessed on April 10, 2021. doi: 10.1002/mnfr.200700157.

[114] Mahady, Gail B, Susan L. Pendland, Gina S. Yun, Zhi-Zhen Lu, and Adina Stoia 2003. "Ginger (*Zingiber officinale* Roscoe) and the gingerols inhibit the growth of Cag A+ strains of *Helicobacter*

pylori." *Anticancer Res.*, 23(5A):3699-3702. Accessed on April 10, 2021. PMID: 14666666.

[115] Yumnam, Vijayalaxmi, Thongam M. Singh, KH Sulochana Devi, and Kananbala Sarangthem 2019. "Antimicrobial activity of ginger (*Zingiber officianale* Roscoe) found in Manipur." *International Journal of Pharmacy and Biological Sciences*, 9(3): 687-693. Accessed on April 10, 2021. https://ijpbs.com/ijpbsadmin/upload/ijpbs_5e246ff0e4cbb.pdf

[116] Kim, Han-Shim, Sang-Hoon Lee, Youngjoo Byun, and Hee-Deung Park 2005. "6-Gingerol reduces *Pseudomonas aeruginosa* biofilm formation and virulence via quorum sensing inhibition. *Sci. Rep.*, 5: 8656. Accessed on April 10, 2021. https://doi.org/10.1038/srep08656.

[117] Oyedemi, Blessing O. M., E. M. Kotsia, Paul D. Stapleton, and Simon Gibbons S 2019. "Capsaicin and gingerol analogues inhibit the growth of efflux-multidrug resistant bacteria and R-plasmids conjugal transfer." *J. Ethnopharmacol.*, 245:111871. Accessed on April 10, 2021. doi:10.1016/j.jep.2019.111871.

[118] Qian, Qiu-Hai, Wang Yue, Yao-Xia Wang, Zhi-Hong Yang, Zhan-Tao Liu, and Wen-Hui Chen WH 2009. "Gingerol inhibits cisplatin-induced vomiting by down regulating 5-hydroxytryptamine, dopamine and substance P expression in minks." *Arch. Pharm. Res.*, 32:565-73. Accessed on April 10, 2021. doi: 10.1007/s12272-009-1413-9.

[119] Qian, Qiu-Hai, Wang Yue, Wen-Hui Chen, Zi-Hong Yang, Zhan-Tao Liu, and Yao-Xia Wang 2010. "Effect of gingerol on substance P and NK1 receptor expression in a vomiting model of mink." *Chin. Med. J. (Engl).*, 123:478-84. Accessed on April 10, 2021.
https://journals.lww.com/cmj/FullText/2010/02020/Effect_of_gingerol_on_substance_P_and_NK1_receptor.18.aspx

[120] Qian, Weibin, Xinrui Cai, Yingying Wang, Xinying Zhang, Hongmin Zhao, Qiuhai Qian, Zihong Yang, Zhantou Liu, and Junichi Hasegawa 2016. "Effect of Gingerol on Cisplatin-Induced Pica Analogous to Emesis Via Modulating Expressions of Dopamine 2

Receptor, Dopamine Transporter and Tyrosine Hydroxylase in the Vomiting Model of Rats. Yonago." *Acta Med.*, 59(2):100-110. Accessed on April 10, 2021. PMID: 27493480.

[121] Tian, Li, Weiban Qian, Quihai Qian, Wei Zhang, and Xinrui Cai 2020. "Gingerol inhibits cisplatin-induced acute and delayed emesis in rats and minks by regulating the central and peripheral 5-HT, SP, and DA systems." *Journal of Natural Medicines* 2020, 4(2):353-370. Accessed on April 10, 2021. doi:10.1007/s11418-019-01372-x.

[122] van Breemen, Richard B., Yi Tao, and Wenkui Li 2011. "Cyclooxygenase-2 inhibitors in ginger (*Zingiber officinale*)." *Fitoterapia*, 82(1):38-43. Accessed on April 10, 2021. doi:10.1016/j.fitote.2010.09.004.

[123] Zhang, Yong-Xin, Jai-Song Li, Li-Hua Chen, Wen-Wen Peng, and Bao-Chang Cai 2012. "Simultaneous determination of five gingerols in raw and processed ginger by HPLC." *Chin. Pharm. J.,* 47:471-474. Accessed on April 10, 2021. https://en.cnki.com.cn/Article_en/CJFDTOTAL-ZGYX201206019.htm.

[124] Teng, Hui, Kemueli T. Seuseu, Won-Young Lee, and Lei Chen 2019. "Comparing the effects of microwave radiation on 6-gingerol and 6-shogaol from ginger rhizomes (*Zingiber officinale* Rosc)." *PLoS ONE*, 14(6): e0214893. Accessed on April 10, 2021. https://doi.org/10.1371/journal.pone.0214893.

[125] Chen, Derrick, Scott A. Cunningham, Nicolynn C. Cole, Peggy C. Kohner, Jayawant N. Mandrekar, and Robin Patel R 2017. "Phenotypic and Molecular Antimicrobial Susceptibility of *Helicobacter pylori*." *Antimicrobial Agents and Chemotherapy*, 61 (4) e02530-16. Accessed on April 10, 2021. doi: 10.1128/AAC.02530-16.

[126] Weir, Connor B., and Jacqueline K. Le 2020. "Metronidazole." [Updated 2020 Jun 28]. In: *StatPearls* [Internet]. Treasure Island (FL): StatPearls Publishing; 2020 Jan-. Accessed on April 12, 2021. https://www.ncbi.nlm.nih.gov/books/NBK539728/.

[127] Thai, Tony, Blake H. Salisbury, and Patrick M. Zito 2020. "Ciprofloxacin." [Updated 2020 Jul 10]. In: *StatPearls* [Internet].

Treasure Island (FL): StatPearls Publishing; 2020 Jan-. Accessed on April 12, 2021. https://www.ncbi.nlm.nih.gov/books/NBK535454/.

[128] Wang, Xin, Yi Shen, Kiran Thakur, Jinzhi Han, Jian-Guo Zhang, Fe Hu and, Zhao-Jun Wei 2020. "Antibacterial Activity and Mechanism of Ginger Essential Oil against *Escherichia coli* and *Staphylococcus aureus*." *Molecules*, 2020;25(17):E3955. Accessed on April 12, 2021. doi:10.3390/molecules25173955.

[129] Feng, X., Q. Cheng, Q. Meng, Y. Yang, and K. Nie 2019. "Effects of ondansetron and [6]-gingerol on pica and gut microbiota in rats treated with cisplatin." *Drug Des. Devel. Ther.*, 13:2633-2641. Accessed on April 12, 2021. doi:10.2147/DDDT.S211845.

[130] Higuchi, Kyuoko, and Takashi Yanagawa T 2019. "Evaluating dose of cisplatin responsible for causing nephrotoxicity." *PLoS ONE*, 14(4): e0215757. Accessed on April 12, 2021. https://doi.org/10.1371/journal.pone.0215757.

[131] Griddine Alexandria, and Jeffrey S. Bush 2020. "Ondansetron." [Updated 2020 Apr 21]. In: *StatPearls* [Internet]. Treasure Island (FL): StatPearls Publishing; 2020 Jan-. Accessed on April 12, 2021. https://www.ncbi.nlm.nih.gov/books/NBK499839/.

[132] Isola, Sasank, Azhar Hussein, Anterpreet Dua, Karanpal Singh and Ninos Adams 2020. "Metoclopramide." [Updated 2020 Apr 21]. In: *StatPearls* [Internet]. Treasure Island (FL): StatPearls Publishing; 2020 Jan-. Accessed on April 12, 2021. https://www.ncbi.nlm.nih.gov/books/NBK519517/.

[133] Zakaria, Z.A., A.S. Mohamad, C.T. Chear, Y.Y. Wong, D.A. Israf, and M.R. Sulaiman 2010. "Antiinflammatory and Antinociceptive Activities of *Zingiber zerumbet* Methanol Extract in Experimental Model Systems." *Med. Princ. Pract.* 19:287-294. Accessed on April 12, 2021. doi: 10.1159/000312715.

[134] Jeena, Kottarapat, Vijayastelter B. Liju, and Ramadasan Kuttan 2013. "Antioxidant, anti-inflammatory and antinociceptive activities of essential oil from ginger." *Indian J. Physiol. Pharmacol.*, 57(1):51-62. Accessed on April 12, 2021. PMID: 24020099.

[135] Sepahvand, Reza, Saeed Esmaeili-Mahani, Ardeshir Arzi, Bahram Rasoulian, and Medhi Abbasnejad 2010. "Ginger (*Zingiber officinale* Roscoe) elicits antinociceptive properties and potentiates morphine-induced analgesia in the rat radiant heat tail-flick test." *J. Med. Food*, 2010;13(6):1397-1401. Accessed on April 12, 2021. doi:10.1089/jmf.2010.1043.

[136] Dedov, Vadim N., Van H. Tran, Colin C. Duke, Mark Connor, MacDonald J. Christie, Sravan Mandadi, and Basil D. Roufogalis 2002. "Gingerols: a novel class of vanilloid receptor (VR1) agonists." *British Journal of Pharmacology*, 137(6):793-798. Accessed on April 12, 2021. doi: 10.1038/sj.bjp.0704925.

[137] Fajrin, Fifteen A., Aguna E. Nugroho, Rina Susilowati, and Arief Nurrochmad 2018. "Molecular Docking Analysis of Ginger Active Compound on Transient Receptor Potential Cation Channel Subfamily V Member 1 (TRPV1)." *Indonesian Journal of Chemistry,* 18(1): 179-185. Accessed on April 12, 2021. https://doi.org/10.22146/ijc.28172.

[138] Mezey, Éva, Zsuzsannah E. Toth, Daniel N. Cortright, Michelle K. Arzubi, James E. Krause, Robert Elde, Athena Guo, Peter M. Blumberg, and Arpad Szallasi 2000. "Distribution of mRNA for vanilloid receptor subtype 1 (VR1), and VR1-like immunoreactivity, in the central nervous system of the rat and human." *Proc. Natl. Acad. Sci. U.S.A.,* 97:3655–3660. Accessed on April 12, 2021. doi: 10.1073/pnas.060496197.

[139] Andrews, P.L.R., and P. Bhandari 1993. "Resinferatoxin, an ultrapotent capsaicin analogue, has anti-emetic properties in the ferret." *Neuropharmacology*, 32:799-806. Accessed on April 12, 2021. http://dx.doi.org/10.1016/0028-3908(93)90189-A.

[140] Rudd, John A., Eugene Nalivaiko, Norio Matsuki, Christina Wan, and Pail L.R. Andrews 2015. "The role of the TRPV1 receptor in emesis and anti-emesis." *Temperature,* 2(2):258-276. Accessed on April 12, 2021. doi: 10.1080/23328940.2015.1043042.

[141] Shiroshita, Yasuteru, Tomushige Koga, and Hiroyuki Fukuda 1997. "Capsaicin in the 4th ventricle abolishes retching and transmission of

emetic vagal afferents to solitary nucleus neurons." *Eur. J. Pharmacol.*, 339:183-92. Accessed on April 12, 2021. http://dx.doi.org/10.1016/S0014-2999(97)01370-8.

[142] Edwards, Sarah M., Solveig A. Cunningham, Anne L. Dunlop, and Elizabeth J. Corwin 2017. "The Maternal Gut Microbiome During Pregnancy." *MCN Am J Matern Child Nurs.*, 42(6):310-317. Accessed on April 12, 2021. doi:10.1097/NMC.0000000000000372.

[143] Elmassry, Moamen, Rui Wang, Abdul Hamood, Volker Neugebauer, and Chwan-Li Shen 2020. "Two Isomers of Ginger Root Extracts Modify Composition and Function of Gut Microbiota in Rats Treated with Neuropathic Pain." *Current Developments in Nutrition* 4(suppl. 2):394. Accessed on April 12, 2021. https://doi.org/10.1093/cdn/nzaa045_027.

[144] Mishra, Abhay P., Sarla Sakani, and Subhash Chandra 2013. "Estimation of gingerol content in different brand samples of ginger powder and their anti-oxidant activity: A comparative study." *Recent Research in Science and Technology*, 5(1): 54-59. Accessed on April 12, 2021. https://updatepublishing.com/journal/index.php/rrst/article/view/1008.

[145] Ghasemzadeh, Ali, Hawa Z. Jaafar, and Asmah Rahmat 2016. "Changes in antioxidant and antibacterial activities as well as phytochemical constituents associated with ginger storage and polyphenol oxidase activity." *BMC Complement. Altern. Med.*, 16(1):382. Accessed on April 12, 2021. 10.1186/s12906-016-1352-1.

[146] Koo, Karen L. K., Alaina J. Ammit, Van H. Tran, Colin C. Duke, and Basil D. Roufogalis 2001. "Gingerols and related analogues inhibit arachidonic acid-induced human platelet serotonin release and aggregation." *Thromb. Res.*, 103(5):387-397. Accessed on April 12, 2021. doi:10.1016/s0049-3848(01)00338-3.

[147] Morera, Enrico, Luciano Petrocellis, Ludovica Morera, Aniello S. Moriello, Marianna Nalli, Vincenzo DiMarzo, and Georgio Orar 2012. "Synthesis and biological evaluation of [6]-gingerol analogues as transient receptor potential channel TRPV1 and TRPA1

modulators." *Biorg. Med. Chem. Lett.*, 22:1674-1677. Accessed on April 12, 2021. doi: 10.1016/j.bmcl.2011.12.113.

[148] Kumboonm, Pakit, Thanaset Senawong, Somprasong Saenglee, Chavi, Venjai, and Chanokbhorn Phaosiri C 2017. "Identification of phenolic compounds from *Zingiber offinale* and their derivatives as histone deacetylase inhibitors and antioxidants." *Med. Chem. Res.*, 26:650–661. Accessed on April 12, 2021. https://doi.org/10.1007/s00044-017-1785-1.

[149] Luna-Dulcey, Liany, Rebeka Tomasin, Marina A. Naves, James A. da Silva JA, and Marcia R. Cominetti 2018. "Autophagy-dependent apoptosis is triggered by a semi-synthetic [6]-gingerol analogue in triple negative breast cancer cells." *Oncotarget*, 9(56):30787-30804. Accessed on April 12, 2021. doi:10.18632/oncotarget.25704.

[150] Zhu, Yingdong, Pei Wang, Yantao Zhao, Chun Yang, Anderson Clark, TinChung Leung, Xiaoxin Chen, and Shengmin Sang S 2016. "Synthesis, evaluation, and metabolism of novel [6]-shogaol derivatives as potent Nrf2 activators." *Free Radical Biology and Medicine*, 95: 243-254. Accessed on April 12, 2021. https://doi.org/10.1016/j.freeradbiomed.2016.03.026.

[151] Zhuang, Xiaoying, Zhong-Bin Deng, Jingyao Mu, Lifeng Zhang, Jun Yan, Donald Miller, Wenke Feng, Craig J. McClain, and Huang-Ge Zhang 2015. "Ginger-derived nanoparticles protect against alcohol-induced liver damage." *Journal of Extracellular Vesicles*, 4:1. Accessed on April 12, 2021. doi: 10.3402/jev.v4.28713.

[152] Zhang, Mingzhen, Emilie Viennois, Meena Prasad, Yunchen Zhang, Lixen Wang, Zhen Zhang, Moon K. Han, Bo Xiao, Chanlong Xu, Shanthi Srinivasan, and Didier Merlin 2016. "Edible ginger-derived nanoparticles: A novel therapeutic approach for the prevention and treatment of inflammatory bowel disease and colitis-associated cancer." *Biomaterials*, 101:321-340. Accessed on April 12, 2021. doi:10.1016/j.biomaterials.2016.06.018.

[153] Zhang, Mingzhen, Xiauyu Wang, Moon K. Han, James F. Collins, and Didier Merlin 2017. "Oral administration of ginger-derived

nanolipids loaded with siRNA as a novel approach for efficient siRNA drug delivery to treat ulcerative colitis." *Nanomedicine*, 12: 1927–1943. Accessed on April 12, 2021. doi: 10.2217/nnm-2017-0196.

[154] Kalarikkal, Sreeram P., Durga Prasad, Ravi Kasiappan, Sachin R. Chaudhari, and Gopinath M. Sundaraam 2020. "A cost-effective polyethylene glycol-based method for the isolation of functional edible nanoparticles from ginger rhizomes." *Sci. Rep.*, 10: 4456. Accessed on April 12, 2021. https://doi.org/10.1038/s41598-020-61358-8.

[155] Pais, Joana M., Bruna Pereira, Felipe A. A. Paz, Susana M. Cardoso SM, and Susana S. Braga 2020. "Solid γ-cyclodextrin inclusion compound with gingerols, a multi-component guest: preparation, properties and application in yogurt." *Biomolecules*, *10*(2): 344. Accessed on April 12, 2021. https://doi.org/10.3390/biom10020344.

[156] Manatunga, Danushika C., Rohini M. de Silva, K.M. Nalin de Silva, Dulharie T. Wijaratne, Gathsaurie N. Malavige, and Gareth Williams 2018. "Fabrication of 6-gingerol, doxorubicin and alginate hydroxyapatite into a bio-compatible formulation: enhanced anti-proliferative effect on breast and liver cancer cells." *Chemistry Central Journal*, 12:19. Accessed on April 12, 2021. https://doi.org/10.1186/s13065-018-0482-6.

[157] Yang, Chunghua, Mingzhen Zhang, Sudeep Lama, Lixin Wang, and Didier Merlin 2020. "Natural-lipid nanoparticle-based therapeutic approach to deliver 6-shogaol and its metabolites M2 and M13 to the colon to treat ulcerative colitis." *Journal of Controlled Release*, 323: 293-310. Accessed on April 12, 2021. https://doi.org/10.1016/j.jconrel.2020.04.032.

[158] Kemkar, Kerin, L. Sathiyanarayanan, Arimmothi Sathiyanarayanan, and Kaksaheb Mahadik 2018. "6-Shogaol rich ginger oleoresin loaded mixed micelles enhances in vitro cytotoxicity on MCF-7 cells and in vivo cancer activity against DAL cells." *International Journal of Pharmacy and Pharmaceutical Sciences,* 10(1): 160-168. Accessed on April 12, 2021. doi:10.22159/ijpps.2018v10i1.23077.

[159] Zhang, Huiyun, Qilong Wang, Congyong Sun, Yuan Zhu, Qiuxuan Yang, Qiuyu Wei, Jiaxin Chen, Wenwen Deng, Michael Adu-Frimpong, Jiangnan Yu, and Ximing Xu 2019. "Enhanced Oral Bioavailability, Anti-Tumor Activity and Hepatoprotective Effect of 6-Shogaol Loaded in a Type of Novel Micelles of Polyethylene Glycol and Linoleic Acid Conjugate." *Pharmaceutics*, 11(3):107. Accessed on April 12, 2021. doi:10.3390/pharmaceutics11030107.

[160] Eckschlager, Tomas, Johana Plch, Marie Stiborova, and Jan Hrabeta 2017. "Histone Deacetylase Inhibitors as Anticancer Drugs." *Int. J. Mol. Sci.*, 18(7):1414. Accessed on April 12, 2021. doi:10.3390/ijms18071414.

[161] Richon, V.M. 2006. "Cancer biology: mechanism of antitumour action of vorinostat (suberoylanilide hydroxamic acid), a novel histone deacetylase inhibitor." *Br. J. Cancer*, 95(Suppl 1): S2-S6. Accessed on April 12, 2021. doi:10.1038/sj.bjc.6603463.

[162] Dodson, Matthew, Montserrat de la Vega, Aram B. Cholanians, Cody J. Schmidlin, Eli Chapman, and Donna D. Zhang 2019. "Modulating NRF2 in Disease: Timing Is Everything." *Annu. Rev. Pharmacol. Toxicol.*, 59:555-575. Accessed on April 12, 2021. doi:10.1146/annurev-pharmtox-010818-021856.

[163] Nguyen, Hang T., Guillaume Dalmasso, Leif Torkvist, Jonas Halfvarson, Yutao Yan, Hamed Laroui, Doron Schmerling, Tiziano Tallone, Mauro D'Amato, Shanthi Sitamaran, and Didier Merlin 2011. "CD98 expression modulates intestinal homeostasis, inflammation, and colitis-associated cancer in mice." *J. Clin. Invest.*, 121(5):1733-1747. Accessed on April 14, 2021. doi:10.1172/ JCI44631.

[164] Maeng, Jin H., Don-Haeng Lee, Kyung H. Jung, You-Han Bae, In-Suh Park, Seok Jeong, Yong-Sun Jeon, Chang-Koo Shim, Wooyoung Kim, Jungahn Kim, Jeongmi Lee, Yoon-Mi Lee, Ji-Hee Kim, Won-Hong Kim, and Soon-Sun Hong 2010. "Multifunctional doxorubicin loaded superparamagnetic iron oxide nanoparticles for chemotherapy and magnetic resonance imaging in liver cancer." *Biomaterials*

31(18): 4995-5006. Accessed on April 14, 2021. https://doi.org/10.1016/j.biomaterials.2010.02.068.

[165] Lee, Hyun S., Eun Y. Seo, Nam E. Kang, and Woo K. Kim 2008. "[6]-Gingerol inhibits metastasis of MDA-MB-231 human breast cancer cells." *The Journal of Nutritional Biochemistry* 19(5):313-319. Accessed on April 14, 2021. https://doi.org/10.1016/j.jnutbio.2007.05.008.

[166] Kapoor, Vaishani, Sadya Aggarwal, and Satya Das 2016. "6-Gingerol Mediates its Anti Tumor Activities in Human Oral and Cervical Cancer Cell Lines through Apoptosis and Cell Cycle Arrest." *Phytother. Res.*, 30: 588– 595. Accessed on April 14, 2021. doi: 10.1002/ptr.5561.

[167] Lv, Lishuang, Huadong Chen, Dominique Soroka, Xiaoxin Chen, TinChung Leung, and Shenmin Sang 2012. "6-gingerdiols as the major metabolites of 6-gingerol in cancer cells and in mice and their cytotoxic effects on human cancer cells." *J. Agric. Food Chem.*, 60(45):11372-11377. Accessed on April 14, 2021. doi:10.1021/jf303879b.

[168] Ling, H., H. Yang, S.H. Tan, W. K. Chui, and E.H. Chew 2010. "6-Shogaol, an active constituent of ginger, inhibits breast cancer cell invasion by reducing matrix metalloproteinase-9 expression via blockade of nuclear factor-κB activation." *Br. J. Pharmacol.*, 161(8):1763-1777. Accessed on April 14, 2021. doi:10.1111/j.1476-5381.2010.00991.x.

[169] Bawadood, Azizah S., Fahad A. Al-Abbasi, Firoz Anwar, Ali M. El-Halawany, and Ahmed M. Al-Abd 2020. "6-Shogaol suppresses the growth of breast cancer cells by inducing apoptosis and suppressing autophagy via targeting notch signaling pathway." *Biomedicine & Pharmacotherapy*, 128: 110302. Accessed on April 14, 2021. https://doi.org/10.1016/j.biopha.2020.110302.

[170] Liu, Qun, Yong-Bo Peng, Lian-Wen Qi, Xiao-Lan Cheng, Xiao-Jun Xu, Le-Le Liu, E-Hu Liu, and Ping Li 2012. "The cytotoxicity mechanism of 6-shogaol-treated HeLa human cervical cancer cells revealed by label-free shotgun proteomics and bioinformatics

analysis." *Evidence-Based Complementary and Alternative Medicine,* Volume 2012: Article ID 278652. Accessed on April 14, 2021. https://doi.org/10.1155/2012/278652.

[171] Qi, Lian-Wen, Zhiyu Zhang, Chun-Feng Zhang, Samantha Anderson, Qun Liu, Chun-Su Yuan, and Chong-Zhi Wang 2015. "Anti-colon cancer effects of 6-shogaol through G2/M cell cycle arrest by p53/p21-cdc2/cdc25A crosstalk." *The American Journal of Chinese Medicine*, 43(4): 743-756. Accessed on April 14, 2021. https://doi.org/10.1142/S0192415X15500469.

[172] Liu, Qun, Yong-Bo Peng, Ping Zhou, Lian-Wen Qi, Mu Zhang, Ning Gao, E-Hu Liu, and Ping Li 2013. "6-Shogaol induces apoptosis in human leukemia cells through a process involving caspase-mediated cleavage of eIF2α." *Mol. Cancer*, 12, 135. Accessed on April 14, 2021. https://doi.org/10.1186/1476-4598-12-135.

[173] Kim, Myoung O., Mee-Hyun Lee, Naomi Oi, Sung-Hyun Kim, Ki B. Bae, Zunnan Huang, Dong J. Kim, Kanamata Reddy, Sung-Young Lee, Si-Jun Park, Jae Y. Kim, Hua Xie, Joydeb K. Kundu, Zae Y. Ryoo, Ann M. Bode, Young-Joon Surh, and Zigang Dong 2014. "Z[6]-Shogaol inhibits growth and induces apoptosis of non-small cell lung cancer cells by directly regulating Akt1/2." *Carcinogenesis*, 35(3): 683–691. Accessed on April 14, 2021. https://doi.org/10.1093/carcin/bgt365.

[174] Saha, Achinto, Jorge Blanda, Eric Silver, Linda Beltran, Jonathan Sessler, and John DiGiovanni 2014. "6-shogaol from dried ginger inhibits growth of prostate cancer cells both *in vitro* and *in vivo*." *Cancer Prev. Res.*, 7(6):627-638. Accessed on April 14, 2021. doi: 10.1158/1940-6207.CAPR-13-0420.

[175] Zhong, Weilong, Wendong Yang, Yuan Qin, Wenguang Gu, Yinyin Xue, Yuanho Tang, Henwei Xu, Hongzi Wang, Changhua Zhang, Bo Sun, Yanrong Liu, Huijuan Liu, Honggang Zhou, Shuang Chen, Tao Sun, and Cheng Yang 2019 C. "6-Gingerol stabilized the p-VEGFR2/VE-cadherin/β-catenin/actin complex promotes microvessel normalization and suppresses tumor progression." *J. Exp.*

Clin. Cancer Res., 38: 285. Accessed on April 14, 2021. https://doi.org/10.1186/s13046-019-1291-z.

[176] Kim, Eok-Chon, Jeong-Ki Min, Tae-Yoon Kim, Shin-Jeong Lee, Hyun-Ok Yang, Sanghwa Han, Young-Myeyong Kim, and Young-Guen Kwon 2005. "[6]-Gingerol, a pungent ingredient of ginger, inhibits angiogenesis *in vitro* and *in vivo*." *Biochemical and Biophysical Research Communications*, 335(2): 300-308. Accessed on April 14, 2021. https://doi.org/10.1016/j.bbrc.2005.07.076.

[177] Brown, Amy C., Chirag Shah, Jesse Liu, Jimmy T. Pham, Jian G. Zhang, and Martin R. Jadus 2009. "Ginger's (*Zingiber officinale* Roscoe) inhibition of rat colonic adenocarcinoma cells proliferation and angiogenesis *in vitro*." *Phytother. Res.*, 23(5):640-5. Accessed on April 14, 2021. doi: 10.1002/ptr.2677.

[178] Mukkavilli, Rao, Chunhua Yang, Reenu S. Tanwar, Roopali Saxena, Sushma R. Gundula, Yingyi Zhang, Ahmed Gareeb, Stephen D. Floyd, Subrahmanayam Vangala, Wei-Wen Kuo, Padmashree C.G. Rida, and Ritu Aneja 2018. "Pharmacokinetic-pharmacodynamic correlations in the development of ginger extract as an anticancer agent." *Sci. Rep.*, 8; 3056. Accessed on April 14, 2021. https://doi.org/10.1038/s41598-018-21125-2.

[179] Wu, Hou, Min-Chi Hsieh, Chih-Yu Lo, Cheng B. Liu, Shengmin Sang, Chi-Tang Ho, and Min-Hsiung Pan 2010. "6-Shogaol is more effective than 6-gingerol and curcumin in inhibiting 12-*O*-tetradecanoylphorbol 13-acetate-induced tumor promotion in mice." *Mol. Nutr. Food Res.*, 54: 1296-1306. Accessed on April 14, 2021. doi:10.1002/mnfr.200900409.

[180] Zhang, Feng, Na Ma, Yong-Feng Gao, Li-Li Sun, and Ji-Guo Zhang 2017. "Therapeutic Effects of 6-Gingerol, 8-Gingerol, and 10-Gingerol on Dextran Sulfate Sodium-Induced Acute Ulcerative Colitis in Rats." *Phytother. Res.*, 31(9):1427-1432. doi:10.1002/ptr.5871.

[181] Ajayi, B. O., I. A. Adedara, and E. O. Farombi 2018. "Protective mechanisms of 6-gingerol in dextran sulfate sodium-induced chronic

ulcerative colitis in mice." *Hum. Exp. Toxicol.*, 37(10):1054-1068. Accessed on April 14, 2021. doi:10.1177/0960327117751235

[182] Sheng, Yingue, Tielong Wu, Yuanyuan Dai Y, Ke Ji, Yao Zhong, and Yuzheng Xue 2020. "The effect of 6-gingerol on inflammatory response and Th17/Treg balance in DSS-induced ulcerative colitis mice." *Annals of Translatable Medicine*, 8(7):442. Accessed on April 14, 2021. doi: 10.21037/atm.2020.03.141.

[183] Seyedian, Seyed S., Forogh Nokhostin, and Mehrdad D. Malamir 2019. "A review of the diagnosis, prevention, and treatment methods of inflammatory bowel disease." *J. Med. Life*, 12(2):113-122. Accessed on April 14, 2021. doi:10.25122/jml-2018-0075.

[184] Guan, Qingong. "A Comprehensive Review and Update on the Pathogenesis of Inflammatory Bowel Disease." *J. Immunol. Res.*, 2019:7247238. Accessed on April 14, 2021. doi:10.1155/2019/7247238.

[185] Mizoguchi, Atshushi, and Emiko Mizoguchi 2020. "Animal models of IBD: linkage to human disease." *Curr. Opin. Pharmacol.*, 10(5):578-587. Accessed on April 14, 2021. doi:10.1016/j.coph.2010.05.007.

[186] Fujino, S., A. Andoh, S. Bamba, A. Ogawa, K. Hata, Y. Araki, T. Bamba, and Y. Fujiyama 2003. "Increased expression of interleukin 17 in inflammatory bowel disease." *Gut*, 52(1): 65–70. Accessed on April 14, 2021. doi: 10.1136/gut.52.1.65.

[187] Hardenberg G, Steiner TS, Levings MK 2011. "Environmental influences on T regulatory cells in inflammatory bowel disease." *Seminars in Immunology*, 23(2):130–138. Accessed on April 14, 2021. doi: 10.1016/j.smim.2011.01.012.

[188] Magro, Daniela O., Andrey Santos, Dioze Guadagnini, Flavia M. de Godoy, Silvia H.M Silva, Wilson J.F. Lemos, Nicola Vitulo, Sandra Torriani, Lilian V. Pinheiro, Carloz A.R. Martinez, Mario J. A. Saad, and Claudio S.R. Coy 2019. "Remission in Crohn's disease is accompanied by alterations in the gut microbiota and mucins production." *Sci. Rep.*, 9: 13263. Accessed on April 14, 2021. https://doi.org/10.1038/s41598-019-49893-5.

[189] Shen, J., Z.X. Zuo, and A.P. Mao 2014. "Effect of probiotics on inducing remission and maintaining therapy in ulcerative colitis, Crohn's disease, and pouchitis: meta-analysis of randomized controlled trials." *Inflammatory Bowel Disease*, 20:21–35. Accessed on April 14, 2021. doi: 10.1097/01.mib.0000437495.30052.be.

[190] Ahmadmehrabi, Shadi, and W.H. Wilson Tang 2017. "Gut microbiome and its role in cardiovascular diseases." *Curr. Opin. Cardiol.*, 32(6):761-766. Accessed on April 14, 2021. doi:10.1097/HCO.0000000000000445

[191] Bu, Jin, and Zhaohui Wang Z 2018. "Cross-Talk between Gut Microbiota and Heart via the Routes of Metabolite and Immunity." *Gastroenterology Research and Practice*, 2018: Article ID 6458094. Accessed on April 14, 2021. https://doi.org/10.1155/2018/6458094.

[192] Wu, Ping, Fangyuan Jia, Bao Zhang, and Peiying Zhang 2017. "Risk of cardiovascular disease in inflammatory bowel disease." *Exp. Ther. Med.*, 13(2):395-400. Accessed on April 14, 2021. doi:10.3892/etm.2016.3966.

In: Ginger's Antimicrobial …
Editor: Diana R. Cundell
ISBN: 978-1-68507-117-2

Chapter 2

GINGER AS AN ANTIBACTERIAL AGENT

Manuela Tripepi*, PhD,
Mary-Ann Wagner-Graham, PhD, Madison Bright, Nicholas Wahba and Maithili Patel
College of Life Sciences, Jefferson University, Philadelphia, PA, USA

ABSTRACT

Bacterial infections represent one of the leading causes of death worldwide. With the drastic rise in bacterial-related infections, it has become shockingly apparent that the once effective sources of treatment have begun to lose its potency. The use of antibiotics has been the primary therapy against bacterial infections for years. Unfortunately, many bacteria are developing resistance resulting in the inefficacy of many antibiotics. The race to find a solution to antibiotic resistance has focused in on the potential of plants and their active constituents as novel antimicrobials. Phytochemicals have been used for centuries in alternative medicine in remedies against different malaises. *Zingiber officinale* (ginger) rhizome has been used as a spice and as a health supplement due to its numerous properties. Over the recent years the interest in ginger and its compounds has increase, so scientific research which has generated a great amount of

* Corresponding Author's E-mail: Manuela.Tripepi@jefferson.edu.

data on the efficacy of these chemicals against different diseases. In this review we present an overview of studies conducted on the antibacterial efficacy of ginger against the causative agents of infections in 4 major body systems; skin and joints, respiratory, digestive, and the oral cavity.

Keywords: ginger, Zingiber officinale, antibacterial, medicinal plants, essential oils

INTRODUCTION

The fight against bacterial infections, that would otherwise threaten the life of a patient was made possible through the discovery of antimicrobials, in addition to their incorporation into surgical procedures such us organ transplants, open-heart surgery, and cancer treatment [1-3]. According to the World Health Organization (WHO), and European Commission antibacterial resistance threatens the effective prevention and treatment of an ever-increasing range of infections caused by bacteria [4-6]. It is an increasingly serious threat to global public health that requires action across all government sectors and society [7]. Therefore, in recent years there has been extensive focus on the development of measures and solutions able to ameliorate the antibiotic resistance crisis [1, 8]. Strategies to find alternatives include modifying current antibiotic molecules, searching for new antibiotic targets, creating new molecules, and exploring different niche to find novel natural components [9]. Another possible solution that is being explored are the compounds and dietary supplements derived from plants [10]. Scientists are looking into natural remedies from centuries far before the golden era that were employed in alternative medicine, specifically in traditional Chinese Medicine (TCM), Ayurveda, Kampo, Unani and Siddha [1, 11].

Of particular interest are plants that produce essential oils, secondary volatile metabolites, that are used with various delivery methods in a practice called aromatherapy [13, 14]. Essential oils can be extracted by several processes such as steam distillation, hydro diffusion, or pressure. More than 17,000 plants produce essential oils, but only the products of around 300 plants are currently available in commerce [14]. Essential oils are used by the food and beverage industries, as well as cosmetics. Their efficacy in the pharmaceutical field has been noted, as there is evidence of antioxidant, anti-inflammatory, antibacterial, antiviral, antidiabetic and anticancer activity [15]. Furthermore, even if scattered, there have been reports of the immunomodulatory activities that essential oils possess [16, 17]. Immunostimulation is an immunomodulation process that consists of the enhancement of immune response through secondary mechanisms that are not the usual mechanisms that stimulate an immune response [15].

Zingiber officinale Rosc. (ginger), member of Zingiberaceae family, is commonly used as a spice and a medicinal plant in non-traditional western medicine against a range of diseases [16]. Ginger is the most common condiment in the world, as it is available as fresh, powder, or dry, and its rich aroma is due to its bioactive components [18, 19]. It is cultivated in various tropical locations where temperatures range between 28°C and 35°C, with India being the biggest producer worldwide and China the number one exporter [20]. Ginger is used in many cuisines for its flavoring, especially in Indian, Chinese, Japanese, Korean, Vietnamese, and many other South Asian cuisines. It is also used as a food preservative, in candy, and in alcoholic beverages [21].

Ginger has a broad and well explored therapeutic role, with recognition from various regulatory authorities as a safe herbal supplement [22]. It is reported to be effective against many ailments because of its properties as an antioxidant, anti-inflammatory, antiviral, antimicrobial, anticancer, antidiabetic, antinausea agent [23, 24, 25]. The medicinal properties of ginger come from the constituents that can be extracted from the rhizome. These compounds are divided into two groups: volatile essential oils and fragrant or harsh phenol compounds [26]. Gingerol and shogaols are phenolic compounds that are obtained from the terpenes of ginger, whereas paradol and zingerone derive from gingerols [26].

In this chapter we examine the available data on the efficacy of ginger's components as antimicrobial. We will begin by defining the compounds and then report studies by group of diseases and when appropriate the microbes for which ginger showed antimicrobial efficacy.

Antibacterial Compounds of Ginger

Recent and extensive reviews [27, 28, 29, 30] summarize the rich chemical profile of ginger oil, and present relative percent composition of chemical species varies by geographic location of the source plants, along with the plant tissue used as starting material and whether or not the plant material was dried prior to processing. A comprehensive historical, qualitative/semi-quantitative overview of the varied compositions of ginger oils and extracts of different source plants and preparation methods is presented by Govindarajan (1982), in which one- and three-dimensional thin-layer chromatograms and GC elution profiles of oils/extracts from multiple sources are presented. For ease of reference, representative components of ginger oil and extracts are shown in Figure 1 [31].

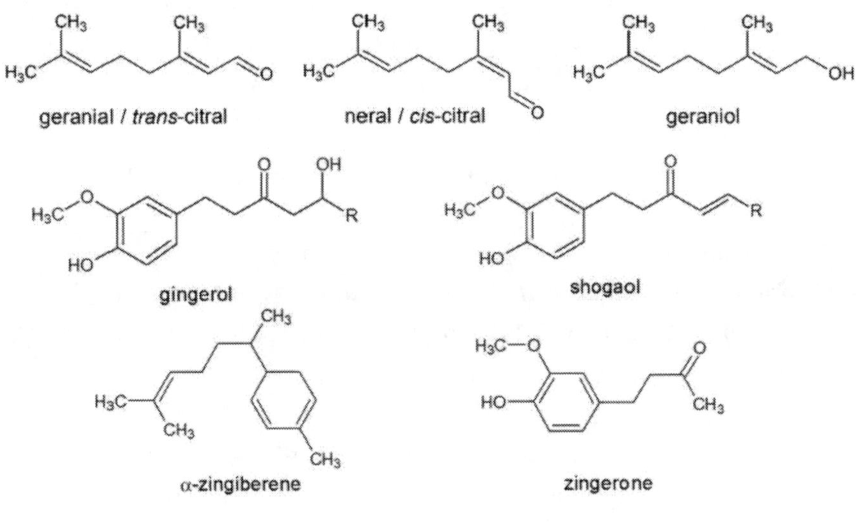

Figure 1. Representative components of ginger oils and extracts. Variable substituents of gingerol and shogaol include: -$(CH_2)_4CH_3$ (6-gingerol, 6-shogaol); -$(CH_2)_6CH_3$ (8-gingerol, 8-shogaol); or -$(CH_2)_8CH_3$ (10-gingerol, 10-shogaol).

Inherent variation in chemical composition of ginger essential oil impedes direct comparison of reports of antibacterial effectiveness of ginger oils, and can explain variation across studies. Use of non-standard nomenclature for chemical constituents of essential oils further complicates comparison of studies.

Comparative transcriptome analysis of multiple plant tissues indicated genes for gingerol synthesis are most highly expressed in rhizome tissue, beginning in early development, and suggest caffeoyl-coenzyme A O-methyl transferase (CCoAOMT) and hydroxycinnamoyl-coenzyme A shikimate/quinate hydroxycinnamoyl transferase (HCT) activities may limit production of gingerols [32]. A concise and updated overview of the gingerol biosynthetic pathway is presented [32].

In addition to bio-active small molecules, water-soluble extracts of ginger contain bio-active proteins. Ginger extracts contain protease activity [33, 34, 35] proteins with antifungal properties [36]. Ginger rhizome juice, extracted via homogenization in a blender, and used at a concentration of 100 ug/mL in agar well diffusion assay, lost all antibacterial activity against *Escherichia coli, Klebsiella pneumoniae, and Staphylococcus aureus* when rhizome tissue was boiled in water for 30 min before homogenization [37]. Note that heating changes the chemical composition of ginger extracts and oils, with heat inducing conversion of gingerols to shogaols [38].

Chemical components of ginger oils can also interfere directly with actions of bacterial toxins to lessen morbidity. For example, 6-gingerol and zingerone block in vitro binding of *E. coli* heat-labile enterotoxin B-subunit to GM1 ganglioside, although 6-gingerol fails to suppress ETEC induced diarrhea in vivo [39]. A synthetic zingerone-like compound (2-[(4-methoxybenzyl)oxy]benzoic acid) shows promise as an anti-diarrheal agent which blocks binding between intestinal epithelial GM1 ganglioside and heat-labile enterotoxin [39]. When applied to Vero and HT-29 cells, zingerone prevents cytopathogenic effects promoted by clostridial toxins in cell-free *Clostridium difficile* culture supernatant [40]. Since this protective effect is seen only if zingerone is applied to Vero and HT-29 cells before the toxin-containing culture supernatant, or if zingerone is added to and pre-incubated with cell-free *C. difficile* culture supernatant before application to the cells, it is likely that zingerone exerts its effects by blocking binding of clostridial toxins to the cells [40].

ANTIBACTERIAL EFFECTS OF *ZINGIBER OFFICINALE* AGAINST SKIN AND JOINT INFECTIONS

Bacterial skin and joint infections have garnered more attention over the past few years due to the significant rise in antibiotic resistance that has been recorded in many clinical settings. Recent studies have identified that approximately 60% of presented cases are caused by either acute bacterial skin and skin structure infections (ABSSSIs) or complicated skin and skin structure infections (cSSSIs) [41]. Strains of bacteria found to cause skin and joint infections include *Staphylococcus aureus, Streptococcus pyogenes, Enterococcus faecalis*, and Gram-negative bacteria [42]. Patients who are diagnosed with ABSSSIs or cSSSIs often exhibit comorbidities, such as diabetes, that impede treatment and ultimately elevates the rate of mortality [41]. As the efficacy of several broad-spectrum antibiotics are weakening, components of *Zingiber officinale* has exhibited anti-bacterial properties that have showed promise for future application in treating bacterial skin and joint infections.

Staphylococcus aureus

S. aureus is a gram-positive bacterium that is notorious for its ability to develop a mechanism for antibiotic resistance [43]. Over time, various strains of S. aureus have been identified, most known include methicillin-susceptible S. aureus (MSSA), methicillin-resistant *S. aureus* (MRSA), vancomycin-intermediate S. aureus (VISA), and vancomycin-resistant S. aureus (VRSA) [44]. *S. aureus*, between 2001 and 2003 in the United States, was believed to have been the cause of 11.6 million health visits annually because of its role in various skin and soft tissue infections ranging from abscesses to toxic shock syndrome (TSS) [45, 46]. In 2017, S. aureus reached a peak of around 120,000 bloodstream infections and 20,000 deaths [47]. Six literature studies have examined the effects of ginger extract, or purified gingerol and shogaols on soft tissue isolates of S. aureus [48-53]. The results of these studies are summarized in Table 1.

Table 1. Studies of the efficacy of ginger compounds against *S. aureus*

Study design	Results	Reference
In vitro: Water-ethanol extract of ginger evaluated by disc-diffusion method and MIC.	*S. aureus* and MRSA disc diffusion inhibition was 16 and 9 mm, respectively. MIC for *S. aureus* and MRSA were 52 μg/ml.	[48]
In vitro; ginger, 6-gingerols and 6-shogaols MIC evaluated against 10 strains of *S. aureus* including 6 MRSA strains.	MICs ranged from 8 to 512 mg/L. 6-shogaol displaying the highest potency against the resistant strain RN4220 (8 mg/L). *S. aureus* strains. Tetracycline efflux mutants) were susceptible to gingerol at an MIC of 16 mg/L.	[49]
In vitro: CGE was mixed with media and inoculated. EGE was examined via Kirby-Bauer test and broth dilution test.	Total inhibition at 100% CGE. A 19 mm zone of inhibition at 100 μg/10 μl. The MIC of the EGE against *S. aureus* was 400 μg/ml.	[50]
In vitro: Roots and leaves of ginger were extracted using distilled water and ethanol. A Kirby-Bauer test was performed.	Distilled water and ethanol extracts (100 g/100 mg) produced 30 and 32 mm zones of inhibition, respectively.	[51]
In vitro: Aqueous extract tested by disc diffusion method.	200 mg/ml produced a zone of inhibition of 13.5 mm.	[52]
In vivo: Wistar rats (n = 5) received oral (10 mg/ Kg) daily extract of ginger for 30 days.	Necropsy and analysis of serum liver enzymes revealed elevations in aspartate transaminase (AST) compared with controls. Other liver enzymes were unaffected.	
In vitro: Red ginger ethanolic extract (6.25-50%) disc diffusion assay of *S. aureus* from animal mastitis samples	Zones of inhibition for *S. aureus* ranged from 8-16 mm.	[53]

Abbreviations used in the table: CGE (crude ginger extract), EGE (ethanolic ginger extract), MIC (minimum inhibitory concentration), MRSA (methicillin-resistant *S. aureus*).

A number of different methodologies were used for these, primarily *in vitro* studies [48-53] but good efficacy against *S. aureus* was reported in each. Analysis of aqueous ginger extracts suggest these consist of a mixture of vanillylacetone, 6-gingerol, 6-shogaol, and 1,4-cineol [54] In contrast, ethanolic extracts of are predominantly gingerol mixtures with 6-gingerol being the largest bioactive component [55]. Rahman et al. [50] demonstrated *Z. officinale*'s antibacterial properties through the incubation of *S. aureus* with crude ginger extract (CGE) and ethanolic ginger Extract (EGE). Partial inhibition was noted at 70% GCE media and total inhibition at 100% CGE [50]. From the broth dilution test, the MIC of the EGE against *S. aureus* was found to be 400 μg/ml [50]. Although mixtures of ginger bioactive components were found to produce changes in one of the rodent liver enzymes in the study by Sulaiman et al. [52], these toxicities have not been reported in other animal studies with 6-gingerol or 6-shogaol [56]. Further research with purified bioactive ginger components such as gingerols and shogaols is therefore needed to identify whether these merit development as antibiotics.

Streptococcus pyogenes

S. pyogenes is another gram-positive bacterium that has been known to cause various skin and joint infections, as well as respiratory tract infections. In the United Kingdom specifically, *S. pyogenes* was responsible for 42% of the skin and soft tissue infections reported [57]. S. pyogenes causes a plethora of skin and joint infections that can be easily treated, like impetigo, to more severe and deadly illnesses like rheumatic fever and necrotizing fasciitis [57]. *S. pyogenes* is a major concern to physicians because of its involvement in the development of rheumatic fever and other rheumatic disorders. Rheumatic fever often appears after an individual is infected with scarlet fever or strep throat. This infection not only target's one's skin and joints, but can lead to serious health concerns with the heart and brain as well [58]. Each year, there are an estimated 336,000 new cases of acute rheumatic fever in children between the ages 5 and 14 [58]. Due to the major role *S. pyogenes* plays in rheumatic disorders, two in vitro studies have been performed using *Z. officinale* to identify whether this plant would be an appropriate alternative source of treatment [51, 58]. Sebiomo et al. [51] compared the effect of an ethanolic ginger root extract with three antibiotic (chloramphenicol, ampicillin and tetracycline.) and their abilities to kill *S.*

pyogenes. Both the root and leaf ethanol ginger extracts had the largest zone of inhibition at 30 mm than all three antibiotics when used at a concentration of–100g/100ml.–The ethanol extract yielded more significant results as compared to the water extract for inhibition of S. pyogenes growth [51].

Assegaf et al. [59] utilized eight concentrations of ethanolic red ginger extract (0.625-80%). MIC was determined through a plate count and MBC was calculated through a streaking test [59]. Unfortunately, due to interference with the turbidity, the MIC could not be properly concluded. The MBC of the extract, however, displayed that by a 20% extract concentration, minimum colony growth was recorded. No colony growth of S. pyogenes was evident at concentrations higher than 20% [59]. Assegaf et al. [59] suggested that their findings were due to the gingerol properties from the ginger extract. Gingerol was able to achieve antimicrobial activity through both destroying the cytoplasmic membrane of S. pyogenes and protein denaturation [59].

Other Notable Bacterial Agents in Skin and Joint Infections

There are a number of different bacteria that are causative agents for skin and joint infections. While there is a shortage of clinical research on the use of *Z. officinale* for the following bacteria, in vitro studies present the possibility of using ginger as an effective antibacterial in medicine. *Staphylococcus epidermidis*, *Enterococcus faecalis, and Acinetobacter baumannii* are three strains of bacteria that have been studied specifically for their involvement with skin and joint infections [60-65].

Staphylococcus epidermidis is a gram-positive bacterium known to cause postoperative wound infection and has become more of a concern to physicians with its rising resistance to previously effective antibiotics, such as methicillin. This resistance is partially due to *S. epidermidis'* involvement in biofilms [60]. One *in vitro* study that has garnered attention used *Z. officinale* against *S. epidermidis*, *S. aureus*, and *Streptococcus agalactiae* isolated from cow's with mastitis [53]. Various red ginger rhizome extracts (50, 25, 12.50, and 6.25%) were used in a Kirby-Bauer Test [53]. The results displayed the higher the concentration of ginger extract used, the larger the zone of inhibition present for all three bacteria. *S. epidermidis* was the most susceptible to the ginger extract with an average zone of inhibition of 14.15 mm [53]. This study was successful in demonstrating *Z. officinale* antibacterial properties through the inhibition of these three mastitis causing bacteria, specifically *S. epidermidis*.

Enterococcus faecalis is also a gram-positive bacterium that largely contributes to skin and soft tissue infections worldwide. As a whole, enterococci are the third leading cause in the in US of hospital-acquired infections [61]. Recently, vancomycin-resistant *Enterococcus* (VRE) has been on the rise in hospital environments and causes bacteremia, ulcers, and soft tissue abscesses [62]. With this growing threat, physicians and researchers are scouring for alternative methods of treatment. An in vitro study conducted by Silva et al. [63] examined the use of various plant essential oils with calcium hydroxide to record any antibacterial activity against *E. faecalis*. Of the thirteen test plant extracts, *Z. officinale* (ZO) essential oil was tested independently as well as with calcium hydroxide (ZOH) [63]. The MIC results against *E. faecalis* varied from 5.5 to 223.75 mg/ml, but neither ZO or ZOH were present in the 0 to 100 mg/ml range. Both ZO and ZOH test groups demonstrated bactericidal properties with *E. faecalis* with no bacterial growth present on the plates. This study presents promising results in that combinations of *Z. officinale* essential oil and calcium hydroxide could be used in future research to combat *E. faecalis* [63].

Lastly, *Acinetobacter baumannii* is a gram-negative bacterium that often targets immunocompromised individuals and thrives in hospital settings [64, 65]. With a rise in its multi-drug resistance, *A. baumannii* has taken the globe and has amounted to a 30% mortality rate [64]. This deadly strain of bacteria has been known to cause bacteremia, cSSSIs, and central nervous system infections [64]. An *in vitro* study focused on using *Z. officinale* rhizomes to combat antibiotic resistance in *A. baumannii*, specifically tetracycline [65]. MIC was determined via broth microdilution testing with various ginger components: [6]-dehydrogingerdione, [10]-gingerol, [6]-shogaol, and [6]-gingerol. The ginger compounds were tested both with and without tetracycline in attempts to alter *A. baumannii*'s drug resistance [65]. Results presented that each of the four ginger components tested exhibited antibacterial effects against *A. baumannii*, specifically [6]-dehydrogingerdione being the most inhibitory [65]. When combined with tetracycline, the MIC's of the ginger components dropped [65]. These findings are extremely important in that it is suggestive that tetracycline used in conjunction with components of ginger could restore susceptibility of *A. baumannii* to tetracycline [65].

ANTIBACTERIAL EFFECTS OF *ZINGIBER OFFICINALE* AGAINST RESPIRATORY INFECTIONS

With the respiratory tract being exposed to the environment at all times along with-it displaying properties akin to the preferable habitat for bacteria, the respiratory system is the site for bacterial infection. The most common type of infection is an upper respiratory tract infection (URTI) [66]. URTIs are significant because the bacteria must overcome the bodies innate immune system to begin an infection [66]. The mucosal layer on the upper respiratory tract is designed to reduce the ability of foreign pathogens to bind directly to the epithelial wall linings of the tract [66]. However, bacteria are unique in that it readily can reproduce using the moisture and heat the mucosal layer provides removing the need to bind to the epithelial lining [66]. The most prominent bacterium to induce URTIs are *Haemophilus influenzae*, *Streptococcus pneumoniae*, and *Moraxella catarrhalis*. These species are responsible for ~70% of all URTIs [66]. All three of these species have been treated with penicillin in the past but in recent years all three have developed penicillin-resistant strains [66]. With the eventuality that strains resistant to all known antibiotic treatments for URTIs and respiratory tract infections in general, an alternative treatment for respiratory infections is in high demand. *Zingiber officinale* has shown promise in other bacteria that affect the respiratory tract and could therefore pose a possible solution.

Effects of Ginger on Multiple Respiratory Bacteria

Akoachere et al. [67] investigation of ethanolic extracts of ginger (10 μg) on respiratory isolated of *S. aureus*, *S. pneumoniae*, *H. influenzae*, and *S. pyogenes*. Sampling of respiratory bacteria occurred from three areas of Cameroon, namely Bokwango, Molyko, and Bolifamba [67]. These authors concluded that ginger was not very efficient at inhibiting the growth of the *S. pneumoniae* and *H. influenzae* with zones of inhibition of 2-4 mm and 1-4 mm, respectively [67].

Okiki et al. [68] utilized an aqueous extract of ginger and a methanolic extract to compare the effect of ginger to 13 commonly used antibiotics against 17 hospital isolates of respiratory tract bacteria species. The bacteria were spread on agar plates and then each plate was exposed to one of the antibiotics or the ginger extracts (50-400 mg/ml) [68]. All bacteria were found to be sensitive to both preparations of ginger with the methanolic extract demonstrating greater potency [68]. In contrast, Okiki et al. [68], reported that the gram-positive isolates were resistant to cloxacillin, augmentin and tetracycline with >two-thirds of strains also resistant to erythromycin, streptomycin and cotrimaxazole. Similar antibiotic resistance was seen in the gram-negative respiratory isolates [68]. Interestingly, both gram-negative and gram-positive bacteria showed similar sensitivity to the ginger extracts [68].

Nag et al. [69] reported that individual components of *Zingiber zerumbet* could inhibit the DNA ligase activity of *H. influenzae*. Although, this is a different species of ginger, it shares many of the same phytochemicals as *Zingiber officinale* [69]. This study utilized the phytocompounds humulene, zerumbone, and camphene from *Zingiber zerumbet* as ligands to target the DNA ligase on *H. influenzae* [69]. Nag et al. [69] found that by introducing these phytocompounds, the bacteria's overall activity could be reduced as its DNA replication is halted significantly. With the exception of zerumbone, these phytochemicals are also present in similar amounts in *Zingiber officinale* meaning that these effects could apply to both species of ginger.

Pseudomonas aeruginosa

Diffuse pan bronchiolitis (DPB) is an infection of the lower respiratory tract that is most times chronic if gone untreated [70]. DPB is caused by the bacteria *Pseudomonas aeruginosa* and is typically transmitted in hospital environments as it can be transmitted through droplet contact. *Pseudomonas aeruginosa* is a gram-negative bacterium of the Pseudomonadaceae family [71]. It is commonly known as a nosocomial infection that has achieved substantial antibiotic resistance over the years *P. aeruginosa* makes up 10-20% of all infections received during hospital stays [71]. DPB infections are currently treated with long term erythromycin antibiotic treatment but with increasingly antibiotic-resistant strains developing, new treatments are a necessity [71].

Two studies of the effects of ginger on *in vitro P. aeruginosa* function have reported positive findings [72, 73]. Chakotiya et al. [72] explored the ability of ginger to be both antibacterial in a time-kill study over 24 hours. Agar plates were maintained with a highly-antibiotic resistant strain of *P. aeruginosa* and tested against varying concentrations of both amikacin and *Z. officinale* oil extract [72]. At a concentration of 200 mg/ml, amikacin inhibited the growth to a 30.78 ± 0.1 mm zone and *Z. officinale* inhibited the growth to a 27.09 ± 0.003 mm zone with the same concentration. Other tests at concentrations at 50 mg/ml, 100 mg/ml, and 150 mg/ml also concluded similar results [72]. Kim and Park [73] tested the *in vitro* efficacy of a water extract of *Z. officinale* against *P. aeruginosa* and reported it significantly ($p<0.05$) inhibited the formation of biofilms. Ginger extracts of 1%, 5%, and 10% had similar results of inhibiting the growth of biofilms by 39%-56% [73]. The ginger extract of 1% was also found to reduce the extracellular polymeric substance (EPS) content of the biofilms by ~30%.

Klebsiella pneumoniae

Klebsiella pneumoniae is a species of bacteria that accounts for a significant number of infections acquired from hospital environments, especially pneumonia [74]. This bacterium causes an estimated 7-14% of all hospital acquired pneumonia cases and is currently treated using a multitude of antibiotics as it is highly antibiotic resistant in most patients [74]. Due to both its prevalence and resistance, ginger might provide a possible route of treatment. Karuppiah and Rajaram [75] produced agar plates containing various clinical isolates of multiple antibiotic-resistant bacteria. The plates were exposed to a soaked disc of either *Z. officinale* or *Allium sativum* (garlic) extract oils with varying concentrations (50 mg/ml - 200 mg/ml) [75]. *Z. officinale* was found to be relatively effective against *Klebsiella sp.* at high concentrations with a 7.50 ± 0.50 mm zone of inhibition at 200 mg/ml [75]. This was comparable to garlic [76].

In a clinical study on ICU patients with nosocomial pneumonia and acute respiratory distress syndrome (ARDS) on ventilators, ginger extract was used to measure mortality rate and gastric emptying rate [77]. Despite ginger having antimicrobial properties, there was no decrease in the 15.6% mortality rate between the ginger group and the control group. However, the ginger group did have an overall increase in the amount of food tolerated via the enteral feeding compared to the control group [77].

Mycobacterium tuberculosis

Mycobacterium tuberculosis produces the chronic respiratory infection tuberculosis (TB) that is prevalent in upwards of 20% in some populations [78]. With the historical prevalence of tuberculosis allowing the disease to be the leading cause of death in years past, the need for better treatments is always desired [78]. Along with many other bacteria-based infections, the threat of the bacterium strain causing the strain mutating to become antibiotic-resistant increasing the demand for alternative remedies [78, 79].

Kulkarni et al. [78] evaluated the efficacy of ginger in the treatment of sixty-nine patients with active TB. The study design was placebo-controlled and randomized but single blind [78]. Patients in the control group received 3 g starch capsules and the experimental group received pills with a ginger extract pill of 3g daily for 1 month [78]. After the trial, the experiment was found to significantly reduce the inflammation and necrosis of tissues that TB can cause on patients [78]. However, the study did not evaluate the degree of infection or rate of proliferation of the bacterial cells [78].

ANTIBACTERIAL EFFECTS OF *ZINGIBER OFFICINALE* ON DISEASES OF THE DIGESTIVE SYSTEM

Every year, millions of people in the United States become ill from gastrointestinal infections or foodborne illnesses [80]. The digestive system is an epicenter of microbial growth in humans, as many bacteria are components of normal gut flora [81]. Diseases of the digestive system are commonly caused by bacteria such as *E. coli*, *Salmonella*, *Shigella*, *Pseudomonas aeruginosa*, *Helicobacter pylori*, *Staphylococcus*, and *Campylobacter* which are mainly transmitted through contaminated food sources, overuse of antibiotics, international food trade, international travel, and poor hygiene practices [81]. For many years, antibiotics such as ciprofloxacin, cefotaxime, vancomycin, streptomycin, and meropenem have clinically proven to effectively treat microbial infections of the digestive system [82]. The increased usage of antibiotics has promoted rapid modifications in the composition of gut flora and elicited the emergence of more resistant microorganisms [82]. Specifically, Enterobacteriaceae have acquired antibiotic resistance to third-generation cephalosporins [83]. Also, antibiotic resistance is frequently seen in certain strains of *E. coli*, which is a part of normal intestinal microbiota [84-86]. *E. coli* strains are increasingly becoming more resistant to carbapenems, antibiotics utilized as a last line of therapy for severe nosocomial infections, and 49 countries around the world have reported bloodstream infections due to resistant strains of *E. coli* [84-86].

As a public health crisis, increased antibiotic resistance promotes the exploration of alternative treatment options to optimize and stimulate immunity. *Zingiber officinale* is a conventional medicinal treatment commonly used by many Asian countries as it contains anti-inflammatory, anti-microbial, and antioxidant properties. While ginger is beneficial for alleviating symptoms for a wide spectrum of health conditions, the pungent components of gingerol, shogaol, zingerone, and paradol in *Zingiber officinale* have shown marked effectiveness in treating bacterial diseases of the gastrointestinal tract [87]. Hence, as microorganisms rapidly evolve over time, the future of public health requires an evolution of conventional practices to find therapeutic alternatives to antibiotics. Therefore, it's important to consider and evaluate the efficacy of *Zingiber officinale* as a means for disease management and microbial growth inhibition in the digestive system.

Escherichia coli

E. coli is a gram-negative bacterium of the Enterobacteriaceae family that normally inhabits the lower intestines of healthy people and animals [85]. While most strains of *E. coli* are harmless and helpful in digestive processes, at least six pathogenic variants that can produce gastrointestinal infections [85]. Overall, pathogenic *E. coli* produces a shiga toxin (STEC) that damages the intestinal lining and causes diarrhea and other gastrointestinal symptoms [86]. Common routes of transmission for *E. coli* are from ingesting food sources, drinking water, or touching surfaces that have been contaminated with harmful strains of *E. coli* [86]. STEC accounts for 265,000 reported infections per year in the United States alone [85].

An *in vitro* study by Yassen and Ibrahim [88] examined the minimum inhibitory concentration (MIC) of aqueous and organic extracts of *Zingiber officinale* against gastrointestinal isolates of *E. coli* and *S. aureus* [88]. Aqueous extracts were dissolved in distilled water and the organic extracts were dissolved in dimethyl sulfoxide [88]. Organic (methanol, ethanol and hexane extracts) of *Zingiber officinale* produced MIC of16 mm, 15 mm, and 15 mm, respectively, for *E. coli* [88]. Ethanol, methanol, and hexane extracts produced similar antibacterial effects against *S. aureus* [88]. The highest zone of inhibition for *E. coli* was observed at 10 mm using ethanol extract at 1000 mg/ml and the highest diameter zone of inhibition for *S. aureus* was observed with hexane extract at 20 mm with 1000 mg/ml concentration [88]. Aqueous and acetone extracts were without effect on either bacterium [88].

A second *in vitro* study compared the antimicrobial activity of ethanol and hot water extracts of fresh *Zingiber officinale* to the three antibiotics streptomycin, tetracycline, and penicillin [89]. Specifically, an agar diffusion method was used to compare the effect of ginger extract, antibiotic therapy, as well as ginger extract combined with antibiotics. Ethanolic ginger extracts yielded the greatest inhibitory effects against *E. coli* and *S. aureus* [89].

Helicobacter pylori

Helicobacter pylori is a gram-negative microaerophilic bacterium that inhabits the digestive tract and colonizes the digestive system of more than half of the global population [90]. In the United States alone, there are 1.24 million new *H. pylori* infections each year [91]. This bacterium is often transmitted through direct contact with an infected individual's saliva, vomit, or feces [90, 91]. Also, areas of the world that lack access to clean water sources are at greater risk for this infection 90, 91]. *H. pylori* attacks the stomach lining and the duodenum by releasing an enzyme that decreases the acid produced by the stomach [92]. This, in turn, weakens the stomach lining and leads to sores or ulcers that cause symptoms of abdominal pain, nausea, vomiting and ultimately peptic ulcers [92]. *H. pylori* has also been connected with symptoms of chronic gastritis and functional dyspepsia (FD) [91]. Although these latter conditions are not life threatening, they fracture a healthy individual's quality of life through gastric discomfort [91]. *H. pylori* infection is typically treated with antibiotics such as clarithromycin, metronidazole, or amoxicillin, but its ability to develop resistance has posed a few challenges in its treatment [92]. For example, clarithromycin resistance is prevalent in China, Turkey, and Italy at 50%, 40% and 30%, respectively [92]. Thus, the growing antibiotic resistance of *H. pylori* demands the new treatments for alleviating symptoms of a gastrointestinal disease [92]. Three studies of ginger's efficacy against *H. pylori* have appeared in the literature as described in Table 2 below.

Table 2. Studies of the efficacy of ginger compounds against *Helicobacter pylori*

Study design	Results	Reference
In vitro: Boiled water extract of ginger evaluated for bactericidal activity using standard kill-curve and a viable colony count. Anti-adhesive properties of extract evaluated using four strains of FITC-labeled *H. pylori* strains and their ability to bind to isolated stomach biopsy sections.	Bactericidal effects observed within 30 minutes as100% inhibition of growth for all *H. pylori* clinical strains used in the study. The extract had no effect on the adhesion of *H. pylori* to the stomach surface.	[93]
In vitro: MIC of methanol extract of dried ginger rhizome, and individual isolates of 6-, 8- and 10-gingerol and 6 shogaol were determined using19 strains of *H. pylori*, 5 of which were designated *CagA+*. MIC compared with that of the standard medication of amoxycillin.	Methanol extract of the dried ginger rhizome inhibited the growth of *H. pylori* in all 19 strains with an MIC of 6.25-50.0 μg/ml. All three gingerols were also able to inhibit *H. pylori* growth in 5 *CagA+* strains with an MIC of 1.56-12.5 μg/ml. 10-gingerol was the most effective with a mean MIC of 1.56 μg/ml. In comparison, MIC for Amoxicillin was 0.0039-0.25 μg/ml.	[94]
In vivo: Unblinded trial of 15 patients given tablets (1 g ginger powder) t.i.d. for 4 weeks. Questionnaire for symptom reduction and stool analysis for HpSAg.	After 4 weeks of ginger therapy, there were significant improvements in patients' symptoms of FD after consuming ginger namely ↓ gastric fullness ($p<0.02$), early satiety ($p <0.05$), nausea ($p<0.02$), belching ($p<0.02$), gastric pain ($p < 0.005$) and gastric burn ($p <0.05$). Most importantly these correlated with a 53.5% eradication rate of *H. pylori* ($p<0.02$) as assessed by the absence of HpSAg. = 0.019).	[95]

Abbreviations used in the table: *CagA+* (gene present in *H. pylori* that initiates the development of lesions and stomach cancer), FD (functional dyspepsia), FITC (fluorescein isothiocyanate), HpSAg (*Helicobacter pylori* surface antigen), MIC (minimum inhibitory concentration) and t.i.d. (three times a day).

Although the three studies of *H. pylori* utilized different spice preparations, they do demonstrate that ginger may have potential future utility in the treatment of this bacterium. Although the clinical pilot study was small and unblinded, it was able to correlate an impressive reduction in patients' symptoms with the disappearance of the bacterium from their stool samples [95]. Further, the observation that gingerols were able to eliminate *H. pylori*, including *CagA+* strains [94] and that a normal cooking technique (boiling) did not eradicate these effects [93] is promising. As with the other bacteria discussed in this chapter it is now necessary to optimize delivery systems for this spice as well as conduct fully double blind, randomized placebo-controlled trials.

Salmonella typhi

Salmonella enterica serotype typhi (*S. typhi*) is a gram-negative bacterium responsible for food-borne illnesses [96]. This bacterium alone is responsible for 11-21 million infections worldwide each year. It is commonly found in developing countries, especially in Asia, with poor sanitation practices, contaminated water, and undercooked meat [97]. *S. typhi* enters the digestive system after the ingestion of contaminated food and water; it later adheres to the small intestine and proliferates which causes the symptoms. Specifically, it causes severe inflammation of the intestines, nausea, vomiting, constipation, abdominal pain, and diarrhea [97]. Typhoid fever is a fatal complication caused by growth of *S. typhi* and requires antibiotic therapy. However, since *S. typhi* has strains that are multi-drug resistant, it adds to the challenges to finding treatment [97, 98]. Commonly used antibiotics such as ciprofloxacin, fluoroquinolones, and chloramphenicol have shown failure in treatment for certain resistant strains [99]. In 2017, 74% of *S. typhi* infections were found to be resistant to ciprofloxacin therapy [99].

Thus, the alarming rise of antibiotic resistance gives importance to the need for alternative treatment options. Currently only three studies have appeared in the literature that examine the effect of ginger against *S. typhi* [100-102] as shown in Table 3 below.

Table 3. Studies of the efficacy of ginger compounds against *Salmonella typhi*

Study design	Results	Reference
In vitro: methanol extracts of fresh ginger dissolved in DMSO tested against 50 clinical isolates from typhoid fever patients using disc diffusion method.	Extracts at between 10 and 50% dilutions produced between 10 and 23 mm of inhibition of growth of all *S. typhi* strains. All clinical isolates were antibiotic susceptible.	[100]
In vitro: methanol extract (80%) of fresh ground ginger reconstituted in DMSO. Aqueous extract also investigated. Efficacy of standard antibiotics against *S. typhi* with ginger extracts using disc diffusion method.	*S. typhi* was sensitive to the ethanol (9 mm and 10 mm inhibition) and aqueous (8 mm) ginger extracts. These data compared favorably to erythromycin, tetracycline, and chloramphenicol (inhibition of 9 mm, 4 mm, and 5 mm, respectively.	[101]
In vitro: antimicrobial activity of *Zingiber officinale* against gastrointestinal pathogens including *E. coli*, *Pseudomonas aeruginosa*, *Staphylococcus aureus*, *Vibrio cholerae*, *Klebsiella* spp. and *Salmonella* sp. Soybean oil (40 ml) and ginger powder (10 g) were mixed and boiled for 30 minutes before the disc diffusion assay. Discs containing 20 μl of ginger extract, soybean oil or 10 μl of gentamycin (control) were added to filter paper discs of each of the six agar plates.	Zones of inhibition ranged between 8.0±1.73 mm 11.67±1.53 mm for the ginger extract and 12.33±7.09 mm to 19.33±3.51 mm for gentamicin. *Zingiber officinale* showed the greatest antimicrobial activity against Salmonella species and the lowest activity against *E.* coli. This study involved the extraction of ginger in soybean which protected the antibacterial properties of the ginger at higher temperatures.	[102]

Abbreviations used in the table: DMSO (dimethyl sulfoxide) and g (grams).

While the three studies do not identify the active principle in ginger that is effective against *S. typhi* the study by Islam et al. [102] identified that extracting in soybean oil protected the antibacterial properties of the ginger at higher temperatures.

Also, since the ginger was boiled prior to its use, it shows the thermostability of ginger extracts and its wide applicability, especially in cooking [102]. It is to be anticipated that using the individual bioactive principles from these extracts in both pre-clinical animal studies as well as human clinical trials will identify whether ginger may be useful in the treatment of this pathogen.

Other Gastrointestinal Bacterial Pathogens

As discussed on section 3.2 *Pseudomonas aeruginosa* is a gram-negative bacterium that has developed substantial antibiotic resistance that has permitted its high fatality rate in hospital patients [103]. The digestive tract is a major colonization site for *P. aeruginosa*, especially in ICU patients where it is associated with a high mortality rate [104]. *P. aeruginosa* relies on its adherence to the intestinal epithelial barrier and utilizes mechanisms to translocate to various areas of the body to perpetuate gut-derived septicemia [104]. Therefore, it's essential to treat *P. aeruginosa* to prevent its proliferation in the digestive tract and diminish its invasiveness into other regions of the body [104]. As mentioned above ginger has been shown to work against respiratory strain of *P. aeruginosa* [72, 73]. The study conducted by Azadpour et al., discussed in Table 1 for their findings on *S. aureus*, also showed that *Pseudomonas aeruginosa* (ATCC: 27853) was susceptible to antimicrobial effects of ginger extract which was shown through its considerably high MIC of 416 μg/ml. Overall, the antibacterial effects of *Zingiber officinale* inhibited the growth of *P. aeruginosa* and sheds light on a potential therapeutic method to overcome difficulties posed by antibiotic resistance [48].

As discussed in section 2 *Staphylococcus aureus* is a gram-positive staphylococcal bacterium that contributes to skin, lung, heart valve, and bone infections [43, 44]. Certain strains of staphylococci contribute to food poisoning from ingesting meat, fish, or dairy products contaminated with *S. aureus* [105-107].

In the United States, S. aureus food-borne illness accounts for 241,000 reported illnesses annually [107]. While *S. aureus* infections are commonly treated with β-lactams such as penicillin, methicillin, oxacillin, and cloxacillin, methicillin-resistant *S. aureus* (MRSA) has presented a new challenge for treatment [108]. While MRSA is commonly known to be carried on the skin and nose, research has shown that it can be transmitted from livestock to humans through food contamination [108]. Thus, it's important to consider the benefits of *Zingiber officinale* in its use for treating *S. aureus* infections of the digestive system. The study conducted by Rahman et al. [50], showed that the ginger root and leaf ethanol extract produced an inhibition zone on *S. aureus* which adds to the efficacy of *Zingiber officinale* in inhibiting bacterial growth of *S. aureus* that contributes to digestive system diseases. Overall, this study supports the success of *Zingiber officinale* in inhibiting bacterial growth of *S. aureus* compared to increasingly resistant antibiotic therapies currently used [50].

In an *in vivo* study, Yadufashije et al. examined the antibacterial activity of *Zingiber officinale* on different pathogens that contribute to digestive tract infections in patients attending the Muhoza Health Center [109]. This study investigated bacteria isolated from stool samples of 30 patients with digestive tract infections. A bacterial culture of different bacteria and biochemical tests were used to determine the extent of antimicrobial activity exerted by *Zingiber officinale*. Specifically, the study involved isolated bacteria such as *E. coli*, Salmonella species, Enterobacter spp, Shigella spp, and *Citrobacter* [109]. Ethanol and methanol were used for the purpose of ginger oil extraction and to determine the antibacterial activity of *Zingiber officinale* [109]. Ethanol extracts were effective against all but the Enterobacter species (zones of inhibition between 9.5 and 14 mm compared with 0.66 mm, respectively) [109]. As indicated by the zone of inhibition readings, *Zingiber officinale* shows promising results in having antibacterial activity that can be applied in treatment of digestive system infections [109].

ANTIBACTERIAL EFFECTS OF *ZINGIBER OFFICINALE* AGAINST ORAL INFECTIONS

Despite improvement in oral health habits, caries and periodontal disease are found in the majority of the population throughout the world, particularly in disadvantaged and poor communities [110]. The key players associated with both of these oral diseases are the pathogens found in dental biofilms [111]. *Streptococcus mutans* is involved in the development of dental caries [112], meanwhile *Lactobacillus* species play a role in the progression of caries [113]. Periodontal disease is caused by specific bacteria, including *Porphyromonas gingivalis, Tannerella forsythia, Treponema denticola, Fusobacterium nucleatum, Prevotella intermedia*, and *Aggregatibacter actinomycetemcomitans*, that are responsible for the inflammation of the supportive tissue of teeth and subsequential destruction of alveolar bone and connective tissue [114]. Antimicrobial chemicals aid in the prevention of dental caries, but these agents such as chlorhexidine, amoxicillin, and antiseptics can present with side effects like tooth staining or disruption of oral and intestinal flora [115]. This emphasizes the utilization of natural compounds, such as ginger, that could offer a promising alternative to the chemicals currently used as antimicrobials for oral infection and dental caries [116, 117].

Streptococcus mutans

Streptococcus mutans (*S. mutans*) is found in the cultivable flora in biofilms extracted from carious lesions which are visible breakdowns in the tooth surface [118]. Various studies have examined the effect of ginger compounds in helping combat caries adding them to mouthwashes [119]. These findings, summarized in Table 2 [120-124] such as the one reported below suggest the application of ginger in Phyto-pharmaceutical formulations for new prevention and treatment methods to combat tooth decay-causing diseases [121].

Table 4. Studies of the efficacy of ginger compounds to combat dental caries

Study design	Results	Reference
In vitro: Aqueous extract tested by disc diffusion method.	20 gr/ 100ml produced a zone of inhibition of 20 ± 0.7 mm.	[118]
In vitro: Water-ethanol extract of ginger evaluated by disc-diffusion method and MIC.	10% ethanolic ginger extract showed zone of inhibition of 8 mm against *S. mutans*. The MIC against *S. mutants* was at 1.25% concentration.	[119]
In vitro: essential oil from rhizomes of *Zingiber zerumbet (L.) Smith* extracted by hydro-distillation evaluated by MIC.	Essential oil showed a MIC of 250 μg/mL and a minimum bactericidal concentration MBC of 500 μg/mL against S. mutans.	[120]
In vivo: double-blind clinical study (n = 31) assessed the efficacy of 0.5% *Z. officinale* essential oil (ZOEO) mouthwash.	ZOEO mouthwash was an effective antimicrobial agent when used against *S. mutans*. It expressed anti-inflammatory properties through reduction of gingival bleeding. The ZOEO was successful in regulating the growth of oral biofilms.	[122]
In vitro: Ethanol ginger extract evaluated for MIC, MBC.	The MIC of the *Zingiber officinale* extract was 0.02 mg/mL for *S. mutans*. The MBC of *Zingiber officinale* extract was 0.04 mg/mL for *S. mutans*.	[123]
In vitro: Aqueous ginger extract evaluated by disc-diffusion method and MIC.	500 mg/ml of ginger extract showed zone of inhibition of 20mm. The MIC was 31.25 mg/ml of ginger extract.	[124]

Abbreviations used in the table: MIC (minimum inhibitory concentration), MBC (minimum bactericidal concentration).

Lactobacillus

Lactobacillus acidophilus is a beneficial bacterial flora that is present in many digestive tracts, including the mouth [125]. However, at higher levels in the body, it can have undesired effects on the entire human body. High colony counts of *L. acidophilus* can cause endocarditis, the infection and inflammation of the heart [125].

This infection is typically caused by either a vast volume of *L. acidophilus* in the lower gastrointestinal tract or in the oropharynx. Such high volumes in the oropharynx are generally a trademark of poor oral hygiene but can be seen in patients with compromised immune system. As indicated in the name, *L. acidophilus* thrives in an acidic environment, which is exactly what poor hygiene of the mouth allows as decaying carbohydrates decrease the pH levels of the oropharynx [125]. In an evaluation of the efficacy of multiple plant species as antibacterial mouth rinses; ginger, chlorohexidine, and cocoa bean husk were given to patients age 18-25 in a randomized controlled clinical study [126]. The patients all had *L. acidophilus* present in their oropharynx flora at the beginning of the study to measure the change over the course of two months using the different mouth rinses. The results found that the patients that received the cocoa bean husk and chlorohexidine had a slight decrease in oral bacteria but the patients using the ginger mouth rinse had a significant decrease in oral bacteria ($p<0.05$) [126].

To test different plant species on both *L. acidophilus* and *S. mutans*, researchers created methanolic extracts of five different plant species and tested the MIC and MBC of each extract using a disc diffusion assay. The five plant species tested were: ginger, clove, cinnamon, turmeric, and black seed. The results concluded that both cinnamon and clove provided the largest zones of inhibition of 14-18mm for both bacterial species but ginger provided no inhibition [126]. Interestingly, ginger had no effect on the *L. acidophilus* in this study despite proving effective in at least one clinical trial.

In a study using extract human teeth, researchers investigated how ginger and honey affected the populations of bacterial species on the teeth. A total of 250 carious teeth were analyzed for bacterial populations before the experiment showing that a majority of the of bacteria was from *S. mutans* and *L. acidophilus* [127]. The results concluded that the ginger and honey were both equally effective at creating a zone of inhibition with zones varying from 18-27mm. Compared to the antibiotic gentamycin also tested, they were slightly more effective as the zone for this was 18-23mm [127].

CONCLUSION

Ginger is not only used as a spice in many parts of the world but has been used for many centuries as a medicinal herb [128]. Ginger rhizomes and their compounds are harmless and have been recognized as safe for human's use by the FDA [128].

Until the beginning of the 19th century, all medicines were so-called "traditional medicine" [129]. According to the World Health Organization (WHO) more than 80% of the emerging world's population still relies on traditional medicine [130]. Moreover, another study reports that even other country such us Germany and Canada reports that at least 70% of their population have tried alternative medicine (CAM) [131]. Medicinal plants, is based on tradition and the knowledge is passed on from generation to generation [129]. This creates a difficulty in understanding and defining formulations of the active ingredients as well as their molecular interactions [128, 129]. Until these can be standardized, as occurs with classic pharmaceuticals, they will not be acceptable as medications [128, 129].

According to the studies reviewed in this chapter ginger compounds have the potential to be effective antibacterial agents against at least 12 bacteria, 6 Gram-positive and 6 Gram-negative (Figure 2). The mechanisms of action of ginger on bacterial cells have been investigated [132-133]. It has been shown, by scanning electron microscopy, that ginger essential oils destroy the continuity of the cell structure, thus indicating an ability to easily penetrate the lipid layers [132]. It appears that Gram-positive bacteria are slightly more susceptible to the action of ginger which further point to the thick layer of peptidoglycan as a target of their action [134].

It is important to note, that these studies are mostly conducted *in vitro* with the ability to control the environment surrounding the experiments. Moreover, they focus most on the effects of ginger rather than the mechanisms that allow for the results. This has generated lack of knowledge on the molecular interaction and molecular targets that ginger compounds interact with [129].

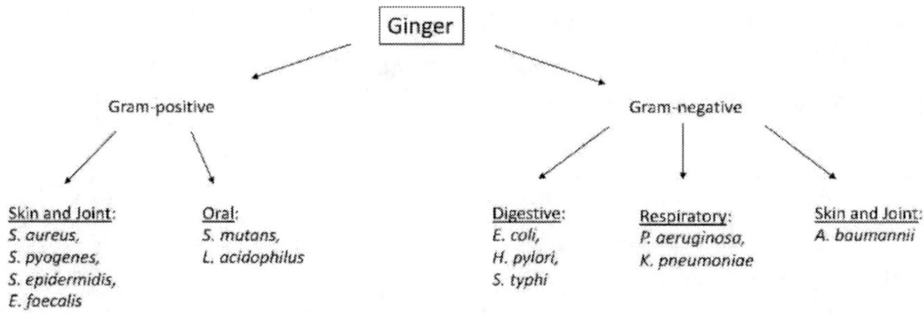

Figure 2. Ginger efficacy on Gram-positive and Gram-negative bacteria based on body system. Figure constructed using the following references: 48-53, 59-65, 72-77, 88, 89, 93-95, 100-102, 118-124, 126, 127.

Several studies have suggested that organic extracts, i.e., ethanol or methanol or hexane extracts of ginger, were more effective as antibacterial agents [132]. This could be correlated to the extraction method isolating the gingerols, rather than the shogaols that are isolated when water extraction is used. Interestingly to note is that there is no difference between dry versus fresh ginger extract when in solvent [135].

In terms of lead directions, some studies have assessed the use of ginger in animals, reporting good outcome in leech infestation in cattle, ulcer treatment in horses and upper respiratory infection in poultry [129, 136]. Animal studies require less in terms of approval procedures and would therefore be an easier route for ginger-derived medications [129, 136].

These authors would also suggest two human directions for development, namely ginger as mouthwash and ginger as an oral medication. We have reported the efficacy of ginger against oral bacteria, in particular against *S. mutans* and *L. acidophilus* (Figure 2). The use of ginger in mouthwash showed great results, especially it was successful in regulating the growth of oral biofilms [122]. The importance of good oral hygiene is highlighted by Nazir especially in correlation with association of periodontal diseases with systemic diseases such as cardiovascular disease, diabetes, and adverse pregnancy outcomes [137]. The author explain that periodontal diseases and their ramifications are a serious issue in adulthood for individuals living developed nations, and can lead to tooth loss even in young adult [137].

A second strategy to use the property of ginger as an antibacterial could be as an oral medication. We have reported that ginger is effective against several important gastrointestinal pathogens namely *E. coli, H. pylori and S. typhi* (Figure 2).

Chapter 1 details the possibility of delivery ginger under a nanoparticle form. These applications could not only help with nausea and vomiting but, finding the right extract could provide an aid in fighting bacterial infections caused of the digestive system.

More *in vivo* large clinical trials are needed to define the right protocols and dosage for these phytochemical compounds. Further there is the need to understand what components are available in the delivery options used in humans and if these components can work alone or need other chemicals to for inter-reactivity or dependency to exert their functions. The rhizome extract from ginger is valuable candidate to be part of the solution to the crisis due to antibiotic resistance but ultimately more standardized studies are needed to make sure these phytochemicals don't remain in the "alternative medicine" section but gain a primary spot in everyday medicine.

References

[1] Aminov, Rustam I. 2010. "A brief history of the antibiotic era: lessons learned and challenges for the future." *Frontiers in microbiology*. 1, 134. Accessed on April 26, 2021. https://doi.org/10.3389/fmicb.2010.00134.

[2] Hutchings, Matthew I., Andrew W. Truman, and Barrie Wilkinson 2019. "Antibiotics: past, present and future." *Curr Opin Microbiol.* 51:72-80. Accessed on April 26, 2021. doi: 10.1016/j.mib.2019.10.008.

[3] Prescott, John F. 2014. "The resistance tsunami, antimicrobial stewardship, and the golden age of microbiology." *Vet microbiol.* 171(3-4): 273-278. Accessed on April 26, 2021. doi: 10.1016/j.vetmic.2014.02.035.

[4] Aslam, Bilal, Wei Wang, Muhammad Imran Arshad, Mohsin Khurshid, Saima Muzammil, Muhammad Hidayat Rasool, Muhammad Atif Nisar, et al. 2018. "Antibiotic Resistance: A Rundown of a Global Crisis." *Infection and Drug Resistance* 11: 1645–58. Accessed on April 26, 2021. doi: 10.2147/IDR.S173867.

[5] Livermore, D. M. 2004. "The Need for New Antibiotics." *Clinical Microbiology and Infection: The Official Publication of the European Society of Clinical Microbiology and Infectious Diseases* 10 Suppl 4: 1–9. Accessed on April 26, 2021. https://doi.org/ 10.1111/j.1465-0691.2004.1004.x.

[6] *WHO|WHO Global Strategy for Containment of Antimicrobial Resistance*. 2016. Accessed on April 26, 2021. https://www.who. int/drugresistance/WHO_Global_Strategy.htm/en/.

[7] Laxminarayan, Ramanan, Adriano Duse, Chand Wattal, Anita K. M. Zaidi, Heiman F. L. Wertheim, Nithima Sumpradit, Erika Vlieghe, et al. 2013. "Antibiotic Resistance—the Need for Global Solutions." *The Lancet Infectious Diseases* 13 (12): 1057–98. Accessed on April 26, 2021. https://doi.org/10.1016/s1473-3099(13)70318-9.

[8] Chemical Sciences Roundtable, Board on Chemical Sciences and Technology, Division on Earth and Life Studies, and National Research Council. 2014. *Challenges in Overcoming Antibiotic Resistance*. Washington, D.C., DC: National Academies Press.

[9] Hayashi, Mirian A., Fernando C. Bizerra, and Pedro Ismael Da Silva Jr. 2013. "Antimicrobial Compounds from Natural Sources." *Frontiers in Microbiology* 4: 195. Accessed on April 26, 2021. doi:10.3389/fmicb.2013.00195.

[10] Cowan, M. M. 1999. "Plant products as antimicrobial agents." *Clin Microbiol Rev*. 1999;12(4):564-582. Accessed on April 26, 2021.

[11] Gupta, Pooja D., and Tannaz J. Birdi. 2017. "Development of Botanicals to Combat Antibiotic Resistance." *Journal of Ayurveda and Integrative Medicine* 8 (4): 266–75. Accessed on April 26, 2021. doi: 10.1016/j.jaim.2017.05.004.

[12] Wińska, Katarzyna, Wanda Mączka, Jacek Łyczko, Małgorzata Grabarczyk, Anna Czubaszek, and Antoni Szumny. 2019. "Essential

Oils as Antimicrobial Agents-Myth or Real Alternative?" *Molecules (Basel, Switzerland)* 24 (11): 2130. Accessed on April 26, 2021. doi:10.3390/molecules24112130.

[13] Yap, Polly Soo Xi, Beow Chin Yiap, Hu Cai Ping, and Swee Hua Erin Lim. 2014. "Essential Oils, a New Horizon in Combating Bacterial Antibiotic Resistance." *The Open Microbiology Journal* 8 (1): 6–14. Accessed on April 26, 2021. doi: 10.2174/1874285801408010006.

[14] Peterfalvi, Agnes, Eva Miko, Tamas Nagy, Barbara Reger, Diana Simon, Attila Miseta, Boldizsár Czéh, and Laszlo Szereday. 2019. "Much More than a Pleasant Scent: A Review on Essential Oils Supporting the Immune System." *Molecules (Basel, Switzerland)* 24 (24). Accessed on April 26, 2021. https://doi.org/10.3390/molecules24244530.

[15] Carrasco, Fábio Ricardo, Gustavo Schmidt, Adriano Lopez Romero, Juliano Luiz Sartoretto, Silvana Martins Caparroz-Assef, Ciomar Aparecida Bersani-Amado, and Roberto Kenji Nakamura Cuman. 2009. "Immunomodulatory Activity of *Zingiber Officinale* Roscoe, *Salvia Officinalis* L. and *Syzygium Aromaticum* L. Essential Oils: Evidence for Humor- and Cell-Mediated Responses." *The Journal of Pharmacy and Pharmacology* 61 (7): 961–67. Accessed on April 26, 2021. doi:10.1211/jpp/61.07.0017.

[16] Mahboubi, Mohaddese. 2019. "*Zingiber Officinale* Rosc. Essential Oil, a Review on Its Composition and Bioactivity." *Clinical Phytoscience* 5 (1). Accessed on April 26, 2021. https://doi.org/10.1186/s40816-018-0097-4.

[17] Sandner, Georg, Mara Heckmann, and Julian Weghuber. 2020. "Immunomodulatory Activities of Selected Essential Oils." *Biomolecules* 10 (8): 1139. Accessed on April 26, 2021.

[18] Bode, A. M., and Z. Dong. 2011. *Chapter 7: The Amazing and Mighty Ginger.* Edited by Eds Benzie Iff and Wachtel-Galor S, 2nd ed. Boca Raton (FL: CRC Press/Taylor & Francis).

[19] Yumnam, V., T. N. Singh, K. H. S. Devi, and K. Sarangthem. 2019. "Antimicrobial Activity of Ginger (*Zingiber Officinale* Roscoe)

Found in Manipur." *International Journal of Pharmacy and Biological Sciences* 9 (3): 687–693. Accessed on April 26, 2021.

[20] Madan, M. S. 2016. "Production, Marketing, and Economics of Ginger." In *Ginger*, 455–88. CRC Press. Accessed on April 26, 2021. doi:10.1201/9781420023367-16, ISBN 9781420023367.

[21] Nair, K. P., Turmeric, and Ginger. 2019. - *World's Invaluable Medicinal Spices: The Agronomy and Economy of Turmeric and Tinger*. Switzerland AG: Springer Nature.

[22] Wei, Chien-Kei, Yi-Hong Tsai, Michal Korinek, Pei-Hsuan Hung, Mohamed El-Shazly, Yuan-Bin Cheng, Yang-Chang Wu, Tusty-Jiuan Hsieh, and Fang-Rong Chang. 2017. "6-Paradol and 6-Shogaol, the Pungent Compounds of Ginger, Promote Glucose Utilization in Adipocytes and Myotubes, and 6-Paradol Reduces Blood Glucose in High-Fat Diet-Fed Mice." *International Journal of Molecular Sciences* 18 (1): 168. Accessed on April 26, 2021. doi:10.3390/ijms18010168.

[23] Masuda, Yuki, Hiroe Kikuzaki, Masashi Hisamoto, and Nobuji Nakatani. 2004. "Antioxidant Properties of Gingerol Related Compounds from Ginger." *BioFactors (Oxford, England)* 21 (1–4): 293–96. Accessed on April 26, 2021.

[24] Young, Haw-Yaw, Yen-Lin Luo, Hao-Yuan Cheng, Wen-Chiuan Hsieh, Jung-Chun Liao, and Wen-Huang Peng. 2005. "Analgesic and Anti-Inflammatory Activities of [6]-Gingerol." *Journal of Ethnopharmacology* 96 (1–2): 207–10. Accessed on April 26, 2021. doi: 10.1016/j.jep.2004.09.009.

[25] Chung, Won-Yoon, Yeon-Joo Jung, Young-Joon Surh, Sang-Sup Lee, and Kwang-Kyun Park. 2001. "Antioxidative and Antitumor Promoting Effects of [6]-Paradol and Its Homologs." *Mutation Research. Genetic Toxicology and Environmental Mutagenesis* 496 (1–2): 199–206. Accessed on April 26, 2021. doi:10.1016/s1383-5718(01)00221-2.

[26] Rahmani, Arshad H., Fahad M. Al Shabrmi, and Salah M. Aly. 2014. "Active Ingredients of Ginger as Potential Candidates in the Prevention and Treatment of Diseases via Modulation of Biological

Activities." *International Journal of Physiology, Pathophysiology and Pharmacology* 6 (2): 125–36. Accessed on April 26, 2021.

[27] Koch, Wojciech, Wirginia Kukula-Koch, Zbigniew Marzec, Elwira Kasperek, Lucyna Wyszogrodzka-Koma, Wojciech Szwerc, and Yoshinori Asakawa. 2017. "Application of Chromatographic and Spectroscopic Methods towards the Quality Assessment of Ginger (*Zingiber Officinale*) Rhizomes from Ecological Plantations." *International Journal of Molecular Sciences* 18 (2): 452. Accessed on April 26, 2021. https://doi.org/10.3390/ijms18020452.

[28] Sharifi-Rad, Mehdi, Elena Varoni, Bahare Salehi, Javad Sharifi-Rad, Karl Matthews, Seyed Ayatollahi, Farzad Kobarfard, et al. 2017. "Plants of the Genus Zingiber as a Source of Bioactive Phytochemicals: From Tradition to Pharmacy." *Molecules (Basel, Switzerland)* 22 (12): 2145. Accessed on April 26, 2021. doi:10.3390/molecules22122145.

[29] Mbaveng, A. T., and V. Kuete. 2017. "*Zingiber Officinale*, In: Medicinal Spices and Vegetables from Africa." *Kuete* V: 627–639. Accessed on April 26, 2021. https://doi.org/10.1016/B978-0-12-809286-6.00030-3.

[30] Kieliszek, Marek, Amr Edris, Anna Maria Kot, and Kamil Piwowarek. 2020. "Biological Activity of Some Aromatic Plants and Their Metabolites, with an Emphasis on Health-Promoting Properties." *Molecules (Basel, Switzerland)* 25 (11): 2478. Accessed on April 26, 2021. doi: 10.3390/molecules25112478.

[31] Mahboubi, Mohaddese 2016. "*Zingiber officinale* Rosc. essential oil, a review on its composition and bioactivity." *Clin Phytosci* 5: 6. Accessed on April 26, 2021. https://doi.org/10.1186/s40816-018-0097-4.

[32] Govindarajan, V. S. 1982. "Ginger-Chemistry, Technology, and Quality Evaluation: Part 2." *Critical Reviews in Food Science and Nutrition* 17 (3): 189–258.

[33] Jiang, Yusong, Mengjun Huang, Michael Wisniewski, Honglei Li, Meixia Zhang, Xiang Tao, Yiqing Liu, and Yong Zou. 2018. "Transcriptome Analysis Provides Insights into Gingerol

Biosynthesis in Ginger (*Zingiber officinale*).” *The Plant Genome* 11 (3): 1–11. Accessed on April 26, 2021. https://doi.org/10.3835/plantgenome2018.06.0034.

[34] Thompson, E. H., I. D. Wolf, and C. E. Allen. 1973. “Ginger Rhizome: A New Source of Proteolytic Enzyme.” *Journal of Food Science* 38 (4): 652–55. Accessed on April 26, 2021. https://doi.org/10.1111/j.1365-2621.1973.tb02836.x.

[35] Choi, K. H., and R. A. Laursen. 2000. “Amino-Acid Sequence and Glycan Structures of Cysteine Proteases with Proline Specificity from Ginger Rhizome *Zingiber officinale*: Primary Structure of Ginger Proteases.” *European Journal of Biochemistry* 267 (5): 1516–26. Accessed on April 26, 2021. https://doi.org/10.1046/j.1432-1327.2000.01152.x.

[36] Huang, X. W., L. J. Chen, Y. B. Luo, H. Y. Guo, and F. Z. Ren. 2011. “Purification, Characterization, and Milk Coagulating Properties of Ginger Proteases.” *Journal of Dairy Science* 94 (5): 2259–69. Accessed on April 26, 2021. https://doi.org/10.3168/jds.2010-4024.

[37] Wang, Hexiang, and Tzi Bun Ng. 2005. “An Antifungal Protein from Ginger Rhizomes.” *Biochemical and Biophysical Research Communications* 336 (1): 100–104. Accessed on April 26, 2021. doi: 10.1016/j.bbrc.2005.08.058.

[38] Pankaj, Sah, Al Tamimi Balqees, Al Nassri Najat, and Al Mamari Rahma. 2012. “Effect of Temperature on Antibiotic Properties of Garlic (*Allium sativum* L.) and Ginger (*Zingiber officinale* Rosc.).” *African Journal of Biotechnology* 11 (95): 16192–95. Accessed on April 26, 2021. doi:10.5897/AJB12.1402.

[39] “Ginger: *Zingiber Officinale* R (Zingiberaceae).” 2017. In *Natural Food Flavors and Colorants*, 209–14. Chichester, UK: John Wiley & Sons, Ltd. https://doi.org/10.1002/9781119114796.ch57.

[40] Chen, Jaw-Chyun, Li-Jiau Huang, Shih-Lu Wu, Sheng-Chu Kuo, Tin-Yun Ho, and Chien-Yun Hsiang. 2007. “Ginger and Its Bioactive Component Inhibit Enterotoxigenic *Escherichia Coli* Heat-Labile Enterotoxin-Induced Diarrhea in Mice.” *Journal of Agricultural and*

Food Chemistry 55 (21): 8390–97. Accessed on April 26, 2021. https://doi.org/10.1021/jf071460f.

[41] Roshan, Niloufar, Thomas V. Riley, Daniel R. Knight, and Katherinc A. Hammer. 2018. "Effect of Natural Products on the Production and Activity of *Clostridium Difficile* Toxins in Vitro." *Scientific Reports* 8 (1): 15735. Accessed on April 26, 2021. https://doi.org/10.1038/s41598-018-33954-2.

[42] Pulido-Cejudo, Abraham, Mario Guzmán-Gutierrez, Abel Jalife-Montaño, Alejandro Ortiz-Covarrubias, Jose Luis Martínez-Ordaz, Héctor Faustino Noyola-Villalobos, and Luis Mauricio Hurtado-López. 2017. "Management of Acute Bacterial Skin and Skin Structure Infections with a Focus on Patients at High Risk of Treatment Failure." *Therapeutic Advances in Infectious Disease* 4 (5): 143–61. Accessed on April 26, 2021. doi:10.1177/2049936117723228.

[43] Pantosti, Annalisa, Andrea Sanchini, and Monica Monaco. 2007. "Mechanisms of Antibiotic Resistance In *Staphylococcus Aureus*." *Future Microbiology* 2 (3): 323–34.

[44] Foster, Timothy J. 2004. "The *Staphylococcus Aureus* 'Superbug.'" *The Journal of Clinical Investigation* 114 (12): 1693–96. Accessed on April 26, 2021. https://doi.org/10.1172/JCI23825.

[45] Rehm, Susan J., and Alan Tice. 2010. "*Staphylococcus Aureus*: Methicillin-Susceptible *S. Aureus* to Methicillin-Resistant *S. Aureus* and Vancomycin-Resistant *S. Aureus*." *Clinical Infectious Diseases: An Official Publication of the Infectious Diseases Society of America* 51 Suppl 2 (S2): S176-82. Accessed on April 26, 2021. doi:10.1086/653518.

[46] McCaig, Linda F., L. Clifford McDonald, Sanjay Mandal, and Daniel B. Jernigan. 2006. "*Staphylococcus Aureus*-Associated Skin and Soft Tissue Infections in Ambulatory Care." *Emerging Infectious Diseases* 12 (11): 1715–23. Accessed on April 26, 2021. https://doi.org/10.3201/eid1211.060190.

[47] Kourtis, Athena P., Kelly Hatfield, James Baggs, Yi Mu, Isaac See, Erin Epson, Joelle Nadle, et al. 2019. "Vital Signs: Epidemiology and

Recent Trends in Methicillin-Resistant and in Methicillin-Susceptible *Staphylococcus Aureus* Bloodstream Infections - United States." *MMWR. Morbidity and Mortality Weekly Report* 68 (9): 214–19. Accessed on April 26, 2021. http://dx.doi.org/10.15585/mmwr.mm6809e1.

[48] Azadpour, M., N. Azadpour, M. Bahmani, H. Hassanzadazar, M. Rafieian-Kopaei, and N. Naghdi. 2016. "Antimicrobial Effect of Ginger Antimicrobial effect of ginger (*Zingiber officinale*) and mallow (*Malva sylvestris*) hydroalcoholic extracts on four pathogen bacteria'. *Der Pharmacia Lettre*. 8(1): 181-187. Accessed on April 26, 2021.

[49] Oyedemi, Blessing Om, E. M. Kotsia, Paul D. Stapleton, and Simon Gibbons. 2019. "Capsaicin and Gingerol Analogues Inhibit the Growth of Efflux-Multidrug Resistant Bacteria and R-Plasmids Conjugal Transfer." *Journal of Ethnopharmacology* 245 (111871): 111871. Accessed on April 26, 2021. https://doi.org/10.1016/j.jep.2019.111871.

[50] Rahman, Md Abdur, Shyamal Kumar Shaha, Syed Didarul Haque, Refat Zahan, Tarifat Alam, Subir Kumar Mandal, and Md Shamsul Huda Mamun. 2020. "Antibacterial Effect of Ginger (*Zingiber Officinale*) against *Staphylococcus Aureus*." *Mediscope* 7 (1): 31–37. Accessed on April 26, 2021. https://doi.org/10.3329/mediscope.v7i1.47137.

[51] Sebiomo, A., A. D. Awofodu, A. O. Awosanya, F. E. Awotona, and A. J. Ajayi. 2010. "Comparative Studies of Antibacterial Effect of Some Antibiotics and Ginger." *Journal of Microbiology and Antimicrobials*. 3(1), 18-22. Accessed on April 26, 2021.

[52] Sulaiman, F. A., M. O. Kazeem, A. M. Waheed, S. O. Temowo, I. O. Azeez, F. I. Zubair, T. A. Adeyemi, A. Nyang, and O. S. Adeyemi. n.d. "Antimicrobial and Toxic Potential of Aqueous Extracts of *Allium Sativum, Hibiscus Sabdariffa* and *Zingiber Officinale* in Wistar Rats." Accessed on April 26, 2021. https://doi.org/10.1016/j.jtusci.2014.05.004.

[53] Poeloengan M. 2011. "The effect of red ginger (*Zingiber officinale Roscoe*) extract on the growth of mastitis causing bacterial isolates." *African Journal of Microbiology Research*. 5(4): 382-389. Accessed on April 26, 2021. doi:10.5897/AJMR10.776.

[54] Hwang, Jie H., Hyo W. Jung, Seung Y. Oh, Jong-Seong Kang, Jong-Pil Kim, and Yong-Ki Park 2017. "Effects of *Zingiber officinale* extract on collagen-induced arthritis in mice and IL-1β-induced inflammation in human synovial fibroblasts. *European Journal of Inflammation*, 168-178. Accessed on April 20, 2021. doi:10.1177/1721727X17727997.

[55] Nguyen, Sinh T., Phuc H. Vo, Thao D. Nguyen, Nghia M. Do, Bao H. Le, Duong T Dinh, Kiet D. Truong, and Phuc D. Pham. "Ethanol extract of Ginger *Zingiber officinale* Roscoe by Soxhlet method induces apoptosis in human hepatocellular carcinoma cell line." *Biomedical Research and Therapy*, 2019; 6(11): 3433-3442. Accessed on May 21, 2021. https://doi.org/10.15419/bmrat.v6i11.572.

[56] Zick, Suzanna M., Zora Djuric, Mack T. Ruffin, Amie J. Litzinger, Daniel P. Normolle, Sara Alrawi, Meihua R. Feng, and Dean E. Brenner 2017. "Pharmacokinetics of ginger phytochemicals." *Molecules*, 17:1930-1936. Accessed on April 7, 2021. doi:10.1158/1055-9965.EPI-07-2934.

[57] Efstratiou, A., and T. Lamagni. 2016. *Streptococcus Pyogenes: Basic Biology to Clinical Manifestations* [Internet. Oklahoma City, OK: University of Oklahoma Health Sciences Center.

[58] CDC. 2021. *Staphylococcal (Staph) Food Poisoning.* Cdc.Gov. Accessed on April 15, 2021. https://www.cdc.gov/foodsafety/diseases/staphylococcal.html.

[59] Assegaf, Samira, Arthur Pohan Kawilarang, and Retno Handajani. 2020. "Antibacterial Activity Test of Red Ginger Extract (*Zingiber Officinale* Var. Rubrum) Against *Streptococcus Pyogenes in Vitro*." *Biomolecular and Health Science Journal* 3 (1): 24.

[60] Lowy, F. D., and S. M. Hammer. 1983. "*Staphylococcus Epidermidis* Infections." *Annals of Internal Medicine* 99 (6): 834–39. Accessed on April 26, 2021. https://doi.org/10.7326/0003-4819-99-6-834.

[61] Rajkumari, Nonika, Purva Mathur, and Mahesh Chandra Misra. 2014. "Soft Tissue and Wound Infections Due to *Enterococcus* Spp. Among Hospitalized Trauma Patients in a Developing Country." *Journal of Global Infectious Diseases* 6 (4): 189–93. Accessed on April 26, 2021. doi:10.4103/0974-777X.145253.

[62] Levitus M., Rewane A., Perera T. B. 2020. "Vancomycin-Resistant *Enterococci*." *StatPearls* [Internet]. Treasure Island (FL): StatPearls Publishing; 2021 Jan–. PMID: 30020605.

[63] Silva, Silmara, Nayane Alves, Priscila Silva, Thalita Vieira, Panmella Maciel, Lúcio Roberto Castellano, Paulo Bonan, Christianne Velozo, and Diana Albuquerque. 2019. "Antibacterial Activity of *Rosmarinus Officinalis*, *Zingiber Officinale*, *Citrus Aurantium Bergamia*, and *Copaifera Officinalis* Alone and in Combination with Calcium Hydroxide against *Enterococcus Faecalis*." *BioMed Research International* 2019: 8129439. Accessed on April 26, 2021. doi:10.1155/2019/8129439.

[64] Perez, Federico, Andrea M. Hujer, Kristine M. Hujer, Brooke K. Decker, Philip N. Rather, and Robert A. Bonomo. 2007. "Global Challenge of Multidrug-Resistant *Acinetobacter Baumannii*." *Antimicrobial Agents and Chemotherapy* 51 (10): 3471–84. Accessed on April 26, 2021. doi:10.1128/AAC.01464-06.

[65] Wang, Hui-Min, Chung-Yi Chen, Hsi-An Chen, Wan-Chun Huang, Wei-Ru Lin, Tun-Chieh Chen, Chun-Yu Lin, et al. 2010. "*Zingiber Officinale* (Ginger) Compounds Have Tetracycline-Resistance Modifying Effects against Clinical Extensively Drug-Resistant *Acinetobacter Baumannii*." *Phytotherapy Research: PTR* 24 (12): 1825–30. Accessed on April 26, 2021. doi:10.1002/ptr.3201.

[66] Cappelletty, Diane. 1998. "Microbiology of Bacterial Respiratory Infections." *The Pediatric Infectious Disease Journal* 17 (Supplement): S55–61. Accessed on April 26, 2021. doi:10.1097/00006454-199808001-00002.

[67] Akoachere, J. F. T. K., R. N. Ndip, E. B. Chenwi, L. M. Ndip, T. E. Njock, and D. N. Anong. 2002. "Antibacterial Effect of *Zingiber Officinale* and *Garcinia Kola* on Respiratory Tract Pathogens." *East African Medical Journal* 79 (11): 588–92. Accessed on April 26, 2021. https://doi.org/10.4314/eamj.v79i11.8804.

[68] Okiki, P. A., O. Oluwadunsin, and O. Benjamin. 2015. "Antibacterial Activity of Ginger (*Zingiber Officinale*) against Isolated Bacteria from the Respiratory Tract Infections." *Journal of Biology, Agriculture and Healthcare* 5: 131–13.

[69] Nag, A., R. Roy-Chowdhury, and N. Shrivastav. 2019. "Phytocompounds from *Zingiber Zerumbet* Can Inhibit the DNA Ligase Activity of the Pathogen *Haemophilus Influenzae*, An *in silico* approach." *Journal of Emerging Technologies and Innovative Research.* 6(2), 646-651.

[70] Nagata, Towako, Hiroshi Mukae, Junichi Kadota, Tomayoshi Hayashi, Takeshi Fujii, Misuzu Kuroki, Ryo Shirai, et al. 2004. "Effect of Erythromycin on Chronic Respiratory Infection Caused by *Pseudomonas Aeruginosa* with Biofilm Formation in an Experimental Murine Model." *Antimicrobial Agents and Chemotherapy* 48 (6): 2251–59. Accessed on April 26, 2021. doi:10.1128/AAC.48.6.2251-2259.2004.

[71] Bodey, G. P., R. Bolivar, V. Fainstein, and L. Jadeja. 1983. "Infections Caused by *Pseudomonas Aeruginosa*." *Clinical Infectious Diseases: An Official Publication of the Infectious Diseases Society of America* 5 (2): 279–313. Accessed on April 26, 2021. https://doi.org/10.1093/clinids/5.2.279.

[72] Chakotiya, Ankita Singh, Ankit Tanwar, Alka Narula, and Rakesh Kumar Sharma. 2017. "*Zingiber Officinale*: Its Antibacterial Activity on *Pseudomonas Aeruginosa* and Mode of Action Evaluated by Flow Cytometry." *Microbial Pathogenesis* 107: 254–60. Accessed on April 26, 2021. https://doi.org/10.1016/j.micpath.2017.03.029.

[73] Kim, Han-Shin, and Hee-Deung Park. 2013. "Ginger Extract Inhibits Biofilm Formation by *Pseudomonas Aeruginosa* PA14." *PloS One* 8

(9): e76106. Accessed on April 26, 2021. https://doi.org/10.1371/journal.pone.0076106.

[74] Podschun, R., and U. Ullmann. 1998. "*Klebsiella* Spp. as Nosocomial Pathogens: Epidemiology, Taxonomy, Typing Methods, and Pathogenicity Factors." *Clinical Microbiology Reviews* 11 (4): 589–603.

[75] Karuppiah, Ponmurugan, and Shyamkumar Rajaram. 2012. "Antibacterial Effect of *Allium Sativum* Cloves and *Zingiber Officinale* Rhizomes against Multiple-Drug Resistant Clinical Pathogens." *Asian Pacific Journal of Tropical Biomedicine* 2 (8): 597–601. Accessed on April 26, 2021. doi:10.1016/S2221-1691(12)60104-X.

[76] Shariatpanahi, Zahra Vahdat, Fourogh Azam Taleban, Majid Mokhtari, and Shaahin Shahbazi. 2010. "Ginger Extract Reduces Delayed Gastric Emptying and Nosocomial Pneumonia in Adult Respiratory Distress Syndrome Patients Hospitalized in an Intensive Care Unit." *Journal of Critical Care* 25 (4): 647–50. Accessed on April 26, 2021. doi:10.1016/j.jcrc.2009.12.008.

[77] Zaman, K. 2010. "Tuberculosis: A Global Health Problem." *Journal of Health, Population, and Nutrition* 28 (2): 111–13. Accessed on April 26, 2021. doi:10.3329/jhpn.v28i2.4879.

[78] Kulkarni, Rashmi Anant, and Ajit Ramesh Deshpande. 2016. "Anti-Inflammatory and Antioxidant Effect of Ginger in Tuberculosis." *Journal of Complementary & Integrative Medicine* 13 (2): 201–6. Accessed on April 26, 2021. doi:10.1515/jcim-2015-0032.

[79] Seung, Kwonjune J., Salmaan Keshavjee, and Michael L. Rich. 2015. "Multidrug-Resistant Tuberculosis and Extensively Drug-Resistant Tuberculosis." *Cold Spring Harbor Perspectives in Medicine* 5 (9): a017863. Accessed June 1, 2021. https://doi.org/10.1101/cshperspect.a017863.

[80] Scallan, Elaine, Patricia M. Griffin, Frederick J. Angulo, Robert V. Tauxe, and Robert M. Hoekstra. 2011. "Foodborne Illness Acquired in the United States--Unspecified Agents." *Emerging Infectious*

Diseases 17 (1): 16–22. Accessed June 1, 2021. doi:10.3201/eid1701.P21101.

[81] Hills, Ronald, Benjamin Pontefract, Hillary Mishcon, Cody Black, Steven Sutton, and Cory Theberge. 2019. "Gut Microbiome: Profound Implications for Diet and Disease." *Nutrients* 11 (7): 1613. Accessed June 1, 2021. doi:10.3390/nu11071613.

[82] Langdon, Amy, Nathan Crook, and Gautam Dantas. 2016. "The Effects of Antibiotics on the Microbiome throughout Development and Alternative Approaches for Therapeutic Modulation." *Genome Medicine* 8 (1): 39. Accessed on April 26, 2021. https://doi.org/10.1186/s13073-016-0294-z.

[83] Carlet, Jean. 2012. "The Gut Is the Epicentre of Antibiotic Resistance." *Antimicrobial Resistance and Infection Control* 1 (1): 39. Accessed on April 26, 2021. https://doi.org/10.1186/2047-2994-1-39.

[84] Levy, J. 2000. "The Effects of Antibiotic Use on Gastrointestinal Function." *The American Journal of Gastroenterology* 95 (1): S8–10. Accessed on April 26, 2021. doi:10.1016/s0002-9270(99)00808-4.

[85] "*E. Coli*." 2020. Who.Int. Accessed May 25, 2021. https://www.who.int/news-room/fact-sheets/detail/e-coli.

[86] *E. Coli: What Is It, How Does It Cause Infection, Symptoms & Causes.* n.d. Clevelandclinic.Org. Accessed May 25, 2021. https://my.clevelandclinic.org/health/diseases/16638-e-coli-infection.

[87] Malu, S. P., G. O. Obochi, E. N. Tawo, and B. E. Nyong. 2009. "Antibacterial Activity and Medicinal Properties of Ginger (*Zingiber Officinale*." *Global Journal of Pure and Applied Sciences* 15 (3–4): 365–368. Accessed April 26, 2021. doi:10.4314/gjpas.v15i3-4.48561.

[88] Yassen D., Ibrahim A. E. "Antibacterial Activity of Crude Extracts of Ginger (*Zingiber Officinale* Roscoe) on *Escherichia Coli* and *Staphylococcus Aureus*: A Study *in Vitro*. *Indo American Journal of Pharmaceutical Research* 2016; 6: 5830-5835." n.d. Sciepub.Com. Accessed May 25, 2021. http://www.sciepub.com/reference/276301.

[89] Harmalkar, M. N., and P. Desai. 2011. "Comparative Assessment of Antibacterial Activity of Ginger Extracts with Antimicrobial Agents." *International Journal of Pharmacology and Biological Sciences* 5 (2): 33–38.

[90] Institute of Medicine (US) Committee to Study Priorities for Vaccine Development, Kathleen R. Stratton, Jane S. Durch, and Robert S. Lawrence. 2000. *Helicobacter Pylori*. Washington, D.C., DC: National Academies Press. Accessed April 26, 2021. https://www.ncbi.nlm.nih.gov/books/NBK233297/.

[91] Zullo, Angelo, Cesare Hassan, Vincenzo De Francesco, Alessandro Repici, Rafaelle Manta, Silverio Tomao, Bruno Annibale, and Dino Vaira. 2014. "*Helicobacter pylori* and functional dyspepsia: an unsolved issue?" *World J Gastroenterol*, 20(27):8957-63. Accessed April 26, 2021. doi:10.3748/wjg.v20.i27.8957.

[92] Diaconu, S., A. Predescu, A. Moldoveanu, C. S. Pop, and C. Fierbințeanu-Braticevici. 2017. "*Helicobacter Pylori* Infection: Old and New." *Journal of Medicine and Life* 10 (2): 112–17. Accessed April 26, 2021. PMID: 28616085.

[93] O'Mahony, Rachel, Huda Al-Khtheeri, Deepaka Weerasekera, Neluka Fernando, Dino Vaira, John Holton, and Christelle Basset. 2005. "Bactericidal and Anti-Adhesive Properties of Culinary and Medicinal Plants against *Helicobacter Pylori*." *World Journal of Gastroenterology: WJG* 11 (47): 7499–7507. Accessed April 26, 2021. https://doi.org/10.3748/wjg.v11.i47.7499.

[94] Mahady, Gail B., Susan L. Pendland, Gina S. Yun, Zhi-Zhen Lu, and Adina Stoia. 2003. "Ginger (*Zingiber Officinale* Roscoe) and the Gingerols Inhibit the Growth of Cag A+ Strains of *Helicobacter Pylori*." *Anticancer Research* 23 (5A): 3699–3702.

[95] Ebrahimzadeh Attari, Vahideh, Mohammad Hosein Somi, Mohammad Asghari Jafarabadi, Alireza Ostadrahimi, Seyed-Yaghob Moaddab, and Neda Lotfi. 2019. "The Gastro-Protective Effect of Ginger (*Zingiber Officinale* Roscoe) in *Helicobacter Pylori* Positive Functional Dyspepsia." *Advanced Pharmaceutical Bulletin* 9 (2): 321–24. Accessed April 26, 2021. 10.15171/apb.2019.038.

[96] Ashurst, John V., Justina Truong, and Blair Woodbury. 2020. "*Salmonella Typhi*." In *Stat Pearls*. Treasure Island (FL): StatPearls Publishing.

[97] Deng, Wen, Shian-Ren Liou, Guy Plunkett III, George F. Mayhew, Debra J. Rose, Valerie Burland, Voula Kodoyianni, David C. Schwartz, and Frederick R. Blattner. 2003. "Comparative Genomics of *Salmonella enterica* Serovar Typhi Strains Ty2 and CT18." *Journal of Bacteriology* 185 (7): 2330–37. Accessed April 26, 2021. https://doi.org/10.1128/jb.185.7.2330-2337.2003.

[98] Hirose, K., K. Tamura, H. Sagara, and H. Watanabe. 2001. "Antibiotic Susceptibilities of *Salmonella Enterica* Serovar Typhi and *S. Enterica* Serovar Paratyphi A Isolated from Patients in Japan." *American Society for Microbiology* 45 (3): 956–958. Accessed April 26, 2021. doi:10.1128/AAC.45.3.956-958.2001.

[99] CDC. 2018. *Salmonella serotype typhi.* Cdc.Gov. Accessed June 1, 2021. https://www.cdc.gov/drugresistance/pdf/threats-report/salmonella-typhi-508.pdf.

[100] Kadum, H. 2019. "Effect of Ginger (*Zingiber Officinale*) Extract on *Salmonella Typhi*." *Plant Archives* 19: 708–711. Accessed April 26, 2021.

[101] Ekwenye, U. N., Elegalam N. N. 2005. "Antibacterial Activity Ginger Roscoe, and Garlic. 2005. "Extracts on *Escherichia Coli* and *Salmonella Typhi*." *International Journal of Molecular Medicine and Advance Sciences* 1 (4): 411–417.

[102] Islam, K., A. A. Rowsni, M. Khan, and S. Kabir. 2014. "Antimicrobial Activity of Ginger (*Zingiber Officinale*) Extracts against Food-Borne Pathogenic Bacteria." *International Journal of Science* 3. Accessed April 26, 2021.

[103] Lister, Philip D., Daniel J. Wolter, and Nancy D. Hanson. 2009. "Antibacterial-Resistant *Pseudomonas Aeruginosa*: Clinical Impact and Complex Regulation of Chromosomally Encoded Resistance Mechanisms." *Clinical Microbiology Reviews* 22 (4): 582–610. Accessed April 26, 2021. doi:10.1128/CMR.00040-09.

[104] Okuda, Jun, Naoki Hayashi, Masashi Okamoto, Shinji Sawada, Shu Minagawa, Yoshitaka Yano, and Naomasa Gotoh. 2010. "Translocation of *Pseudomonas Aeruginosa* from the Intestinal Tract Is Mediated by the Binding of ExoS to an Na, K-ATPase Regulator, FXYD3." *Infection and Immunity* 78 (11): 4511–22. Accessed April 26, 2021. doi:10.1128/IAI.00428-10.

[105] *Staphylococcus Aureus Infections - Infections - Merck Manuals Consumer Version.* n.d. Merckmanuals.Com. Accessed May 25, 2021. https://www.merckmanuals.com/home/infections/bacterial-infections-gram-positive-bacteria/staphylococcus-aureus-infections.

[106] Principato, Maryann, and Bi-Feng Qian. 2014. "Staphylococcal Enterotoxins in the Etiopathogenesis of Mucosal Autoimmunity within the Gastrointestinal Tract." *Toxins* 6 (5): 1471–89. Accessed April 26, 2021. doi:10.3390/toxins6051471.

[107] Kadariya, Jhalka, Tara C. Smith, and Dipendra Thapaliya. 2014. "*Staphylococcus Aureus* and Staphylococcal Food-Borne Disease: An Ongoing Challenge in Public Health." *BioMed Research International* 2014: 827965. Accessed April 26, 2021. https://doi.org/10.1155/2014/827965.

[108] Silva, Anderson Clayton da, Marjory Xavier Rodrigues, and Nathália Cristina Cirone Silva. 2020. "Methicillin-Resistant *Staphylococcus Aureus* in Food and the Prevalence in Brazil: A Review." *Brazilian Journal of Microbiology* 51 (1): 347–56. Accessed April 26, 2021. https://doi.org/10.1007/s42770-019-00168-1.

[109] Yadufashije, Callixte, Adolyne Niyonkuru, Emanuel Munyeshyaka, Sibomana Madjidi, and Joseph Mucumbitsi. 2020. "Antibacterial Activity of Ginger Extracts on Bacteria Isolated from Digestive Tract Infection Patients Attended Muhoza Health Center." *Asian Journal of Medical Sciences* 11 (2): 35–41. Accessed April 26, 2021. https://doi.org/10.3126/ajms.v11i2.27449.

[110] Petersen, Poul Erik, Denis Bourgeois, Hiroshi Ogawa, Saskia Estupinan-Day, and Charlotte Ndiaye. 2005. "The Global Burden of Oral Diseases and Risks to Oral Health." *Bulletin of the World Health Organization* 83 (9): 661–69.

[111] Sanz, Mariano, David Beighton, Michael A. Curtis, Jaime A. Cury, Irene Dige, Henrik Dommisch, Roger Ellwood, et al. 2017. "Role of Microbial Biofilms in the Maintenance of Oral Health and in the Development of Dental Caries and Periodontal Diseases. Consensus Report of Group 1 of the Joint EFP/ORCA Workshop on the Boundaries between Caries and Periodontal Disease." *Journal of Clinical Periodontology* 44: S5–11. Accessed April 26, 2021. doi:10.1111/jcpe.12682.

[112] Selwitz, Robert H., Amid I. Ismail, and Nigel B. Pitts. 2007. "Dental Caries." *Lancet* 369 (9555): 51–59. Accessed April 26, 2021. doi:10.1016/S0140-6736(07)60031-2.

[113] Ahirwar, S. S., Gupta Mk, and S. K. Snehi. 2019. "Dental Caries and Lactobacillus: Role and Ecology in the Oral Cavity." *Int J Pharm Sci & Res* 10 (11): 4818–29. Accessed April 26, 2021. doi:10.13040/IJPSR.0975-8232.10(11).4818-29.

[114] Dahiya, Parveen, and Reet Kamal. 2013. "Hyaluronic Acid: A Boon in Periodontal Therapy." *North American Journal of Medical Sciences* 5 (5): 309–15. Accessed April 26, 2021. doi:10.4103/1947-2714.112473.

[115] Porto, Thiago S., Rander Rangel, Niege A. J. C. Furtado, Tatiane C. de Carvalho, Carlos H. G. Martins, Rodrigo C. S. Veneziani, Fernando B. Da Costa, et al. 2009. "Pimarane-Type Diterpenes: Antimicrobial Activity against Oral Pathogens." *Molecules (Basel, Switzerland)* 14 (1): 191–99. Accessed April 26, 2021. doi:10.3390/molecules14010191.

[116] Kanth, M. Rajini, A. Ravi Prakash, G. Sreenath, Vikram Simha Reddy, and S. Huldah. 2016. "Efficacy of Specific Plant Products on Microorganisms Causing Dental Caries." *Journal of Clinical and Diagnostic Research: JCDR* 10 (12): ZM01–3. Accessed April 26, 2021. doi:10.7860/JCDR/2016/19772.9025.

[117] Rashmi, K. J., and Ritu Tiwari. 2016. "Pharmacotherapeutic Properties of Ginger and Its Use in Diseases of the Oral Cavity: A Narrative Review." *Journal of Advanced Oral Research* 7 (2): 1–6. Accessed April 26, 2021. doi:10.2047/joaor-07-02-001.

[118] Premkishore, K., T. Umapathy, M. D. Kathariya, A. Agrawal, P. S. P. Kumar, and G. Kallampilly. 2013. "Effect of Honey and Aqueous Ginger Extract against *Streptococcus Mutans* Isolated from Extracted Carious Deciduous Teeth." *Journal of Indian Academy of Oral Medicine and Radiology* 25(4). Accessed April 26, 2021.

[119] Giriraju, Anjan, and G. Y. Yunus. 2013. "Assessment of Antimicrobial Potential of 10% Ginger Extract against *Streptococcus Mutans, Candida Albicans*, and *Enterococcus Faecalis*: An *in Vitro* Study." *Indian Journal of Dental Research: Official Publication of Indian Society for Dental Research* 24 (4): 397–400. Accessed April 26, 2021.

[120] Moreira da Silva, Thiago, Carlos Danniel Pinheiro, Patricia Puccinelli Orlandi, Carlos Cleomir Pinheiro, and Gemilson Soares Pontes. 2018. "Zerumbone from *Zingiber Zerumbet* (L.) Smith: A Potential Prophylactic and Therapeutic Agent against the Cariogenic Bacterium *Streptococcus Mutans*." *BMC Complementary and Alternative Medicine* 18 (1): 301. Accessed April 26, 2021. https://doi.org/10.1186/s12906-018-2360-0.

[121] Saffari, Fereshteh, Mohammad Danesh Ardakani, Hengameh Zandi, Hamed Heidarzadeh, and Mohammad Hassan Moshafi. 2015. "The Effects of Chlorhexidine and Persica Mouthwashes on Colonization of *Streptococcus Mutans* on Fixed Orthodontics O-Rings." *Journal of Dentistry (Shiraz, Iran)* 16 (1): 54–57. Accessed April 26, 2021.

[122] Tr, Bauer Faria, Furletti-Goes Vf, Franzini Cm, Aro AA, Andrade TAM, Sartoratto A, and Menezes CC. 2021. "Anti-Inflammatory and Antimicrobial Effects of *Zingiber Officinale* Mouthwash on Patients with Fixed Orthodontic Appliances." *Am J Orthod Dentofacial Orthop* Jan;159(1):21-29. Accessed April 26, 2021. doi:10.1016/j.ajodo.2019.10.025.

[123] Azizi, Arash, Shabnam Aghayan, Saeed Zaker, Mahdieh Shakeri, Navid Entezari, and Shirin Lawaf. 2015. "In Vitro Effect of *Zingiber Officinale* Extract on Growth of *Streptococcus Mutans* and Streptococcus Sanguinis." *International Journal of Dentistry* 2015: 489842.

[124] Patel, Roopal V., Vidhi T. Thaker, and V. K. Patel. 2011. "Antimicrobial Activity of Ginger and Honey on Isolates of Extracted Carious Teeth during Orthodontic Treatment." *Asian Pacific Journal of Tropical Biomedicine* 1 (1): S58–61. Accessed April 26, 2021. https://doi.org/10.1016/S2221-1691(11)60124-X.

[125] Encarnacion, Carlos Omar, Austin Mitchell Loranger, A. G. Bharatkumar, and G. Hossein Almassi. 2016. "Bacterial Endocarditis Caused by *Lactobacillus Acidophilus* Leading to Rupture of Sinus of Valsalva Aneurysm." *Texas Heart Institute Journal* 43 (2): 161–64. Accessed April 26, 2021. https://doi.org/10.14503/THIJ-15-5121.

[126] Shrimathi, S., Umesh Kemparaj, Sangeeta Umesh, Muthu Karuppaiah, Palanivel Pandian, and Krishnaveni A. 2019. "Comparative Evaluation of Cocoa Bean Husk, Ginger and Chlorhexidine Mouth Washes in the Reduction of *Steptococcus Mutans* and Lactobacillus Count in Saliva: A Randomized Controlled Trial." *Cureus* 11 (6): e4968. Accessed April 26, 2021. doi: 10.7759/cureus.4968.

[127] Elgamily, Hanaa, Rehab Safy, and Rabab Makharita. 2019. "Influence of Medicinal Plant Extracts on the Growth of Oral Pathogens *Streptococcus Mutans* and *Lactobacillus Acidophilus*: An *in-Vitro* Study." *Open Access Macedonian Journal of Medical Sciences* 7 (14): 2328–34. Accessed April 26, 2021. https://doi.org/10.3889/oamjms.2019.653.

[128] Semwal, Ruchi Badoni, Deepak Kumar Semwal, Sandra Combrinck, and Alvaro M. Viljoen. 2015. "Gingerols and Shogaols: Important Nutraceutical Principles from Ginger." *Phytochemistry* 117: 554–68. Accessed June 1, 2020. doi: 10.1016/j.phytochem.2015.07.012.

[129] Mekuriya, Wondale, and Berhanu Mekibib. 2018. "Review on the Medicinal Values of Ginger for Human and Animal Ailments." *Journal of Veterinary Science & Technology* 09 (02). Accessed June 2, 2021. https://doi.org/10.4172/2157-7579.1000519.

[130] *WHO global report on traditional and complementary medicine 2019*. Geneva: World Health Organization; 2019. Accessed June 1, 2021.

[131] Gurib-Fakim, Ameenah. 2006. "Medicinal Plants: Traditions of Yesterday and Drugs of Tomorrow." *Molecular Aspects of Medicine* 27 (1): 1–93. Accessed June 2, 2021.

[132] Abdullahi, A., A. Khairulmazmi, S. Yasmeen, I. S. Ismail, A. Norhayu, M. R. Sulaiman, O. H. Ahmed, and M. R. Ismail. 2020. "Phytochemical Profiling and Antimicrobial Activity of Ginger (*Zingiber Officinale*) Essential Oils against Important Phytopathogens." *Arabian Journal of Chemistry* 13 (11): 8012–25. Accessed June 27, 2021.

[133] Wang, Xin, Yi Shen, Kiran Thakur, Jinzhi Han, Jian-Guo Zhang, Fei Hu, and Zhao-Jun Wei. 2020. "Antibacterial Activity and Mechanism of Ginger Essential Oil against *Escherichia Coli* and *Staphylococcus Aureus*." *Molecules (Basel, Switzerland)* 25 (17): 3955. Accessed June 26, 2021.

[134] Mara Teles, Amanda, Bianca Araújo dos Santos, Cleidiane Gomes Ferreira, Adenilde Nascimento Mouchreck, Kátia da Silva Calabrese, Ana Lucia Abreu-Silva, and Fernando Almeida-Souza. 2020. "Ginger (*Zingiber Officinale*) Antimicrobial Potential: A Review." In *Ginger Cultivation and Its Antimicrobial and Pharmacological Potentials*. Intech Open. Accessed June 26, 2021.

[135] Gao, Demin, and Yingying Zhang. 2010. "Comparative Antibacterial Activities of Extracts of Dried Ginger and Processed Ginger." *Pharmacognosy Journal* 2 (15): 41–44. Accessed June 26, 2021.

[136] Sutardi, Lina N., Ietje Wientarsih, Ekowati Handharyani, M. Andriani, and Agus. Setiyono. 2015. "Indonesian Wild Ginger (*Zingiber* Sp) Extract: Antibacterial Activity against *Mycoplasma Gallisepticum*." *IOSR J Pharmacy* 5: 59–64. Accessed June 1, 2021.

[137] Nazir, Muhammad Ashraf. 2017. "Prevalence of Periodontal Disease, Its Association with Systemic Diseases and Prevention." *International Journal of Health Sciences* 11 (2): 72–80. Accessed June 26, 2021.

In: Ginger's Antimicrobial …
Editor: Diana R. Cundell
ISBN: 978-1-68507-117-2

Chapter 3

GINGER AS AN ANTIFUNGAL AGENT

Anne H. Bower*[*], *Tyler Savage, Irene Cooper and Brianne Spellman
College of Life Sciences, Jefferson University, Philadelphia, PA, USA

ABSTRACT

Fungal infections are on the rise globally with an increase in immunocompromised populations and a corresponding decrease in effectiveness of selective pharmaceuticals for treatment due to cost, availability and resistance. Ginger *(Zingiber officinale* Roscoe) has been used for centuries in both the Traditional Chinese Medicine (TCM) and Ayurvedic traditional systems for a wide range of uses including as an antifungal agent and as an immunomodulator. This review explores ginger's production of antifungal enzymes and chemicals in the soil environment, the physiological and biochemical mechanism of how ginger changes cell membranes and inhibits hyphal growth in comparison to other antifungal plant species. The antifungal effectiveness of ginger essential oils to other plant species are systematically reviewed based on chemical constituents, geographic range, and mechanism of action. The cumulative scientific evidence establishes the potential of ginger as an adjuvant treatment in an integrative medicine system to address the two leading fungal pathogens *Candida* and *Aspergillus*.

[*] Corresponding Author's E-mail: Anne. Bower@jefferson.edu.

Keywords: phytotherapy, antifungal, *Zingiberaceae*

INTRODUCTION

Many of the 52 genera of aromatic perennial plants in the *Zingiberaceae* family have long established ethnopharmaceutical and medicinal properties that have been used since ancient times in Traditional Chinese Medicine (TCM), Ayurvedic practitioners as well as many other predominately Asian traditional medical systems [1, 2, 3]. Of the 1,587 species in the family, 144 are in the genus *Zingiber* [4]. Ginger (*Zingiber officinale* Roscoe), turmeric (*Curcuma longa*) and cardamon (*Eletteria cardamomum*) are the most well-documented species with antimicrobial, anti-inflammatory, antioxidant, anti-emetic, anticancer, antihypercholesterolemic, antispasmodic, antithrombotic, carminative, cardioprotective, cholagogue, diaphoretic, and stimulant properties ([1, 2, 3, 5].

Ginger is endemic to northeastern India where its historic use has resulted in decreased genetic diversity of wild cultivars so that use of a cultigen propagated from rhizomes is the most common agricultural production method ([6,7]). Modern cultivation was a $5.3 billion market in 2018 with China dominating in global exports at nearly 70% followed by Thailand (10%), Peru (5%) and India (5%) [8, 9]. Ginger is widely used in food, beverages, flavorings, traditional cuisine and medicine globally. The United States Food & Drug Administration (FDA) classifies it as Generally Recognized as Safe (GRAS) [10] because of its wide use for centuries with little to no observed safety concerns or side effects. It is listed as an approved remedy medicinally by Germany Commission E [11], as well by the World Health Organization [12]. The fresh rhizome dose ranges from 500 to 1000 mg three times per day, 2 to 4 g as a tea; whereas the dried rhizome is 500 mg two to four times per day or 0.5 to 1 g as a tea [1, 3]. It is also available as a capsule in 100 mg to 1000 mg, a 67.5 mg chewable tablet and as a 1:1 extract [13]. The essential oil (EO) is used primarily in food, perfume and for aromatherapy [14]. It has low acute toxicity with an Oral $LD_{50} > 5$ g/kg (rat) and a Dermal $LD_{50} > 5$ g/kg (rabbit) [14, 15].

Two of the most widely used traditional medicine systems both use ginger effectively in many forms to treat patients. In the 240 BC *Yellow Emperor's Classic of Medicine* five element practice of TCM, ginger (Chinese: Sheng jiang *fresh*, Gan jiang *dried*) is the balancing pungent herb associated with the metal element in the autumn season [1, 2, 16]. Ginger is found in over half of all herbal TCM preparations today [17].

In Ayurvedic traditional medicine practiced predominately in India, ginger is considered the universal medicine (Sanskit: Singabera or Ardhrakam) [1, 2, 18]. The fresh root, dried root, juice and essential oil are all used [19]. The root was boiled and then applied to topical fungal infections [20]. Both turmeric (*Curcuma longa*) and cardamom (*Elettaria cardamomum* (L.) Maton) were used as topical antiseptics and antifungal agents in traditional practice [19].

Fungal infections have often been least understood with challenges to both accurate diagnosis and effective treatment. The Leading International Fungal Education Portal (LIFE) has facilitated the ability of public health professionals to have country specific data to strategically coordinate care and outreach planning [21]. Globally, it is estimated that over 1 billion people contract fungal infections with 1.5 million resulting in death [22]. In the United States, direct healthcare costs alone for fungal infections were calculated at $7.2 billion in 2014 with hospitalizations due to invasive *Candida* and *Aspergillus* accounting for $2.6 billion [23]. Health-care related mucormycosis is on the increase from medical devices and the hospital environment during prolonged steroid therapy, surgery, organ transplant, premature birth or as co-morbidity with chronic disease such as diabetes mellitus [24, 25]. It is highly invasive, and was the most expensive of all fungal infections for both inpatient and outpatient settings [23] due the long length of stay and complexity of treatment [26]. In contrast, dermatophyte infections such as vaginal and oral candidiasis were most common for outpatient treatment at the lowest cost per visit ($123-287) [23]. The most prevalent fungal infections globally are aspergillosis, candidiasis, with mucormycosis less frequent, but more lethal [22].

With both the rise in resistance to antifungal pharmaceutics and increase in the immunocompromised proportion of the population, ginger holds much promise. The purpose of this systematic review is to explore the use and efficacy of ginger as an antifungal agent for a range of pathogenic fungal infections with an emphasis on immunocompromised patients.

Ecological Relationships Underpin Mechanisms of Fungal Action

A comparison of selected medicinally active plants in the *Zingiberaceae* family provides an overview of current research findings of the ecological relationships under which plants develop antifungal mechanisms. Mutualism is a common occurrence between a majority of plants and the endophytic fungi that reside in their various organs. Because plants like *Zingiber officinale* are a living environment for the endophytic fungi, the fungi will release bioactive compounds when the plant is in danger. This includes threats from drought, parasites, and diseases like pathogenic fungi [27]. It is believed that the mechanism of action against pathogenic fungi in ginger is from the ability of the endophytic fungi to outcompete the pathogenic fungi while also synthesizing antifungal chemicals, similar to how the endophytic fungi *Paraconiothyrium variabile* in the Japanese Plum Yew (*Cephalotaxus harringtonia*) combats the common pathogenic fungi *Fusarium oxysporum* through inhibition of mycotoxin production with the bioactive compound 13-oxo-9,11-octadecadienoic acid [28]. As shown in Table 1, some specific endophytic fungi found in ginger (*Zingiber officinale* Rosc.) sampled from Indonesia like *Talaromyces*, *Glomerella cingulata*, *Curvularia*, *Fusarium solani*, and *Acremonium* are shared amongst several agricultural plant species including cupuassu (*Theobroma grandiflorum*), cacao (*Theobroma cacao*), and maize (*Zea mays*), suggesting shared antifungal properties and antagonistic action against pathogens [27, 29].

In wild ginger (*Amomum siamense*) rhizomes, leaves, and pseudostems sampled from Thailand during both the wet and dry seasons, the most common endophytic fungi found were *Colletotrichum gloeosporioides* and *Glomerella spp.* (telomorph stage), which were also discovered in ginger (*Zingiber officinale* Rosc) leaves, stem and rhizomes, indicating shared endophytic fungi and similar antifungal mechanisms in the *Zingiberaceae family* [30]. In one example, the endophytic fungi responsible for ginger's antifungal response to *Fusarium oxysporum* were *Collectotrichum gloeosporioides* and *Glomerella cingulata*, where *G. cingulata* as an extract has potential to treat *Rhizopusoryzae*, *Beauveriabassiana*, and *Chrysoporium tropicum* [27, 31]. The mechanism for this action may be explained by the fact that some endophytic fungi, like *G. cingulata*, have the ability to produce secondary metabolites that perform a range of natural functions in the host plant. In particular, the ascomycetes fungi class are recognized for their antimicrobial metabolites [31]. *G. cingulata* as an ascomycetes fungi biotransforms bioactive compounds with the action of a biocatalyst into novel terpenoids, one example being the transformation of (–)-Isolongifolol (1) to (–)-3-hydroxy-isolongifolol and (–)-9-hydroxy-isolongifolol (Miyazawa et al., 2010). It is possible through mechanisms like the biotransformation of terpenoids in *G. cingulata* that metabolites of endophytic fungi possess antifungal properties [31].

Turmeric (*Curcuma longa*), which is in the *Zingiberaceae* family along with ginger, contains three curcuminoids: curcumin, demethylated curcumin and bisdimethyl curcumin. These curcuminoids possess varying levels of antifungal ability in a variety of pathogenic fungi including *Phomopsis obscurans*, *Botrytis cinerea*, *Plasmopara viticola* and *Colletotrichum* species [32]. As an essential oil derived from the leaf and root, turmeric has the ability to disrupt the cell membrane and mitochondria of the pathogenic fungi, *Aspergillus flavus*, while also regulating the expression of mycotoxin genes in the pathogenic fungi [33]. Turmeric also contains a variety of endophytic fungi such as *Trichoderma harzianum* and *Trichoderma asperellum*, which show *in vitro* inhibition for common pathogenic fungi in turmeric like *Pythium aphanidermatum* and *Rhizoctonia solani* [34].

In mechanisms similar to ginger, in the host turmeric plant these endophytic fungi inhibit pathogenic fungi through antibiosis, competition, or triggering the plant's natural response system [34]. On a molecular level, antibiosis responses of endophytic fungi range from the creation of hydrolytic and cellulase-like enzymes to metabolites [34].

Small cardamon (*Elettaria cardamomum* (L.) Maton), also a member of the *Zingiberaceae* family, has been proven to contain endophytes that fight common fungal pathogens. One example includes the endophytes *Hedychium coronarium*, *Amomum subulatum* and *Aframomum melegueta*, which occur naturally in cardamon's roots, rhizomes, petioles and leaves, and have the ability to fight fungal infections such as *Pythium vexans*, *Rhizoctonia solani*, and *Fusarium oxysporum* shown in an *in vitro* study using the endophyte's isolates [35]. It has also been reported in a novel study concerning small cardamom grown in India and an entomopathogenic fungus, *Lecanicillium psalliotae* that biochemical mechanisms from the fungi promote plant growth through creation of ammonia and indole-3-acetic acid and solubilization of minerals, and also produce enzymes like cellulases, α-amylases, and proteases that degrade cell walls [36]. Further evidence is needed to establish *Lecanicillium psalliotae* as an endophytic fungus, however it is important to note that the mechanisms reported are similar to other endophytic fungi that disrupt pathogenic fungi cell walls and with the added ecological advantage of promoting plant growth in cardamom.

Understanding how ginger and related species interact with pathogenic fungi from an ecological standpoint provides insight into how these antifungal constituents are created in the plants' organs. When harvested and processed, the plants continue to carry the antifungal properties of the chemicals that they have manufactured themselves as well as the accompanying endophytic fungi. Therefore, the medicinal applications for both animals and humans, which includes antifungal health applications, are attributed to the natural relationships that are present ecologically.

As shown in Table 2, the antifungal properties of selected plant species are compared emphasizing the key antifungal constituent and the mechanism of action against specific fungal species. The majority of this research is laboratory studies from agricultural scientists and mycologists focused on understanding the complex symbiotic and pathogenic relationships of plants to the soil environment.

Table 1. Selected *Zingiberaceae* species with known endophytic fungal species impacting pathogenic fungal species

Endophytic Fungi	Pathogenic Fungi	Reference
Ginger (*Zingiber officinale*) *Talaromyces spp.* *Collectotrichum gloeosporioides* *Glomerella cingulata* *Curvularia spp.* *Fusarium solani* *Acremonium spp.* *Cryptocoryne affinis*	*Fusarium oxysporum* *Rhizopusoryzae spp.* *Beauveriabassian spp.* *Chrysoporium tropicum*	[27, 31]
Wild Ginger (*Amomum siamense*) *Colletotrichum gloeosporioides Glomerella* spp. *Phomopsis* spp. *Gaeumannomyces amomi* *Leiosphaerella amomi*	*Rhizopusoryzae spp.* *Beauveriabassiana spp.* *Chrysoporium tropicum*	[30, 31]
Turmeric (*Curcuma longa*) *Trichoderma harzianum, Trichoderma asperellum*	*Phomopsis obscurans Botrytis cinerea Plasmopara viticola Colletotrichum spp. Aspergillus flavus,* *Pythium aphanidermatum,* *Rhizoctonia solani*	[32, 33]
Small Cardamon (*Elettaria cardamomum*) *Hedychium coronarium, Amomum subulatum, Aframomum melegueta*	*Pythium vexans* *Rhizoctonia solani* *Fusarium oxysporum*	[35]

It is important to note that the chemical constituents in a given plant determine the exact mechanism and antagonistic action on a specific pathogenic fungus. However, most of the mechanisms analyzed are similar in that they act to either lessen the integrity of the pathogenic fungi's membrane structure, cell wall or inhibit growth of the fungi's hyphae or mycelium. Particular emphasis is on the three medicinally active plants in the family *Zingiberaceae*.

A novel N-terminal sequence protein from ginger rhizome disrupted hyphal formation for multiple fungal species [37]. Ginger oleoresin proved effective in inhibiting *in vitro* spore germination and mycelial growth of *Pestalotiopsis microspora* through a membrane-targeted mechanism alongside membrane permeability alteration, membrane lipid peroxidation, and membrane integrity collapse [38].

Table 2. A comparison of antifungal constituents and their actions

Antifungal Constituent	Action	Pathogenic Fungi	Reference
Ginger (*Zingiber officinale*) Novel N-terminal Sequence protein	Disrupts hyphal formation	*Botrytis cinerea* *Fusarium oxysporum* *Mycosphaerella arachidicola* *Physalospora piricola*	[37]
Ginger (*Zingiber officinale*) Oleoresin	Inhibits spore germination Inhibits mycelial growth Disrupts membrane	*Pestalotiopsis microspore*	[38]
Ginger (*Zingiber officinale*) Sesquiterpenes Monoterpenes	Disrupts plasma membrane	*Fusarium moniliforme* *Candida albicans* *Aspergillus spp.*	[39]
Turmeric (*Curcuma longa*) Curcuminoids	Disrupts cell membrane and mitochondria Controls regulation of mycotoxin genes	*Phomopsis obscurans* *Botrytis cinerea* *Plasmopara viticola* *Colletotrichum spp.*	[32]
Small Cardamon (*Elettaria cardamomum*) Phenolics	Synergistic action of phenolic	*Aspergillus flavus Aspergillus niger* *Aspergillus solani* *Aspergillus oryzae*	[40]

Ginger's constituent sesquiterpenes and monoterpenes are responsible for the antifungal properties of ginger due to their capability in altering the fluidity and permeability of a microorganism's plasma membrane [39]. Ginger oleoresin destroyed mycelia morphology which increased intercellular electrolyte, nuclein of *P. misctospore*, sugar and protein leakage which proved to be lethal [38]. Ginger essential oil (EO) has been shown to inhibit *Fusarium moniliforme, Candida albicans, and Aspergillus* species [39].

Table 3. Constituent variation by geographic source of ginger essential oil (EO) and corresponding antifungal activity

EO Source **Antifungal Constituents**	**Test Method**	**Result**	**Refer**
African [6], [8] and [10]-gingerols,[6]-gingerdiol	Sabouraud's dextrose agar culture	Effective on 13 fungal pathogens: *Fusarium oxysporum, Aspergillus fumigatus, accharomyces cerevisiae, Candida albicans, Rhizopus* spp.	[48]
Algerian citral (30.8%), zingiberene (17.1%), Geranyl acetate (6.7%), 1,8-cineol (6.1%) β-Sesquiphellandrene(6%)	Disk diffusion assay (mm), Control: sulfamethoxazole, penicillin G, ampicillin, gentamicin	*Candida koseri* (inactive) *Aspergillus niger* (inactive) *Salmonella typhi* (10 mm)	[44]
Australian EO citral (2, 6-octadienal, 3, 7-dimethyl) (76.94%) geranic acid (2.57%) verbenyl ethyl ether (4%), artemiseole (1.12%)	Agar dilutions PDA plates used No EO as control	*Botrytis cinerea, Alternaria panax, Fusarium oxysporum, Cylindrocarpon destructans Sclerotinia nivalis, Sclerotinia sclerotiorum* Inhibition 0.3%	[49]
Brazilian EO zingiberene (37.65%) δ-amorphene (19.8%) α-curcumin (11.3%) α-bisabolene (10.4%)	Microbroth dilution assay	*Fusarium verticillioides* (MIC 2.5 mg/ml)	[46]
Indian EO Camphene, Geranial Neral, Borneol β-Sesquiphellandrene β-phellandrene, ar-cucumene α-zingiberene, 1,8-cineol	Inverted petri plate	*Fusarium moniliforme* at 6 μL dose	[50]
Thailand EO Camphene, α-pinene 1,8-Cineole, β-Thujene Geranial, Neral	Disk diffusion	*Fusarium* spp (14.5 mm) *Rhodoturola* spp(13.5 mm)	[51]
Vietnamese EO ar-cucumene β-bisabolene α-zingiberene β-sesquiphellandrene	Agar Diffusion Cup Method (mm)	*Salmonella abony* (11.0 mm) *Saccharomycesrevisiae* (16.0), *Candida albicans* (13-14.1), *Aspergillus niger* (32.3), *Rhizopus nigricans* (17) *Penicillium* sp. (39), *Botrytis cinerea* (30.0)	[43]
EO no origin zingiberene (37.65%) δ-amorphene (19.8%) α-curcumin (11.3%) α-bisabolene (10.4%)	Antifungal activity Antiaflatoxigenic activity	Significant effects on *Aspergillus flavus* and aflatoxin B_1 and B_2	[52]
EO no origin gingerols, eugenol, shogaols, gingerdiols, zingerone, monoterpenes, sesquiterpenes	Hot and open-air drying; Broth dilution	*Aspergillus flavus, Candida albicans, Fusarium oxysporum, Geotrichum candidum,* (hot drying); *Candida albicans* (open-air); *Fusarium verticillioides*	[39]

Antifungal Activity of Ginger Essential Oil (EO)

Commercial ginger food and beverages may vary widely in concentrations of gingerol and shogaol based on differences in manufacturing [41] as do dietary supplements or nutraceuticals [42]. Ginger is chemically complex by plant form with oleoresins of acrid gingerols the principal constituent in fresh rhizome with shogoals dominating as it is dried into powdered form. The volatile oil is typically 1-3% with zingiberene the most common. As shown in Table 3, constituent concentration for ginger essential oil (EO) varies widely by geographic location, harvest date and extraction method [14]. The antimicrobial activity of ginger essential oil (EO) has been extensively confirmed in laboratory studies and attributed to its chemical components, mainly consisting of monoterpene and sesquiterpene hydrocarbons such as α-zingiberene, ar-curcumene, β-bisabolene and β-sesquiphellandrene [5]. It is important to note that the geographic location of the ginger's origin along with how the essential oil is extracted and manufactured alters the level and range of effectiveness of the plant's antifungal compounds. Therefore, each variation of ginger displays different interactions and antifungal results vary widely between studies. Biochemical pathways and antifungal mechanisms may differ as well due to this variable level and composition of constituents. In a medical context, this variation is imperative to consider when choosing an essential oil treatment since one variety may be more effective than another. For example, when treating *Candida spp.*, Vietnamese or Algerian EO is most effective, compared to sources from other geographic regions which show little to no inhibition [43, 44, 45]. Additionally, the synergism present between compounds in a particular variation of EO determines its ability to disrupt fungal cell membranes, which is a common antifungal mechanism of ginger essential oil [46]. One possible mechanism for fungal inhibition includes the disruption of ergosterol synthesis and the decrease in integrity of membrane-bound proteins like observed in the interaction between Brazillian EO and *Fusarium verticillioides* [46]. In that specific interaction, the lack of ergosterol combined with the additional effect of reduced fumonisin B1 and B2 production results in a decrease of fungal biomass. Another example of effective synergism includes combined ginger and turmeric (*Curcuma longa*) EO which showed antifungal action against dermatophytes *Trichophyton rubrum* and *Microsporum gypseum* [47]. Singularly, each EO displayed antifungal characteristics, but together showed increased effectiveness and promise for dermatophytic infection treatment, further confirming the importance of present chemical compounds. With further analysis, the versatility of ginger EO is apparent through numerous studies and is valuable for assessing treatment of specific fungal infections.

Pathogenic Human Disease: Ginger as Antifungal Agent for Immunocompromised Populations

Immunocompromised Populations at Risk for Fungal

The proportion of the population that is immunocompromised is increasing. It is estimated that there are 1.8 million new cancer cases in 2020 [53]. By 2040, it is projected that there will be 27.5 million new cancer cases [54]. As of 2019, there are 38 million individuals globally living with HIV, and this number could be as high as 44.5 million with 690,000 individuals dying from AIDS-related illnesses [55]. Approximately one in ten babies born are premature and there is currently a rise in preterm birth rates [56]. In the United States, in 2018, 34.2 million individuals had diabetes, with this chronic disease listed as a contributing or underlying cause of death for 270,702 [57]. These are a few conditions that can leave people immunocompromised and susceptible to potentially deadly fungal infections.

At risk populations for fungal infections include those with pre-existing conditions including cancer, AIDS, organ transplantation, corticosteroid therapies, diabetes, and asthma [22, 58, 59, 60]. The rise in invasive fungal infections due to *Candida* species presents a formidable problem to immunocompromised individuals [61]. There is an increase in disease produced by filamentous fungal human pathogens (FFHP) [59].

Aspergilli, *Fusarium*, and *Mucor* species were able to be isolated in a large variety of foods, encompassing baked goods to vegetables [59]. Aflatoxins are commonly found in cereal, maize, nuts, dairy products, and eggs while fumonisins are commonly found in cereals, maize, and figs [62]. The most popular food groups where FFHP were tested positive were corn, rice, fruits, nuts, beans, and vegetables [59]. Fungi can contaminate crops under certain environmental conditions such as temperature, humidity, and pH [62]. Although cooking will eliminate pathogenic fungi from unprocessed foods, many foods are consumed raw and fresh [59]. Infection from contaminated foods is not restricted to consumption but can occur if exposed for an extended period of time [59]. Essential oils of Zingiber rhizomes have been used for food preservation due to their antimicrobial and antioxidant properties, and have also shown significant antifungal properties against C. albicans, *Aspergillus niger*, and *Candida glabrata* [63]. Ginger was effective against Fusarium spp. fungal strains and inhibited growth of resistant to amphotericin B and ketoconazole fungi [64].

Mucormycosis is an emerging invasive severe fungal infection which occurs as a result of environmental exposure [58]. This exposure can be from inhalation, ingestion, or inoculation via trauma or puncture wounds [65]. Mucorales species responsible regarding healthcare-associated mucormycosis include *Rhizopus spp.*, *Mucor spp.*, *Lichthmemia corymblfera*, *Cunninghamella bertholletiae*, *Rhizomucor spp.*, *Apophysomyces elegans*, *Sakenaea vasiformis*, and non-speciated Mucorales [58]. Common localization is in the skin and gastrointestinal tract [58]. Outbreaks have been associated with adhesive bandages, ineffective anti-fungal treatment, and increased usage of immunosuppressive drugs [58]. At risk populations are those with underlying conditions such as hematologic malignancies, diabetes, and organ transplant recipients [58, 65]. Mucormycosis has increased in immunocompromised individuals, which is caused by Mucor species and mortality rates for gastrointestinal and severe neutropenia developed mucormycosis can be 85% with a range between 68% and 100%, respectively [59].

Mycoses is a fungal disease that can be categorized in two groups: systemic mycoses, infection occurs when fungi is inhaled, and implantation mycoses, infection usually occurs through wounds [66]. Progressive mycoses can occur in individuals with a compromised immune system such as those undergoing chemotherapy, undergone organ transplantation, and with AIDS [59, 66]. Mycotoxins can lead to detrimental health hazards such as carcinogenic, neurotoxic, hepatotoxic, and immunotoxic effects [62]. FFHP is prevalent in a variety of foods, which makes it a likely source of mycoses infection [59]. Fusarium species are on the rise as an infection agent in humans [59*]. F. oxysporum*, *F. verticilliodes* (previously known as *F. moniliforme*), and *F. solani* among others were specifically detected in various food samples [59]. *F. verticilliodes* has negative effects on animals, it is acutely toxic to ducks and causes liver and cardiovascular issues in rats [67]. *Fusarium monoliforme* is associated with high rates of human esophageal cancer, with highest rates in the southwestern districts of Transkei, Africa [67]. Corn is a dietary staple in Transkei, and *F. monoliforme* causes corn diseases including stalk rot, ear rot, and kernel infection due to toxic production [67]. Warehouse storage, shipping, and handling of food should be carefully monitored to reduce risk. Toxins produced by this fungus are fusarium acid, gibberellins, fusarins, monoiliormin (little to no production, but is highly toxic causing rapid death & pathological lesions), and fumonisins [67]. Fumonisin B1 is found to have cancer-promoting activity in rats, equine leukoencephalomalacia, and porcine pulmonary edema [67].

Resistance and Side Effects of Current Pharmaceutical Treatments

Immunocompromising treatments and medical conditions are considered to be a reason for the increase in invasive candidiasis cases [22]. The mortality and rate of infection in intensive care units demand new treatment methods due to ineffectiveness or resistance to current treatments like fluconazole [60, 61]. Two main drug classes for antifungal treatment are echinocandins and azoles [68]. Azoles (fluconazole, voriconazole, posaconazole) and echinocandins (caspofungin, anidulafungin, and micafungin) are both first-line treatments for fungal infections [68, 69]. Amphotericin B is usually a last-resort option for treatment [68]. Amphotericin B is a treatment included in the Polyene drug class [69]

Increasing drug resistance is due to an epidemiological shift in evolutionary less susceptible species and acquired resistance [69]. There is currently a rising threat of superbug fungal infections [68]. Multiple *Candida* species have shown resistance to azole and echinocandin treatment [68]. *C. auris* is multidrug-resistant and in India, a third of *C. auris* isolates are resistant to amphotericin B, most are resistant to fluconazole, and nearly half are resistant to voriconazole. Resistance to echinocandins is increasing [68]. Multidrug resistance has been reported for *Aspergillus lentulus*, *A. calidoustus*, *Fusarium* species, *Scedosporium* species. and several *Candida* species [69]. Many molds are intrinsically resistant to the azole fluconazole. *Candida krusei* and *C. glabrata* demonstrate azole drug treatment resistance [70].

While echinocandins are usually very active against a majority of *candida* species, they show less activity against *Candida parapsilosis*, and *Candida gulliermondii*, and *C. glabrata* has shown resistance to this treatment [68, 69]. Azole-resistant fungi include: *Candida* and *Aspergillus* species namely *A. fumigatus* and *C. auris. Aspergillus lentus*, *A. fumigatiaffinis*, *A. viridinutans*, *A. pseudofischeri*, *A calidoustus*, *A. fumigatus*, *Candida auris*, *Fusarium solani* and other species, *Scefosporium apiospermum* complex, *Scedosporium* species *Lamentospora prolificans*, and mucolares, [69]. Resistance to fluconazole, itraconazole has been found in oropharyngeal candidiasis patients with HIV [70]. Azole low-intermediate effecting fungi include: *Aspergillus udagawae*, *A. lentus*, *A. fumigatiaffinis*, *Scefosporium apiospermum* complex, *Fusarium* species, and mucolares [69]. Resistance to amphotericin B varies across *Aspergillus* species [70]. *Candida* species resistance has increased with use of amphotericin B [70]. Amphotericin B resistant fungi include: *Aspergillus calidoustus*, *A. lentulus*, *A. fumigatiaffinis. Lamentospora prolificans*,

Mucolares *Fusarium* species, *Candida albicans*, *C. glabrata*, *C. rugosa*, *C. lusiniae*, and *C. tropicalis* [69].

Adverse effects of all azoles are hepatoxicity, and some specifically include irritation at site application, vomiting, abdominal pain, nausea, and diarrhea [71]. Adverse reactions of Amphotericin B include hypotension, anemia, abnormalities in renal function, fever, chills, and nephrotoxicity [71]. Adverse effects of echinocandins include hepatoxicity, while some have specifically been associated with hypotension, peripheral edema, fever, insomnia, rash, and respiratory failure [71].

Ginger as an Effective Antifungal Agent for *Aspergillosis*

Immunocompromised hosts are especially at risk for invasive aspergillosis, an aggressive and severe fungal disease [22]. Aspergillosis is currently one of the top common infectious diseases that affect both animals and humans [72]. In a 2009 study in China, invasive aspergillosis has been found to complicate lung cancer [22].

Table 4. Ginger (EO) effectiveness against *Aspergillus* species

Fungi	Method	Result	Reference
A. flavus	Counting colony forming units HPLC/fluorescence	↑Antifungal activity ↓ Aflatoxin production	[73]
A. flavus	RT-qPCR	↓ Aflatoxin production ↑ Inhibition zone	[74]
A. flavus *A. fumigatus*	Agar dilution technique	↑ Inhibition zone	[75]
A. niger	Disc agar diffusion *Zingiber nimmonii* rhizome volatile oil	↑ Inhibition zone	[63]

Aspergillus niger and *Aspergillus fumigatus* are top causes of infection, and other Aspergillus species can be life-threatening and cause economic damage [72]. Aspergillus fumigatus comprises 80-95% of cases of invasive aspergillosis, which makes it the top FFHP [59]. Other Aspergillus species are top FFHP as well, with *A. flavus*, *A. niger*, *A. terrus*, and *A. nidulans* following behind *A. fumigatus* in importance [59]. Asian countries have a higher prevalence of invasive aspergillosis [22]. Specific risk factors associated with aspergillosis include HIV infection, smoking, age, high ammonia concentration, and abuse of cortisone [72]. As shown in Table 4, ginger demonstrates antifungal properties against *A. niger*, and *A. fumigatus*. and anti-aflatoxigenic activity against *A. flavus*.

Ginger as an Effective Antifungal Agent for Candidiasis

Candida infections are divided into two types: invasive candidiasis and local infections [60]. Globally, *Candida albicans* is the most frequently associated Candida species related to nosocomial invasive candidiasis [22]. High morbidity mucosal Candida infections include oropharyngeal candidiasis, chronic mucocutaneous, and vulvovaginal candidiasis [60]. *Candida albicans* is often the cause of fungal infections in people with diabetes [76].

Vaginal Candidiasis

Vaginal candidiasis is an infection of the vagina caused by the yeast species of *Candida*. This infection occurs when there is a change in the vaginal environment that promotes the growth of *Candida*. Vaginal candidiasis is most commonly caused by *Candida albicans* with the remaining cases being caused by *Candida glabrata* [77]. *Candida glabrata* infection is common in those that are immunosuppressed and the infection can be mucosal or systemic [78]. There is a high mortality rate in compromised, at-risk hospitalized patients [78]. Those infected with *Candida glabrata* present with less severe symptoms [77]. The infection is typically known as a vaginal yeast infection with other names including "candidal vaginitis" and "vulvovaginal candidiasis". A vaginal yeast infection occurs when *Candida* species penetrates the lining of the vagina resulting in an inflammatory response [77].

Candida is already present in the vagina and so for vaginal candidiasis to be diagnosed both *Candida* and symptoms such as inflammation, itching, irritation, or dysuria have to be present [77]. Vaginal candidiasis can be complicated or uncomplicated and this impacts treatment [77]. Complicated means that the patient is immunosuppressed or pregnant and so it requires different treatment than normal [77]. Treatment is typically completed with azole antifungals such as fluconazole taken orally or intravaginally [77]. An infection with *Candida glabrata* is difficult to treat as it is resistant to azole antifungal agents, primarily fluconazole [78]. Treatment for *Candida glabrata* includes Amphotericin B and flucytosine [78]. Normal treatment would be completed in one to three days and may include over the counter treatments [77]. Treatment for complicated vaginal candidiasis would be completed over a period of at least a week [77]. The continued use of these azole antifungals results in a phenomenon known as multidrug resistance [79]. In azole resistance, the typical mechanism is overexpression of ATP binding Cassette and major facilitator superfamily efflux pumps [79].

As shown in Table 5, ginger exhibits anti-fungal activity against *Candida albicans*, *C. dubliniensis*, and *C. glabrata*.

Table 5. Ginger effectiveness against *Candida* species

Fungi	Method	Result	Reference
C. albicans	Disk Diffusion Ginger powder	↑ Inhibition zone	[80]
C. albicans	Biofilm assay Ginger EO	↑ Anti-biofilm activity	[81]
C. glabrata and Fluconazole susceptible and resistant *C. dubliniensis*	Susceptibility test M27-A2 Method Ginger EO	↑ Anti-fungal activity	[82]
C. glabrata *C. albicans*	Disc agar diffusion *Zingiber nimmonii* rhizome oil	↑ Inhibition zone	[63]

Zingiber officinale has shown limited success as a treatment for vaginal candidiasis. An exploratory double blind, but not placebo controlled clinical trial with 67 women compared 1% ginger-clotrimazole cream to clotrimazole cream alone once per day indicated a significant decrease in seven days itching ($P > 0.05$), burning ($P > 0.05$), and cheesy secretion ($P < 0.05$) for the ginger treatment. Recurrence at one month follow up was high (48 to 51%) and not statistically significant between the two groups [83]. In comparison, a RCT for 94 women ages 18 to 45 years of a 10% curcumin-based vaginal cream compared to 1% clotrimazole at 5 g per day for seven days indicated significantly decreased symptoms (discharge, itching) ($P < 0.001$) [84]. Curcumin was as effective as clotrimazole. After treatment, there was a trend of slightly higher recovery for curcumin (66%) to clotrimazole (48.5%) ($P = 0.09$).

Oral Candidiasis

Oral candidiasis is a common oral infection affecting the oral mucosa [79]. It is also known as oral thrush or oropharyngeal candidiasis and is caused by *Candida albicans* [79, 85]. *Candida albicans* is a normal component of oral microflora and infection occurs when overgrowth occurs [79]. Symptoms include white patches in the mouth, loss of taste, pain while swallowing or eating, cotton feeling in mouth, cracking and redness at the corners of the mouth [85]. This is uncommon in healthy adults but, those that have weakened immune systems are at a higher risk [85]. Those that wear dentures, take medications that cause dry mouth, smoke, and take antibiotics or corticosteroids [85]. Diagnosis occurs when the doctor looks inside or takes a swab [85]. Typically, treated with topical antifungal creams but, if chronic these may not be effective [79]. Treatment for mild to moderate infections is clotrimazole, miconazole, or nystatin applied for 7 to 14 days [85]. For severe infections, fluconazole is given through a vein or taken by mouth and if no improvement then another antifungal is given [85].

As shown in Table 6, two studies have shown *Zingiber officinale* as a promising treatment for oral candidiasis. The first found a decrease in *Candida albicans* growth using ethanolic ginger extract at a concentration of 1:5 [86]. (The second study tested 10% ethanolic ginger extract against *Candida albicans*, *Streptococcus mutans*, and *Enterococcus faecalis* [87]. The study found a maximum zone of inhibition of 14 mm against *Candida albicans* which is larger than the maximum zone of inhibition of the other two pathogens tested [87]. Giriraju and Yunus also found a minimum inhibitory concentration of 2.5% against *Candida albicans* [87].

Table 7 illustrates a comparison of antifungal capabilities against *Candida* species of *Zingiber officinale*, *Curcuma longa*, and *Elettaria cardamomum* in the *Zingiberaceae* family [88]. *Zingiber officinale* extract at 10 mg/ml and 5 mg/ml showed reduced biofilm formation and increased minimum inhibitory biofilm concentrations in *Candida albicans* and *Candida krusei* respectively [89]. *Curcuma longa* and *Elettaria cardamomum* extracts show increased antifungal activity at 800 µl and 100% concentration respectively against *Candida albicans* [90, 91]. *Curcuma longa* extract at 800 µl showed decreased growth and less fungal colonies in *Candida albicans* ([90]. *Elettaria cardamomum* extract at 100% concentration showed decreased adhesion ability and germ tube formation in *Candida albicans* [91].

As shown in Table 8, other plants have shown more effective anti-*Candida* activity than *Zingiber officinale*. One study found that *Origanum vulgare* and *Satureja montana* essential oils were the most effective at inhibiting growth and producing cell damage in azole-susceptible and azole-resistant *Candida glabrata* of the tested essential oils [92]. The study also found that *Origanum vulgare* and *Satureja montana* essential oils have a medium-high toxicity for human keratinocytes [92]. Another study found that *Cinnamomum zeylanicum*, *Lippia graveolens*, and *Origanum vulgare* essential oils at less than or equal to 3200 µg/ml exhibited antimicrobial activity against fluconazole-resistant and fluconazole-susceptible *Candida glabrata* [45]. *Lippia graveolens* and *Origanum vulgare* showed a high amount of antifungal activity against the fluconazole-susceptible *Candida glabrata* [45]. *Cinnamomum zeylanicum* showed antifungal activity against the fluconazole-resistant *Candida glabrata* [45]. Another study found that *Eucalyptus globulus* and *Mentha piperita* essential oils were the most effective at reducing biofilm formation by 80.87% and 74.16% respectively in highly fluconazole-resistant *Candida albicans* [93].

Table 6. Oral *Candida* effectiveness of ginger ethanolic extract

Fungi	Method	Result	Reference
C. albicans	Agar dilution & disk diffusion	↓ *C. albicans* growth	[86]
C. albicans	Agar disk diffusion & serial broth dilution	↑Maximum inhibition zone ↑ MIC	[87]

Table 7. Comparison of anti-*Candida* action of ethanolic extracts from *Zingiberaceae* species

Species	Method	Result	Reference
Zingiber officinale	Microdilution method	↓ biofilm formation ↑ minimum inhibitory biofilm concentrations	[89]
Curcuma longa	Sabouraud's agar medium & dilutions	↑ antifungal activity ↓ growth ↓ fungal colonies	[90]
Elettaria cardamomum	Modified ages diffusion method & germ tube	↑ antifungal activity ↓ adhesion ↓ germ tube formation	[91]

Table 8. Comparison of anti-*Candida* action of plant EO

Species	Fungi	Method	Result	Reference
Origanum vulgare	Azole-susceptible & azole- resistant *C. glabrata*	Disk diffusion assay	↑growth inhibit ↑ fungal cell damage	[92]
Satureja montana	Azole-susceptible & azole- resistant *C. glabrata*	Disk diffusion assay	↑growth inhibit ↑ fungal cell damage	[92]
Cinnamomum zeylanicum	Fluconazole-resistant & fluconazole-susceptible *C. glabrata*	Broth microdilution	↑fluconazole-resistant antifungal activity	[45]
Lippia graveolens	Fluconazole-resistant & fluconazole-susceptible *C. glabrata*	Broth microdilution	↑fluconazole-susceptible antifungal activity	[45]
Origanum vulgare	Fluconazole-resistant & fluconazole-susceptible *C. glabrata*	Broth microdilution	↑ luconazole-susceptible antifungal activity	[45]
Eucalyptus globulus	Highly fluconazole-resistant *C. albicans*	Disk diffusion assay & XTT reduction assay	↓ biofilm formation	[93]
Mentha piperita	Highly fluconazole-resistant *C. albicans*	Disk diffusion assay & XTT reduction assay	↓ biofilm formation	[93]

Traditional Use to Clinical Trial: An Example

Traditional medicine is still used by approximately 80% of the global population, and nearly 50% of new chemical molecules discovered from 2002 to 2006 originated from natural products [61]. A systematic, evidence-based, collaborative and interdisciplinary research process to successfully move Japanese Hangeshashinto to clinical trial for chemotherapy-induced oral mucosis (OM) is a case study worth examining.

Patients undergoing chemotherapy are immunocompromised during treatment resulting in chemotherapy induced complex and multifaceted oral mucosis (OM) that creates severe pain, inhibits eating and drinking, interrupts treatment, prolongs hospitalization, and slows recovery [94]. Research has indicated that chemotherapy induced OM develops due to the cyclooxygenase pathway that regulated pain and tissue injury through upregulation proinflammatory cytokines and PGE2 with concomitant microbial infections exacerbating the condition [95]. A meta-analysis of 28 RCT with 1861 patients for nine oral mouth rinses for OM found that curcumin and honey were as effective as the currently recommended chlorhexidine or benzydomine [96]. The Multinational Association of Supportive Care in Cancer/International Society of Oral Oncology (MASCC/ISOO) strongly recommended further exploration of traditional ethnobotanical compounds [97].

Hangeshashinto is a traditional Japanese or Kampo medicine based on historic TCM that is approved for use by the Japanese Ministry of Health and composed of seven herbs (*Pinnelliae tuber*, *Scutellariae radix*, *Zingiberis rhizome*, *Ginseng radix*, *Glycyrrhizae radix*, *Zizphi fructus and Coptidis rhizome*)[98]. Hangeshashinto as a mouth rinse was effective in treating chemotherapy induced OM in colorectal cancer patients [99]. Wounding healing and cell repair functions of Hangeshashinto were documented and then analyzed for each herbal component at different concentrations to establish their mechanism of action. Prostaglandin E2 (PGE2) the inflammatory mediator inducing apoptosis resulting in OM is suppressed by the rhizome constituents of gingerol in Zingiberis spp and baicalin in Coptidis spp. [94, 95]. Studies show that 6-shogaol interfers with the activation PI3K/Akt/IκB kinases IKK and MAPK by inhibiting activation of NFκB which results in downregulating iNOS and COX-2 gene expression [100]. The synergistic action of the phytotherapy components act together through multiple mechanisms for wound healing, tissue repair, pain relief, anti-inflammatory and antimicrobial action that are different than a single targeted drug.

An exploratory randomized, double-blind, placebo-controlled trial for 16 patients (88% male, age range 49-79) with diagnosed squamous cell carcinoma who were treated with the chemotherapy regime docetaxel-cisplatin-5-fluorouracil (TPF) were simultaneously administered 2.5 g of TJ-14 or lactose placebo dissolved in 100 ml of drinking water to create an oral rinse solution that was used three times per day after meals for 30 seconds each time for a period of 14 consecutive days. Chemotherapy induced oral mucositis (OM) was monitored. While there were no statistically significant differences in incidence on day of onset of OM between the groups (TJ-14 at 75%, onset day 9.7 and placebo at 87.5%, onset day 6.7), there was a marked reduction in duration of severe infection TJ-14 had 1.3 days of $\geq$ grade 2 OM compared to placebo patients at 3.7 days ($p = 0.039$). There were no differences in adverse effects between the groups with 81% reporting neutropenia and 69% diarrhea [101].

This example underlines the need to examine the combined synergistic mechanism of action for other traditional medicines that have ginger as a component to move from historical observation, clinical promise and *in vivo* laboratory studies of one specific component towards evidence-based treatment understanding the combined effect in clinical settings to improve patient's lives.

CONCLUSION

Drug resistant fungal infections are on the rise globally. Ginger holds promise as an antifungal agent. Ginger contains a wide array of anti-fungal constituents and mechanisms that are useful in a medical context due to geographic location, harvesting technique, and endophytic fungi present.

Because of ginger's variation, further study may confirm a larger range of antifungal specificity and uses in the medical field. There is a need for a global system to standardize origin, extraction methods and quantification of active key active constituents. Additional double-blind, randomized, placebo-controlled trials are needed to established ginger's efficacy and cost with particular emphasis on synergistic effect of its antifungal and immunomodulator properties compared to conventional single target pharmaceuticals.

REFERENCES

[1] Bone, K. & Mills, S. (2013). *Principles and practices of phytotherapy: modern herbal medicine.* Australia: Churchill Livingstone.

[2] Chevalier, A. (2000). *Encyclopedia of herbal medicine*. New York: Dorling Kindersley Publishing.

[3] Wyk, B. V. & Wink, M. (2012). *Medicinal plants of the world: An illustrated scientific guide to important medicinal plants and their uses.* Portland: Timber Press.

[4] The Plant List. (2013). *Zingiberaceae.* Version 1.1. Accessed January 1, 2021. http://www.theplantlist.org.

[5] Mahboubi, M. (2019). "*Zingiber officinale* Rosc. essential oil, a review on its composition and bioactivity". *Clin Phytosci*, *5* (6). Accessed April 30, 2021. doi.org/10.1186/s40816-018-0097-4.

[6] Dalby, A. (2000). *Dangerous tastes: The story of spices*. London, British Museum Press.

[7] Ravindran, P. N. & Nirmal Babu, K. (eds). (2016). *Ginger: The Genus Zingiber*. New York; CRC Press.

[8] Global Trade. (2019). *Global Ginger Market 2019 – U.S. Imports Increases Robustly, Turning The Country into the Most Promising Market* Assessed April 30, 2021. https://www.globaltrademag.com/global-ginger-market-2019-u-s-imports-increases-robustly-turning-the-country-into-the-most-promising-market/.

[9] Food and Agricultural Organization (FAO). (2019). *Crop Statistics: Ginger* Assessed April 30, 2021. http://www.fao.org/faostat/en/#data/QC.

[10] Food and Drug Administration (FDA). (2020). *Code of Federal Regulations. Section 182. Substances Generally Recognized as Safe* Assessed April 30, 2021. https://www.accessdata.fda.gov/.

[11] Blumenthal, M., Goldberg, A. & Brinckmann, J. (eds.). (2000). *Herbal Medicine: Expanded Commission E Monographs.* Austin TX: American Botanical Council; Newton MA: Integrative Medicine Communications.

[12] World Health Organization (WHO). (2012). *Monographs of Selected Medicinal Plants Volume 1: Rhizoma Zingiberis* Assessed April 30, 2021. http://digicollection.org/hss/en/d/Js2200e/ 30.html.

[13] Thomson Healthcare. (2007). *Physician's desk reference for herbal medicine*, Montvale, NJ: Thomson Publishers.

[14] Lis-Balchin, M. (2006). *Aromatherapy science: A guide for healthcare professionals* London: Pharmaceutical Press.

[15] Chrubasik, S., Pittler, M. H. & Roufogalis, B. D. (2005). "*Zingiberis rhizoma*: A comprehensive review on the ginger effect and efficacy profiles" *Phytomedicine*, *12*, 684–701. Assessed April 30, 2021.

[16] Farago, P. (1995). *The Yellow Emperor's Classic of Medicine (the Neijing Suwen) ~240 B.C* Accessed April 30, 2021. http://www.five-element.com/graphics/neijing.pdf.

[17] Shahrajabian, M. H., Sunm W. & Cheng, Q. (2019). "Clinical aspects and health benefits of ginger (*Zingiber officinale*) in both traditional Chinese medicine and modern industry" *Acta Agriculturae Scandinavica, Section B — Soil & Plant Science*, *69*(6), 546-556, Assessed April 30, 2021. doi: 10.1080/09064710.2019.1606930.

[18] Nadkarni, K. M. (1991). Reprint of 1908 *Indian Materia Medica Vol 1 & 2*, Bombay, Bombay Popular Prakashan.

[19] Kumar, K. M., Asish, G. R., Sabu, M. & Balachandran, I. (2013). "Significance of gingers (*Zingiberaceae*) in Indian System of Medicine - Ayurveda: An overview" *Ancient Science of Life*, *32*(4),

253–261. Accessed April 30, 2021. https://doi.org/10.4103/0257-7941.131989.

[20] Meena, A. K., Kaur, R., Singh, B., Yadav, A. K., Singh, U., Ayushy Sachan, A., Pal, B. & Rao, M. M. (2009). "Review on antifungal activities of Ayurvedic Medicinal Plants" *Drug Invention Today*, *2*(2), 146-148. Accessed April 30, 2021.

[21] Denning, D. W. (2017). "Calling upon all public health mycologists". *Eur. J. Clin. Microbiol. Infect. Dis.*, *36*, 923–924. Accessed April 30, 2021. doi: 10.1007/s10096-017-2909-8.

[22] Bongomin, F., Gago, S., Oladele, R. O. & Denning, D. W. (2017). "Global and Multi-National Prevalence of Fungal Diseases-Estimate Precision". *Journal of Fungi*, *3*(4), 57. Accessed April 30, 2021. doi.org/10.3390/jof3040057.

[23] Benedict, K., Jackson, B. R., Chiller, T. & Beer, K. D. (2019). "Estimation of Direct Healthcare Costs of Fungal Diseases in the United States". *Clin Infect Dis.*, *68*(11), 1791-1797. Accessed April 30, 2021.doi: 10.1093/cid/ciy776.

[24] Rammaert, B., Lanternier, F., Zahar, J. R., Dannaoui, E., Bougnoux, M. E., Lecuit, M. & Lortholary, O. (2012). "Healthcare-Associated Mucormycosis". *Clinical Infectious Diseases.*, *54*(1), S44–S54. Accessed April 30, 2021. doi.org/10.1093/cid/cir867.

[25] Kontoyiannis, D. P., Yang, H. & Song, J. (2016). "Prevalence, clinical and economic burden of mucormycosis-related hospitalizations in the United States: a retrospective study". *BMC Infectious Diseases.*, *16*(1), 730. Accessed April 30, 2021.

[26] Zilberberg, M. D., Shorr, A. F., Huang, H., Chaudhari, P., Paly, V. F. & Menzin, J. (2014). "Hospital days, hospitalization costs, and inpatient mortality among patients with mucormycosis: a retrospective analysis of US hospital discharge data". *BMC Infectious Diseases*, *14*, 310. Accessed April 30, 2021.

[27] Cinta Badia Ginting, R., Sukarno, N., Widyastuti, U., Kosim Darusman. & Kanaya, S. (2013). "Diversity of endophytic fungi from red ginger (*Zingiber officinale* Rosc.) plant and their inhibitory effect to *Fusarium oxysporum* plant pathogenic fungi". *HAYATI Journal of*

Biosciences, *20*, 127-137. Accessed April 30, 2021. doi 10.4308/hjb.20.3.127.

[28] Combés, A., Ndoye, I., Bance, C., Bruzaud, J., Djediat, C., Dupont, J., Nay, B. & Prado, S. (2012). "Chemical communication between the endophytic fungus *Paraconiothyrium* variable and the phytopathogen *Fusarium oxysporum*". *PLOS One*, *7*, e47313. Accessed April 30, 2021. doi.org/10.1371/journal.pone.0047313.

[29] Eiji Hanada, R., Pomella, V. A., Salazar Costa, H., Luiz Bezerra, J., Loguercio, L. L. & Pereira, O. J. (2010). "Endophytic fungal diversity in *Theobroma cacao* (cacao) and *T. grandiflorum* (cupuaçu) trees and their potential for growth promotion and biocontrol of black-pod disease". *Fungal Biology*, *114*, 901-910. Accessed April 30, 2021. doi.org/10.1016/j.funbio.2010.08.006.

[30] Bussaban, B., Lumyong, S., Lumyong, P., McKenzie, H. C. E. & Hyde, D. K. (2001). "Endophytic fungi from *Amomum siamense". Canadian Journal of Microbiology*, *47*, 943-948. Accessed April 30, 2021. doi 10.1139/cjm-47-10-943.

[31] Kishore, K. H., Misra, S., Chandra, D. R., Prakash, K. V. V. R. & Murty, U. S. (2007). "Antimicrobial efficacy of secondary metabolites from *Glomerella cingulate". Brazilian Journal of Microbiology*, *38*, 150-152. Accessed April 30, 2021. doi.org/ 10.1590/S1517-83822007000100031.

[32] Radwan, M. M., Tabanca, N., Wedge, E. D., Tarawneh, H. A. & Cutler, J. S. (2014). "Antifungal compounds from tumeric and nutmeg with activity against plant pathogens". *Fitoterapia*, *99*, 341-346. Accessed April 30, 2021. doi.org/10.1016/j.fitote.2014.08.021.

[33] Hu, Y., Zhang, J., Kong, W., Zhao, G. & Yang, M. (2017). "Mechanisms of antifungal and anti-aflatoxigenic properties of essential oil derived from turmeric (*Curcuma longa L.)* on *Aspergillus flavus" Food Chemistry*, *220*, 1-8. Accessed April 30, 2021. doi.org/10.1016/j.foodchem.2016.09.179.

[34] Vinayarani, G. & Prakash, S. H. (2018). "Fungal endophytes of turmeric (*Curcuma longa L.*) and their biocontrol potential against pathogens *Pythium aphanidermatum* and *Rhizoctonia solani*". *World*

Journal of Microbiology and Biotechnology, *34*, 49. Accessed April 30, 2021. doi.org/10.1007/s11274-018-2431-x.

[35] Faisal, P. M., Biju, N. C., Praveena, R., Gowri, R. & Ankegowda, J, S. (2018). "Isolation, chacterization, and antagonisic efficacy of fungal endosymbionts from allied genera of cardamom". *Journal of Plantation Crops.*, *46*, 1-7. doi 10.19071/jpc.

[36] Senthil Kumar, M. C., Jacob, K. T., Devasahayam, S., Thomas, S. & Geethu, C. (2018). "Multifarious plant growth promotion by an entomopathogenic fungus *Lecanicillium psalliotae". Microbiological Research*, *207*, 153-160. Accessed April 30, 2021. https://doi.org/10.1016/j.micres.2017.11.017.

[37] Wang, H. & Ng, B. T. (2005). "A new antifungal protein from ginger rhizomes. *Biochemical and Biophysical Research Communications*, *336*, 100–104. Accessed April 30, 2021. doi: 10.1016/j.bbrc.2005.08.058.

[38] Chen, T., Lu, J., Kang, B., Lin, M., Ding, L., Zhang, L., Chen, G., Chen, S. & Lin, H. (2018). "Antifungal activity and action mechanism of ginger oleoresin against *Pestalotiopsis microspora* isolated from Chinese olive fruits". *Front Microbiol.*, *9*, 2583. Accessed April 30, 2021. doi: 10.3389/fmicb.2018.02583.

[39] Teles, A. M., Araújo dos Santos, B., Ferreira, C. G., Mouchreck, A. N., Silva Calabrese, K., Abreu-Silva, A. L. & Almeida-Souza, F. (2019). "Ginger (*Zingiber officinale*) antimicrobial potential: a review". In: Wang, H. (ed). "Ginger Cultivation and its Antimicrobial and Pharmacological Potentials". *IntechOpen*, Accessed April 30, 2021. doi: 10.5772/intechopen.89780.

[40] Kapoor, P. S. I., Singh, B., Singh, G., Isidorov, V. & Szczepaniak, L. (2008). "Chemistry, antifungal and antioxidant activities of cardamom (*Amomum subulatum*) essential oil and oleoresins". *International Journal of Essential Oil Therapeutics*, *2*, 29-40. Accessed April 30, 2021.

[41] Schwertner, H. A. & Rios, D. C. (2007). "High-performance liquid chromatographic analysis of 6-gingerol, 8-gingerol, 10-gingerol, and 6-shogaol in ginger containing dietary supplements, spices, teas, and

beverages". *J. Chromatograph B Analyst Techno Biomed Life Sci.*, *856*, 41-47. Accessed April 30, 2021.

[42] Schwertner, H. A., Rios, D. C. & Pascoe, J. E. (2006). "Variation in concentration and labeling of ginger root dietary supplements". *Obstet Gynecol.*, *107*(6), 1337-43. Accessed April 30, 2021. doi:0.1097/ 01.AOG.0000217697.33787.8c.

[43] Stoyanova, A., Konakchiev, A., Damyanova, S., Stoilova, I. & Suu, P. T. (2006). "Composition and antimicrobial activity of ginger essential oil from Vietnam." *J Essent Oil Bear Plants.*, *9*(1), 93–8. Accessed April 30, 2021. doi.org/10.1080/ 0972060X.2006.10643478.

[44] Meliani, A., Nair, S. & Bensoltane, A. (2014). "Cyto-biochemical and antimicrobial investigations on essential oil of *Zingiber officinale* Roscoe". *J Essent Oil Bear Plants.*, *7*(6), 1120–9. Accessed April 30, 2021. doi.org/10.1080/0972060X.2014.986540.

[45] Soares, I. H., Loreto, É. S., Rossato, L., Mario, D. N., Venturini, T. P., Baldissera, F., Santurio, J. M. & Alves, S. H. (2015). "*In vitro* activity of essential oils extracted from condiments against fluconazole-resistant and -sensitive *Candida glabrata. Journal de Mycologie Medicale*"., *25*(3), 213–217. Accessed April 30, 2021. doi.org/10.1016/j.mycmed.2015.06.003.

[46] Yamamoto-Ribeiro, M. M., Grespan, R., Kohiyama, C. Y., Ferreira, F. D., Mossini, S. A. & Silva, E. L. (2013). "Effect of *Zingiber officinale* essential oil on *Fusarium verticillioides* and fumonisin production". *Food Chem.*, *141*(3), 3147–52. Accessed April 30, 2021. doi.org/10.1016/j.foodchem.2013.05.144.

[47] Sharma, M. & Sharma, R. (2011). "Synergistic antifungal activity of *Curcuma longa* (turmeric) and *Zingiber officinale* (ginger) essential oils against dermatophyte infections". *J Essent Oil Bear Plants.*, *14*(1), 38–47. Accessed April 30, 2021. doi.org/10.1080/ 0972060X. 2011.10643899.

[48] Ficker, C., Smith, L. M., Akpagana, K., Gbeassor, M., Zhang, J., Durst, T., Assabgui, R. & Arnason, T. J. (20003). "Bioassay-guided isolation and identification of antifungal compounds from ginger". *Phytotherapy Research*, *17*, 897-902. doi 10.1002/ptr.1335.

[49] Hussein, A. K. & Joo, H. J. (2018). "Antifungal activity and chemical composition of ginger essential oil against ginseng pathogenic fungi" *Current Research in Environmental & Applied Mycology*, *8*, 192-203. doi 10.5943/cream/8/2/4

[50] Singh, G., Kapoor, I. P., Singh, P., de Heluani, C. S., de Lampasona, M. P. & Catalan, C. A. (2008). "Chemistry, antioxidant and antimicrobial investigations on essential oil and oleoresins of *Zingiber officinale*". *Food Chem Toxicol.*, *46*(10), 3295-302. Accessed April 30, 2021. doi: 10.1016/j.fct.2008.07.017.

[51] Sa-nguanpuag, K., Srilaong, V., Kanlayanarat, S. & Techavuthiporng, C. (2011). "Ginger (*Zingiber officinale*) Oil as an antimicrobial agent for minimally processed produce: A case study in shredded green papaya". *J. Agric. Biol.*, *13*, 895–901. Accessed April 30, 2021.

[52] Ali, S. E., El-Shaffey, A. A., Selim, M. E., El-massry, K. F. & Sabry, B. A. (2011). "Chemical profile, antioxidant, antifungal and antiaflatoxigenic activity of parsley and ginger volatile and non-volatile extracts". *Journal of Biologically Active Products from Nature*. 1(1):81–96. Accessed April 30, 2021. doi.org/10.1080/22311866.2011.10719074.

[53] American Cancer Society. (2020). *Cancer facts & figures* Accessed Dec. 28, 2020. https://www.cancer.org/research/cancer-facts-statistics/all-cancer-facts-figures/cancer-facts-figures-2020.

[54] American Cancer Society. (2020). *Global cancer facts & figures* Accessed Dec. 28, 2020. https://www.cancer.org/research/cancer-facts-statistics/global.html.

[55] United Nations AIDS. (2020). *Global HIV & AIDS statistics – 2020 fact sheet* Accessed December 28, 2020. https://www.unaids.org/en/resources/fact-sheet#.

[56] Liu, L., Oza, S., Hogan, D., Chu, Y., Perin, J. & Zhu, J. (2016). "Global, regional, and national causes of under-5 mortality in 2000-15: an updated systematic analysis with implications for the Sustainable Development Goals". *Lancet.*, *388*(10063), 3027-35. Accessed April 30, 2021. doi.org/10.1016/S0140-6736(16)31593-8.

[57] Bullard, K. M., Cowie, C. C., Lessem, S. E., Saydah, S. H., Menke, A., Geiss, L. S., Orchard, T. J., Rolka, D. B. & Imperatore, G. (2018). "Prevalence of Diagnosed Diabetes in Adults by Diabetes Type - United States, 2016". *MMWR Morb Mortal Wkly Rep.*, *30*, 67(12), 359-361. doi: 10.15585/mmwr.mm6712a2.

[58] Rammaert, B., Lanternier, F., Zahar, J., Dannaoui, E., Bougnoux, M., Lecuit, M. & Lortholary, O. (2012). "Healthcare-associated mucormycosis" *Clin Infect Dis*, *54*, S44-54. Accessed April 30, 2021. doi: 10.1093/cid/cir867.

[59] Paterson, R. R. M. & Lima, N. (2017). "Filamentous fungal human pathogens from food emphasizing *Aspergillus*, *Fusarium*, and *Mucor". Microorganisms*, *5*(3), 44. Accessed April 30, 2021. doi: 10.3390/microorganisms5030044.

[60] Veerdonk, F. L., Netea, M. G., Joosten, L. A., Meer, J. W. M. & Kullberg, B. J. (2010). "Novel strategies for the prevention and treatment of *Candida* infections: the potential of immunotherapy". *FEMS Microbiol Rev.*, *34*, 1063-1075. Accessed April 30, 2021. doi.org/10.1111/j.1574-6976.2010.00232.x.

[61] Rodrigues, M. E., Silva, S., Azerdo, J. & Henriques, M. (2014). "Novel strategies to fight *Candida* species infection". *Critical Reviews in Microbiology*, *42*(4), 594-606. Accessed April 30, 2021. doi: 10.3109/1040841X.2014.974500.

[62] Pawlowska, A. M., Zannini, E., Coffey, A. & Arendt, E. K. (2012). "Green preservatives: combating fungi in the food and feed industry by applying antifungal lactic acid bacteria". *Advances in Food and Nutrition Research.*, *66*, 217-238. Accessed April 30, 2021. doi: 10.1016/B978-0-12-394597-6.00005-7.

[63] Sabulal, B., Dan, M., Kurup, R., Pradeep, N. S., Valsamma, R. K. & George, V. (2006). "Caryophyllene-rich rhizome oil of *Zingiber nimmonii* from South India: chemical characterization and antimicrobial activity." *Phytochemistry*, *67*, 2469–2473. Accessed April 30, 2021. doi: 10.1016/j.phytochem.2006.08.003.

[64] Sharifi-Rad, M., Varoni, E. M., Salehi, B.; Sharifi-Rad, J., Matthews, K. R., Ayatollahi, S. A., Kobarfard, F., Ibrahim, S. A., Mnayer, D.,

Zakaria, Z. A., Sharifi-Rad, M., Yousaf, Z., Iriti, M., Basile, A. & Rigano, D. (2017). "Plants of the genus *Zingiber* as a source of bioactive phytochemicals: from tradition to pharmacy". *Molecules*, *22*(12), 2145. Accessed April 30, 2021. doi.org/10.3390/molecules22122145.

[65] Reid, G., Lynch, J. P., Fishbein, M. C. & Clark, N. M. (2020). "Mucormycosis". *Semin Respir Crit Care Med*, *41*(1), 99-114. Accessed April 30, 2021. doi: 10.1055/s-0039-3401992.

[66] Queiroz-Telles, F., Fahal, A. H., Falci, D. R., Caceres, D. H., Chiller, T. & Pasqualotto, A. C. (2017). "Neglected endemic mycoses". *Lancet Infect Dis.*, *17*, e367-e377. Accessed April 30, 2021. doi: 10.1016/S1473-3099(17)30306-7.

[67] Nelson, P. E. (1992). "Taxonomy and biology of *Fusarium moniliforme*". *Mycopathologia*, *117*, 29-36. Accessed April 30, 2021. doi.org/10.1007/bf00497276.

[68] Thomas, S. (2020). *Antimicrobial resistance: global challenges and future interventions* Springer, Singapore. Accessed April 30, 2021. doi.org/10.1007/978-981-15-3658-82020.

[69] Perlin, D. S., Rautemaa-Richardson, R. & Alastruey-Izquierdo, A. (2017). "The global problem of antifungal resistance: prevalence, mechanisms, and management. *Lancet Infect Dis*, *17*, e383-e392. Accessed April 30, 2021. doi.org/10.1016/ S1473-3099(17)30316-X.

[70] Eliopulos, G. M., Perea, S. & Patterson, T. F. (2002). "Antifungal resistance in pathogenic fungi". *Clinical Infectious Diseases*, *35*, 1073-1080. Accessed April 30, 2021. doi.org/10.1086/344058.

[71] McKeny, P. T., Nessel, T. A. & Zito, P. M. (2020). Antifungal Antibiotics. In: *StatPearls* [Internet]. Treasure Island (FL): StatPearls Publishing. Accessed April 30, 2021. https://www.ncbi.nlm.nih.gov/books/NBK538168/.

[72] Alwan, D. S. (2019). "Anti-fungal activity of ginger oil against *Aspergillus fumigatus* and *Aspergillus niger* causing aspergillosis". *Indian Journal of Public Health Research & Development*, *10*(10), 847-851. Accessed April 30, 2021. doi.org/10.37506/ijphrd.v10i10.5466.

[73] Nerilo, S. B., Romoli, J. C. Z., Nakasugi, L. S., Zampieri, N. S., Mossini, S. A. G., Rochas, G. H. O., Micotti da Gloria, E., Alves de Abreu Filho, B. & Machinski, M. (2020). "Antifungal activity and inhibition of aflatoxins production by *Zingiber officinale* Roscoe essential oil against *Aspergillus flavus* in stored maize grains". *Ciência Rural*, *50*(6) 1-10. Accessed April 30, 2021. Doi 10.1590/0103-8478cr20190779.

[74] Moon, Y., Lee, H. & Lee, S. (2018). "Inhibitory effects of three monoterpenes from ginger essential oil on growth and aflatoxin production of *Aspergillus flavus* and their gene regulation in aflatoxin biosynthesis". *Applied Biological Chemistry*, *61*(2), 243-250. Accessed April 30, 2021. Doi 10.1007/s13765-018-0352-x.

[75] Nguefack, J., Leth, V., Amvam Zollo, P. H. & Mathur, S. B. (2004). "Evaluation of five essential oils from aromatic plants of Cameroon for controlling food spoilage and mycotoxin producing fungi". *International Journal of Food Microbiology*, *94*, 329-334. Accessed April 30, 2021. doi.org/10.1016/j.ijfoodmicro.2004.02.017.

[76] Zomorodian, K., Kavoosi, F., Pishdad, G. R., Mehriar, P., Ebrahimi, H., Bandegani, A. & Pakshir, K. (2016). "Prevalence of oral Candida colonization in patients with diabetes mellitus". *J Mycol Med.*, *26*(2), 103-110. doi: 10.1016/j.mycmed.2015.12.008.

[77] Jeanmonod, R. & Jeanmonod, D. (2020). "Vaginal Candidiasis" In: *StatPearls* [Internet]. Treasure Island (FL): StatPearls Publishing; 2021 Jan–. PMID: 29083806.

[78] Fidel, P. L., Vazquez, J. A. & Sobel, J. D. (1999). "Candida glabrata: review of epidemiology, pathogenesis, and clinical disease with comparison to C. albicans". *Clin Microbiol Rev.*, *12*(1), 80-96. Accessed April 30, 2021.

[79] Singh, A., Verma, R., Murari, A. & Agrawal, A. (2014). "Oral candidiasis: An overview. *Journal of oral and maxillofacial pathology". JOMFP*, *18*(Suppl 1), S81–S85. Accessed April 30, 2021. doi.org/10.4103/0973-029X.141325.

[80] Supreetha, S., Mannur, S., Simon, S. P., Jain, J., Tikare, S. & Mahuli, A. (2011). "Antifungal activity of ginger extract on *Candida albicans*:

an in-vitro study". *Journal of Dental Sciences and Research*, *2*(2), 1-5. Accessed April 30, 2021.

[81] Rinanda, T., Isnanda, R. P. & Zulfitri. (2018). "Chemical analysis of red ginger (*Zingiber officinale* Roscoe var *rubrum*) essential oil and its anti-biofilm activity against *Candida albicans". Natural Product Communications*, *13*(12), 1587- 1590. Accessed April 30, 2021. doi/pdf/10.1177/1934578X1801301206.

[82] Pozzatti, P., Scheid, L. A., Spader, T. B., Atayde, M. L., Santurio, J. M. & Alves, S. H. I. (2008). "*In vitro* activity of essential oils extracted from plants used as spices against fluconazole-resistant and fluconazole-susceptible *Candida* spp." *Can. J. Microbiol.*, *54*, 950-956. Accessed April 30, 2021.

[83] Shabanian, S., Khalili, S., Lorigooini, Z., Malekpour, A. & Heidari-Soureshjani, S. (2017). "The effect of vaginal cream containing ginger in users of clotrimazole vaginal cream on vaginal candidiasis" *Journal of advanced pharmaceutical technology & research*, *8*(2), 80–84. doi.org/10.4103/japtr.JAPTR_176_16.

[84] Abouali, N., Moghimipour, E., Mahmoudabadi, A. Z., Namjouyan, F. & Abbaspoor, Z. (2019). "The effect of curcumin-based and clotrimazole vaginal cream in the treatment of vulvovaginal candidiasis". *Journal of family medicine and primary care*, *8*(12), 3920–3924. Accessed April 30, 2021. doi.org/10.4103/ jfmpc.jfmpc_584_19.

[85] Centers for Disease Control and Prevention. (2020, June 15). *Candida infections of the mouth, throat, and esophagus* Accessed April 30, 2021. https://www.cdc.gov/fungal/diseases/candidiasis/ thrush/index. html.

[86] Atai, Z., Atapour, M. & Mohseni, M. (2009). "Inhibitory effect of ginger extract on *Candida albicans*". *American Journal of Applied Sciences*, *6*(6), 1067–1069. Accessed April 30, 2021. doi.org/ 10.3844/ajassp.2009.1067.1069.

[87] Giriraju, A. & Yunus, G. Y. (2013). "Assessment of antimicrobial potential of 10% ginger extract against *Streptococcus mutans*, *Candida albicans*, and *Enterococcus faecalis*: an *in vitro* study".

Indian Journal of Dental Research, *24*(4), 397–400. Accessed Apri l30, 2021. doi-org.proxy1.lib.tju.edu/10.4103/0970-9290.118356.

[88] Simpson, M. G. (2019). *Plant Systematics*. California: Academic Press &Elsevier.

[89] Aghazadeh, M., Zahedi Bialvaei, A., Aghazadeh, M., Kabiri, F., Saliani, N., Yousefi, M., Eslami, H. & Samadi Kafil, H. (2016). "Survey of the antibiofilm and antimicrobial effects of *Zingiber officinale* (*in vitro* study". *Jundishapur Journal of Microbiology*, *9*(2), e30167. Accessed April 30, 2021. /doi-org.proxy1.lib.tju.edu/ 10.5812/jjm.30167.

[90] Murugesh, J., Annigeri, R. G., Mangala, G. K., Mythily, P. H. & Chandrakala, J. (2019). "Evaluation of the antifungal efficacy of different concentrations of *Curcuma longa* on *Candida albicans*: An *in vitro* study". *Journal of Oral Maxillofacial Pathology.*, *23*(2), 305. Accessed April 30, 2021. doi.org/10.4103/ jomfp.JOMFP_200_18.

[91] Kadhum, S., Razuqi, N. & Abdul Majeed, S. (2011). "Antifungal efficiency of miswak & cardamom extract on some virulence factors of *Candida albicans* as oral pathogen: *Al-kufa Journal for Biology*., *1*, 3. Accessed April 30, 2021.

[92] Massa, N., Cantamessa, S., Novello, G., Ranzato, E., Martinotti, S., Pavan, M., Rocchetti, A., Berta, G., Gamalero, E. & Bona, E. (2018). "Antifungal activity of essential oils against azole-resistant and azole-susceptible vaginal *Candida glabrata* strains". *Canadian Journal of Microbiology*, *64*(10), 647–663. Accessed April 30, 2021. doi.org/10.1139/cjm-2018-0082.

[93] Agarwal, V., Lal, P. & Pruthi, V. (2010). "Effect of Plant Oils on Candida albicans.". *Journal of Microbiology*, *Immunology and Infection.*, *43*(5), 447-451. Accessed April 30, 2021. doi.org/10.1016/S1684-1182(10)60069-2.

[94] Miyano, K., Eto, M., Hitomi, S., Matsumoto, T., Hasegawa, S., Hirano, A., Nagabuchi, K., Asai, N., Uzu, M., Nonaka, M., Omiya, Y., Kaneko, A., Ono, K., Fujii, H., Higami, Y., Kono, T. & Uezono, Y. (2020). "The Japanese herbal medicine Hangeshashinto enhances oral keratinocyte migration to facilitate healing of chemotherapy-induced

oral ulcerative mucositis". *Sci Rep.*, *10*(1), 625. Accessed April 30, 2021. doi: 10.1038/s41598-019-57192-2.

[95] Kono, T., Kaneko, A., Matsumoto, C., Miyagi, C., Ohbuchi, K., Mizuhara, Y., Miyano, K. & Uezono, Y. (2014). "Multitargeted effects of hangeshashinto for treatment of chemotherapy-induced oral mucositis on inducible prostaglandin E2 production in human oral keratinocytes". *Integr Cancer Ther.*, *13*(5), 435-45. Accessed April 30, 2021. doi: 10.1177/1534735413520035.

[96] Yu, Y. Y., Deng, J. L., Jin, X. R., Zhang, Z. Z., Zhang, X. H. & Zhou, X. (2020). "Effects of 9 oral care solutions on the prevention of oral mucositis: a network meta-analysis of randomized controlled trials". *Medicine*, *99*(16), e19661. Accessed April 30, 2021. doi: 10.1097/MD.0000000000019661.

[97] Yarom, N., Hovan, A., Bossi, P., Ariyawardana, A., Jensen, S. B., Gobbo, M., Saca-Hazboun, H., Kandwal, A., Majorana, A., Ottaviani, G., Pentenero, M., Nasr, N. M., Rouleau, T., Lucas, A. S., Treister, N. S., Zur, E., Ranna, V., Vaddi, A., Barasch, A., Lalla, R. V., Cheng, K. K. F. & Elad, S. (2020). "Mucositis Study Group of the Multinational Association of Supportive Care in Cancer/ International Society of Oral Oncology (MASCC/ISOO). Systematic review of natural and miscellaneous agents, for the management of oral mucositis in cancer patients and clinical practice guidelines - part 2: honey, herbal compounds, saliva stimulants, probiotics, and miscellaneous agents". *Support Care Cancer.*, *28*(5), 2457-2472. Accessed April 30, 2021. doi: 10.1007/s00520-019-05256.

[98] Uezono, Y., Miyano, K., Sudo, Y., Suzuki, M., Shiraishi, S. & Terawaki, K. (2012). "A review of traditional Japanese medicines and their potential mechanism of action". *Curr Pharm Des.*, *18*(31), 4839-53. Accessed April 30, 2021. doi: 10.2174/138161212803216924.

[99] Matsuda, C., Munemoto, Y., Mishima, H., Nagata, N., Oshiro, M., Kataoka, M., Sakamoto, J., Aoyama, T., Morita, S. & Kono, T. (2015). "Double-blind, placebo-controlled, randomized phase II study of TJ-14 (Hangeshashinto) for infusional fluorinated-pyrimidine-based colorectal cancer chemotherapy-induced oral mucositis". *Cancer*

Chemotherapy and Pharmacology, *76*, 97–103. Accessed April 30, 2021. doi.org/10.1007/s00280-015-2767-y.

[100] Pan, M. H., Hsieh, M. C., Hsu, P. C., Ho, S. Y., Lai, C. S., Wu, H., Sang, S. & Ho, C. T. (2008). "6-Shogaol suppressed lipopolysaccharide-induced up-expression of iNOS and COX-2 in murine macrophages". *Mol. Nutr. Food Res.*, *52*, 1467-77. Accessed April 30, 201. doi.org/10.1002/mnfr.200700515.

[101] Taira, K., Fujiwara, K., Fukuhara, T., Koyama, S. & Takeuchi, H. (2020). "The effect of Hangeshashinto on Oral Mucositis Caused by Induction Chemotherapy in Patients with Head and Neck Cancer". *Yonago Acta Medica*, *63*(3), 183–187. Accessed April 30, 2021. doi.org/10.33160/yam.2020.08.007.

In: Ginger's Antimicrobial …
Editor: Diana R. Cundell
ISBN: 978-1-68507-117-2

Chapter 4

GINGER AS AN ANTIVIRAL AGENT

Frank H. Wilkinson*, PhD
College of Life Sciences, Thomas Jefferson University,
Philadelphia, PA, USA

ABSTRACT

Ginger is on a growing list of natural sources under consideration in development of new antiviral compounds. This chapter is a comprehensive review of research investigating the use of ginger as an antiviral agent. Compounds and mixtures isolated from ginger and tested for antiviral activity include 6-gingerols, 6-shogaol, sesquiterpenes, mixed polysaccharides, essential oils, and aqueous or solvent extracts. These compounds appear to exert several activities such as disruption of the viral life cycle, destabilization of the virion, and host immunity support. In some cases, viral proteins were predicted or found to bind to individual ginger compounds resulting in disruption of viral protein activity.

* Corresponding Author's E-mail: Frank.Wilkinson@jefferson.edu.

To evaluate these compounds or extracts, a variety of methods were employed including molecular docking, viral plaque assays, viral titer, gene expression, histopathological score, symptom scoring markers of host immunity, and animal mortality. Viruses that infect a variety of human tissues, animals, and plant species were used as model systems for testing of the ginger compounds. A unifying conclusion from these studies is that ginger exhibits several antiviral activities that can be utilized in further development of new antiviral compounds for therapeutic use.

Keywords: herbal medicine, phytochemical, ginger, antiviral

INTRODUCTION

Converging observations have led to investigating phytochemicals as antiviral agents. Many human societies have a long history of supplementing the diet with specific plant products in response to evident illness [1]. It is now recognized that many plant-derived compounds have antiviral activities. These metabolites include low molecular weight species (e.g., alkaloids, flavonoids, terpenes) and larger compounds (e.g., polyphenols, lignins, and polysaccharides) [2]. The medicinal potential for these naturally sourced remedies is high and remains an area of active investigation.

Ginger joins a growing list of medicinal plants under investigation for antiviral activity. The use of ginger as a dietary supplement in response to viral infections has occurred throughout much of the world for millennia [3, 4]. Most of the studies reviewed herein reported on the use of common ginger, *Zingiber officinale* [5], though one study used pinecone ginger, *Zingiber montanum* [6, 7], and another used torch ginger, *Etlingera elatior* [8]. Some studies used purified compounds. Other studies used partially purified fractions containing sesquiterpenes, essential oils, mixed polysaccharides, or crude aqueous or hexane extracts (see details below). Since many of these compounds or mixtures will demonstrate antiviral activity, whole ginger appears to be a source of multiple antiviral activities.

Evaluation of these activities in ginger used a variety of viral model systems. The viruses chosen are diverse with respect to their genomic material (DNA or RNA), the size of the genome, and the presence of a phospholipid envelope. Given the different compounds tested and methods used (see below), conclusions regarding the efficacy against a particular virus type and not clear. It is, in fact, these differences that lead to the arrangement of this chapter to consider the viruses as separate case studies. Thus, while broad conclusions are desirable, this field has not yet settled on a particular model system or chemical agent to make cross comparisons meaningful.

A logical conclusion of these research efforts is to further develop the compounds present in ginger as medicinal agents. To achieve this goal, identification of active agents, molecular targets, mechanisms of action, delivery routes, and preventative/therapeutic evaluation in situ must be established. Some caution should be maintained in the interpretation of these studies since the bioavailability and pharmacokinetics of these compounds from ginger have not yet been determined. On a more optimistic note, significant progress has been made in this field and justifies continued effort in this direction.

Ginger as an Agent against Human Respiratory Viruses

The first group of viruses evaluated here infect human respiratory tissues including SARS-CoV-2, Influenza viruses, Rhinovirus, and Human Respiratory Syncytial Virus. A summary of the research is presented in Table 1. The authors of these studies employed a combination of purified, partially purified, and crude extracts of ginger. This section will provide background on each of the viruses tested and explore the outcomes of the various studies. I offer my own speculation about potential mechanisms.

Table 1. Research summary of ginger extracts tested against respiratory viruses

Material Used	Virus Studied*	Study Outcome	Reference
6-, 8-, 10-gingerol	SARS-CoV-2	*in silico*, docking to papain-like protease substrate binding site.	[9]
Several compounds	SARS-CoV-2	*in silico*, docking to 3-chymotrypsin-like protease and the spike protein.	[10]
Several compounds	SARS-CoV-2	*in silico*, docking to 3-chymotrypsin-like protease.	[11]
Aqueous extract of whole ginger	Influenza (HP) AIV H5N1	*in vitro*, reduced viral titer in MDCK cells.	[12]
Hexane extract of whole ginger	Influenza (HP) AIV H5N1	*in vitro*, NS1 displaced from RNA, reduced plaques in MDCK cells.	[7]
Aqueous extract of whole ginger	Influenza AIV H9N2	*in vivo* (chick), reduced histologic score; *in vitro*, reduced hemagglutination.	[13]
Allicin, ajoene	Influenza H1N1	*in silico*, docking to NA sialic acid site.	[14]
Mixed polysaccharides	Influenza H1N1	*in vivo* (mouse), increased antibodies; prevention of excessive lung inflammation, promotion of CD19+ and CD278+ cell proportions in lung, elimination of virus in lung, and elevation of IFNγ levels in serum	[15]
Aqueous extract (protector)	Influenza Vaxigrip	*in vivo* (mouse), increased INFγ, IL-12, and HAI antibodies	[16]
Sesquiterpenes	RVIB	*in vitro*, reduced plaques in HeLa cells	[17]
Aqueous extract of whole ginger	HRSV	*in vitro*, reduced plaques in HEp-2 and A549 cells, increased INFβ secretion	[18]

*SARS-CoV-2 (Severe Acute respiratory Syndrome Coronavirus 2), HP (Highly Pathogenic), AIV (Avian Influenza Virus), MDCK (Madin Darby Canine Kidney), NS1 (nonstructural protein 1), INF (Interferon), IL-12 (Interleukin 12), HAI (Hemagglutination Inhibiting Antibody), RVIB (Rhinovirus IB), HSRV (Human Respiratory Syncytial Virus).

SARS-CoV-2

SARS-CoV-2 is a recently identified member of the *Coronaviridae* family [19]. The genome is a ~30 kb, positive-sense, single strand RNA with a 5' cap and polyadenylated 3' end, like cellular mRNAs [20, 21]. The phospholipid envelope contains protein products of the spike (S), hemagglutinin esterase, membrane, and small membrane genes. Within the envelope, the nucleocapsid proteins form a complex with the genomic RNA [22]. The S protein is responsible for receptor binding, membrane fusion, and viral entry into cells [21]. Non-structural proteins (nsp) include two proteases (3-chymotrypsin-like, Mpro, and papain-like, PLpro), a helicase, and an RNA-dependent RNA polymerase [23]. The Angiotensin-converting enzyme 2 (ACE2) protein is the most likely receptor for SARS-CoV-2, like that of SARS-CoV-1 [24, 25]. The ACE2 protein is present on the surface of lung alveolar epithelium [26]. Like other members of the coronavirus family, virions enter through the mucosa of the nose and oropharynx and eventually reach the lungs [27, 28]. Transmission from host to host is mediated by respiratory droplets [29, 30]. SARS-CoV-2 is responsible for the COVID-19 pandemic [31].

Evidence indicates that the host immunological response exacerbates COVID-19 infectious disease. Symptoms of SARS-CoV-2 infection include fever, congestion, body ache, and more severe disorders such as chest pain and breathlessness [27]. Further complications include pneumonia, acute respiratory distress, multiple organ failure, and death [32]. Both innate and adaptive immune cells, such as macrophages and T cells, can respond to this infection. Macrophages can be activated by materials released from dying epithelial cells or those of the pathogen [33-35]. A proinflammatory cytokine burst can follow as ACE2 is downregulated by the virus. This downregulation leads to a four-fold dysfunction of the (i.) renin-angiotensin-aldosterone system, (ii.) downregulation of the angiotensin receptor, MAS (Massey), (iii.) activation of [des-Arg9]-bradykinin, and (iv.) activation of C5a and C5b-9 complement proteins [36]. This dysfunctional axis can itself lead to diminished pulmonary function and lung injury [37, 38]. Further to this pathophysiology, increased release of Interleukin 1b (IL-1b) and IL-6 leads to lung inflammation, fever, and fibrosis [31, 39]. Indeed, the need for mechanical ventilation parallels the levels of IL-6, highlighting the role of this signaling factor [31]. Normal T cell function is essential for viral clearance and suppression of viral infection [40], but T cell-dependent cytokine release can lead to increased tissue inflammation in response to severe viral infections [41]. In COVID-19, apoptotic depletion of T cells following viral clearance and a surviving population of "exhausted," non-responsive T cells, permits viral persistence and better predicts the clinical presentation of patients [34, 42].

Prevention of SARS-CoV-2 transmission changed rapidly through the course of the COVID-19 pandemic. Initially, behavior modification was advised owing to the absence of existing therapies. Many infected individuals were asymptomatic, so defensive measures (e.g., social distancing, mask use) were critical steps to prevent infection [43]. The use of vaccines against COVID-19 has been underway during the preparation of this manuscript. One mRNA vaccine, COMIRNATY ® (BNT162b2), was found to be more than 90% effective in preventing COVID-19 [44]. Another mRNA vaccine, mRNA-1273, has also been developed and shows similar efficacy [45, 46]. Both vaccination strategies target the S protein. While these are certainly exciting advances, vaccine delivery to the global population is expected to take several months. Development of small molecule inhibitors of the SARS-CoV-2 life cycle can supplement vaccine efforts.

Support for anti-SARS-CoV-2 compounds present in ginger has been determined by *in silico* approaches. The first study targeted the S3-S4 substrate binding sites of the papain-like protease, PLpro [9, 47]. This protease is essential for cleavage of the viral polyprotein at the nsp 1/2, nsp 2/3, and nsp 3/4 boundaries recognizing LXGG peptide sequences [48, 49]. Ginger compounds 6-, 8-, and 10-gingerol were predicted to bind into this pocket with high affinity (dissociation constants predicted to be in the 1 to 10 nM range) [9]. It is promising that some compounds that were effective at inhibiting PLpro from SARS-CoV-1 were predicted for inhibiting PLpro from SARS-CoV-2 enabling their rapid development [47, 50]. Two additional *in silico* approaches targeted the SARS-CoV-2 Mpro and the S proteins with ginger compounds [10, 11]. The Mpro cleaves the viral polyprotein at ~11 sites and is essential for the viral life cycle [51, 52]. Fortunately, significant progress in understanding the structure and function of the SARS-CoV-1 Mpro had been underway for several years. High similarity (96% sequence identity and 100% active site conservation) shared between the Mpro proteins led to successful identification and testing of several candidates in a Vero cell plaque reduction assay [52, 53]. The study by Rajagopal et al. [11] furthers this work using ginger-derived compounds. Starting with a crystal structure of the Mpro protein (RCSB PDB - 5R82), the group docked 6-shogaol, 6-, 8-, and 10-gingerol, paradol, zingerone, zingiberene, and phellandrene [11, 54]. Each of these compounds was found to bind to the active site, with 8- and 10-gingerol having amongst the highest affinity (Rajagopal et al. 2020). The study by Ahkam et al. [10] included seven ginger compounds: Gingerenone A, Gingerol, Geraniol, Shogaol, Zingiberene, Zingiberenol, and Zingerone (Ahkam et al. 2020). Each of these compounds was docked to the Mpro protein and all except Gingerenone A was predicted to bind to the same site [10, 52]. Similarly, these compounds were docked to the S protein - ACE2 receptor complex [10, 55]. Further analysis of the ternary S protein - ginger compound - ACE2 interaction suggested structural alterations when compared to the binary S protein - ACE2 complex [10]. Functional studies are needed to determine if this effect would impair the S protein - ACE2 receptor interaction from permitting viral entry into cells.

Influenza Viruses

Influenza A viruses are enveloped and have a negative-sense RNA genome [56-58]. Virions can be elliptical/spherical (80-120 nm diameter), filamentous, or irregular in shape (Noda 2011). The envelope houses the hemagglutinin (HA) and neuraminidase (NA) proteins in an approximately 4:1 ratio. A smaller number of matrix proteins (i.e., M1, M2) also span the envelope [59]. The M1 protein is located inside the envelope and interacts with the inner leaflet. The 8 RNA segments are encapsulated in nucleoprotein (NP) and located at one end of the virion [60]. The HA protein is the receptor-binding protein and is also responsible for membrane fusion and viral entry into cells. HA binds to receptor sites containing sialic acid [61]. Much of the NA and M2 proteins cluster at one end of the virion, opposite the ribonucleoprotein assembly. NA proteins are thought to be important for release of the virions from HA binding sites during budding [60, 62]. The nonstructural protein 1 (NS1) viral gene product is important for blocking the interferon-mediated antiviral response and for inhibiting the processing of cellular mRNA [63]. Immune system evasion results from viral antigenic diversity, which arises from alterations in the HA and NA proteins [64].

There are key species-specific differences in influenza disease observed in mammals and birds. In mammalian hosts, (e.g., humans, pigs, and horses), influenza infects respiratory tissues, whereas in birds, the infection is primarily enteric [61]. The virion binds to α-2,6-linked sialic acid-bearing receptors on the cells of the upper or lower respiratory epithelium, or on the alveolar epithelium [65]. Following attachment, virions are internalized into endosomes, uncoated, and release their viral ribonucleoprotein into the cell [66, 67]. In humans, influenza is a seasonal disease [68] whereas other animals have host-specific epidemiologic factors [69]. Infected persons show a range of respiratory symptoms and can show non-respiratory complications including viral encephalitis, myocarditis, and acute myocardial infarction [70, 71]. Diagnosis of infection starts with symptoms including fever and/or chills, cough, nasal discharge, malaise, muscle pain, and fatigue. Given that patients may not exhibit all these symptoms, laboratory tests (i.e., RT-PCR, virus culture, rapid antigen detection, and serologic detection) are required for definitive diagnosis [68, 72].

Managing influenza has been challenging. Additional small molecule therapies may help fill therapeutic gaps. Current management strategies for influenza include vaccination and antiviral drugs [73]. However, various factors have lessened the efficacy of these strategies. Humans lack pre-existing immunity against antigenically novel strains [65]. Antigenic diversity arises, in part, from the segmented nature of the genome (8 units). Random incorporation of segments, potentially originating from different parent strains, can be combined into progeny [74]. The consequence is a reassortment of allelic combinations of surface antigens into individual virions. Predicting future influenza strains and preparation of vaccines in advance has proven to be problematic [75, 76]. Many adults (~50%) in the US are not vaccinated [77]. Further, influenza strains are developing resistance to the available drugs [78]. Additional drugs are needed to keep pace with the increasing resistance developed by the virus.

Several studies have examined the effects of ginger extracts on different forms of the Influenza A virus. The studies used a variety of virus antigenic variants: H9N2 [13], H5N1 [7, 12], H1N1 [14, 15], and the trivalent Vaxigrip vaccine that has a mixture of H1N1, H3N2, and an influenza B strain, [16, 79]. The ginger was fractionated into either aqueous extract [12, 13, 16] or hexane extract [7] in different studies, but efforts to identify specific components within these crude extracts was not evident. One study used partially purified polysaccharides [15] while another used molecular models for an *in silico* approach [14]. Despite these variations on approach, the studies generally support the evidence for antiviral effects of ginger compounds against influenza viruses, although more work is needed to identify active components and their targets.

The *in silico* approach makes important predictions about the potential anti-influenza mechanisms of action of the compounds present in ginger. The NA protein is one of the key surface antigens. The NA protein's ability to cleave sialic acid from glycans is a critical step for infection [80, 81]. Compounds present in ginger, allicin and ajoene, were predicted to bind to the sialic acid site on the NA protein [14]. If these molecules were to block the sialic acid cleaving activity of the virus, then release of viral progeny would be reduced, presumably resulting in marked decreases in further infection of cells. In fulfillment of this prediction, allicin has been found to have anti-influenza activity in an *in vitro* system [82]. Translation to *in vivo* efficacy should be evaluated. Given that the virion binds and cleaves sialic acid on the extracellular surface, it is not evident that significant antiviral activity found in ginger occurs through this mechanism *in vivo*. Allicin is thought to be absorbed and rapidly transported into cells where it can undergo further transformation [83]. So, despite the presence of the compound in ginger, allicin may not remain active if isolated from the virion and converted to an inactive form. It is possible that a more stable structure can be derived from allicin to block influenza NA activity. Additional work is needed to test this mechanism.

Two studies examined the effects of ginger on host immunity. In one study, mixed polysaccharides isolated from ginger were found to promote vaccine-induced immune responses against H1N1 and attenuate symptoms [15]. Among the immune markers measured, serum Interferon-gamma (IFNγ) was increased, antibodies against H1N1 were increased, CD19+ and CD278+ cells were increased in the lung, and detectable virus and inflammation were greatly reduced. This outcome followed daily intragastric administration of the polysaccharides and two immunizations prior to virus challenge. The extent that intragastric administration of mixed polysaccharides in mice mimics the availability of these molecules in humans following dietary consumption of ginger remains to be determined. This group did not report an experiment where mice were fed ginger (without partial purification of the polysaccharides) to see if the effects of the isolated polysaccharides could be recapitulated. Without these observations, application to antiviral effects in humans is not clear. The second study to examine the effects of ginger on host immunity used an aqueous extract. This extract also contained aqueous-soluble components from pomegranate, red grape, dates, olive, and figs, named "protector." [16]. Oral or intraperitoneal delivery of the extract was reported to increase serum IFNγ, IL-12, and Hemagglutinin Inhibition assay antibodies following an immunization protocol that included oral delivery of protector. These results are consistent with the study by Zhu et al. [15]. A study using human volunteers found that gingerols increase IFNγ from activated T cells [84]. This study determined a measurable increase in gingerols detected in plasma following consumption of an aqueous ginger tea [84]. The increase in IFNγ was determined in an *in vitro* study using purified gingerols [84]. IFNγ was found to have *in vitro* and *in vivo* activity against influenza H5N1 [85]. These studies suggest that ginger can possibly have antiviral effects on the host by increasing the immune response. Yet, other work suggests additional activities directed against the virus.

Activities present in ginger that target the influenza viruses directly are supported by three studies. Two studies used an aqueous extract [12, 13] and one used a hexane extract [7]. Pre-treating the virus suspension with aqueous ginger extract for 10 minutes moderately reduced H5N1 infection of Madin

Darby Canine Kidney (MDCK) cells [12]. In another study, aqueous extract of ginger, pre-mixed with an H9N2 strain and inoculated, was found to reduce hemagglutination activity measured from chick embryo allantoic fluid [13]. Sialidase activity appears to be essential for infection of MDCK cells [86] *in vitro* like *in vivo* infection [80, 81]. It is possible that, in agreement with *in silico* work, a component of ginger may bind to the NA protein and inhibit its enzymatic activity [14]. Lastly, a hexane extract also suggested a distinct anti-influenza activity. Work by Klaywong et al. [7] using an H5N1 strain found that this extract reduced plaque formation in MDCK cells. Using an RNA electrophoretic mobility shift assay, the Nonstructural protein 1 (NS1) was displaced from double stranded RNA by the ginger hexane extract. NS1 is essential for the virus to block cellular antiviral activities [7], therefore, disrupting the activity of this protein could enable the cellular innate response *in vivo* [7].

Collectively, these studies support a role for compounds present in ginger to have potential anti-influenza activity. Future studies should attempt to purify these compounds further (i.e., purified beyond the crude extracts utilized in several of the studies). Further purified compounds can also be tested for antiviral targets (such as the NA or NS1 proteins) in binding studies. Purified compounds can also serve as a starting point for chemical modifications to increase efficacy or stability *in vivo*.

Rhinovirus

Rhinovirus is classified in the *Picornaviridae* family [87]. Rhinoviruses are grouped into 3 species (i.e., A, B, and C) based on sequence analysis [88]. The virion is comprised of a non-enveloped, icosahedral capsid containing a 7.2 kb, positive sense RNA genome. The capsid is composed of 60 copies each of 4 viral proteins. Viral proteins (VP) 1, 2, and 3 are exposed on the surface, and VP4 is on the interior face of the protein shell [87]. A deep surface pocket known as the “canyon” at the fivefold axis of symmetry is the site that binds to cell surface receptor sites [89, 90].

Receptor binding initiates the process of internalization by endocytosis and eventual uncoating inside of the host cell [90, 91].

Rhinovirus infection is estimated to cause as much as 50% of the cases of the "common cold" [92]. Infection is thought to start with the virus entering the nose, transport to the pharynx via mucus, and ultimately migration of the virus to the epithelial cells. The different rhinovirus species exhibit epithelial cell tropism via three receptors. Most rhinoviruses of the A species and all B species viruses use intercellular adhesion molecule 1 (ICAM-1). The remainder of the A types use proteins in the low density lipoprotein receptor family. The C species viruses use Cadherin-related family member 3 (CDHR3) [90]. Antigenic diversity among rhinoviruses makes developing a broadly acting vaccine difficult [87, 93]. Some progress has been reported in a mouse model using a conserved region of the capsid protein and found to promote viral clearance, development of neutralizing antibodies against heterologous subtypes, and the presence of memory T cells in the lung [94]. But the application of these studies in mice has yet to be translated to human medicine. Many of the tested antiviral drugs were found to have limited efficacy in clinical trials despite promising *in vitro* work [90]. So, the search for additional treatments is needed to supplement these efforts.

A hexane extract of ginger containing sesquiterpenes was tested for antiviral activity in a cell culture model system of rhinovirus infection [17]. The four sesquiterpenes isolated and purified included ar-curcumene, β-sesquiphellandrene, α-zingiberene, and β-bisabolene [17]. These molecules are composed of 15 carbon atoms and contain a six-member ring with one or more carbon-carbon double bonds [95]. When tested individually, each of the four compounds was found to reduce plaque formations in Hela cells when infected with rhinovirus species B. The sesquiterpenes were effective when added to the cells at 1-hour post-infection [17]. While sesquiterpenes show cytotoxicity at high concentrations [96], Denyer, et al. were able to apply the compounds at dilutions that did not show these adverse effects during viral challenge [17]. Effective dose values (ED_{50}) showed a ~20-fold concentration range (reported in micrograms (μg)/10 centimeter (cm) dish): ar-curcumene (20.4±7.3), β-sesquiphellandrene (0.90±0.10), α-zingiberene

(1.90±0.41), and β-bisabolene (14.3±1.59) [17]. Work by Rollinger et al. [97] found that sesquiterpene coumarins from non-ginger sources were effective against rhinovirus. Purified extracts of the gum resin asafetida (*Ferula assa-fetida* L. and *F. fetida*) containing farnesiferol C and farnesiferol B were predicted to bind to the hydrophobic canyon in a computational screen and were effective at blocking the cytopathic effect of rhinovirus in a HeLa cell plaque assay [97]. The sesquiterpenes from ginger may act through a similar mechanism, but this question was not addressed by the authors [17].

Additional work is needed to evaluate the antiviral activity of the sesquiterpenes. Since the authors tested the compounds only following infection, it is not possible to determine if they act on a viral target to inhibit the lifecycle or if cellular immunity is enhanced [17]. The target(s) of these compounds should also be determined to see if their action is primarily directed against cellular or viral proteins. It will be interesting to determine if the ED_{50} values reflect differential binding affinity to a common target, or if sufficient structural dissimilarity leads to different targets for one or more of the compounds.

Human Respiratory Syncytial Virus

Human Respiratory Syncytial Virus (HRSV) is an enveloped virus with a 15.2 kb, negative sense RNA genome [98]. It is classified in the *Paramyxoviridae* family [99]. The envelope houses the transmembrane F and G proteins responsible for viral fusion and attachment, respectively. The envelope also houses the SH (small hydrophobic) protein that functions as a viroporin [100]. The F protein can interact with cell surface proteins such as nucleolin, TLR4, or ICAM-1 [101-103]. The G protein can bind to heparin or annexin and may facilitate bringing the F protein to the vicinity of its receptor [98]. Encased by the envelope is the matrix composed of the M protein [104]. The RNA genome is in a complex with the N protein to form the ribonucleoprotein core [98].

Infection begins with binding of the virion to the surface of airway epithelial cells through interactions between the G protein and its binding site [105]. The F protein contacts nucleolin and initiates fusion of the envelope with the host membrane. Following membrane fusion, the nucleocapsid enters the cytoplasm and dissociates from the ribonucleoprotein complex catalyzed by phosphorylation by cellular enzymes [106].

Some successful vaccines and small molecule therapies are being developed to manage HSRV infection. Therapies directed against HRSV have had success targeting viral envelope proteins. The three proteins that project from the envelope, F, G, and SH, are the primary antigenic targets [107]. Prophylaxis with palivizumab (Synagis), a humanized murine monoclonal antibody, has been used to treat pediatric HSRV infection [108, 109]. However, limited efficacy and high costs have limited use of this strategy to high-risk patients [110]. Small molecules that target the F protein to prevent membrane fusion have also been developed and investigated [111, 112]. They were found to be effective in reducing viral load and disease severity when administered within 5 days following a positive test for HRSV [109]. Vaccines, intended for elderly patients and maternal immunization, are an area of active investigation [113].

One study identified that aqueous extracts of ginger had anti-HRSV activity [18]. The authors tested this fraction of ginger for its ability to reduce plaque formation in cell lines that model the upper (HEp-2, [114]) and lower (A549, [115]) respiratory tract. Further, they compared the effects of fresh vs. dried ginger as the source material. The authors found that extracts of fresh ginger were more potent to reduce plaque formation in a dose-dependent manner compared to dried ginger extracts. This result was observed for both cell line model systems tested [18]. Mechanistically, the fresh ginger was able to block attachment and internalization [18], suggesting that an antiviral component of ginger is lost or inactivated during the drying process.

Additional studies will help to further define the anti-HRSV activity in ginger. Standardization of the extraction methods and tests of purified compounds are important next steps. An extract of fresh ginger was analyzed and found to contain 51 compounds, of which 20 were identified for the first time [116]. Starting with commercially dried ginger, the authors reported 88 extracted compounds. In comparison with the fresh ginger extract, 45 compounds were extracted from both sources and 31 were newly reported [117]. Of the 51 compounds identified extracted from fresh ginger, 45 were shared with the inactive, dried ginger preparation [116, 117]. However, there were differences in the methods that may also explain the differences in extraction profile. The fresh ginger was reported to be mixed with methanol [116], but the dried ginger was immediately processed with methylene chloride [117]. So, the solvent differences may partially explain the differences in extracted compounds. Chang et al. [18] used an aqueous extraction method for their ginger sources so there may be yet additional solvent effects on the compounds extracted. Interestingly, Chang et al. [18] reported that 6-gingerol was the major component extracted from both fresh and dried ginger. However, this compound was ineffective at inhibiting HRSV [18]. This result is a contrast to reports that have shown activity of 6-gingerol against other viruses (see elsewhere in this chapter and the original reports) [118-121]. Further work is needed to identify the anti-HRSV activities in ginger.

GINGER AS AN AGENT AGAINST HUMAN NON-RESPIRATORY VIRUSES

In this section, the viruses evaluated infect human tissues outside of the respiratory system including Herpes Simplex Viruses 1 & 2, Norovirus (modeled as Feline Calicivirus), Hepatitis Viruses A and C, Human Papillomavirus, and Dengue Virus. These research efforts are presented in Table 2. Ginger extracts tested in this section include purified compounds (6-gingerol, dodecanal, and n-dodecanol), essential oils, and crude aqueous extracts of ginger. As in section 1, background on the viruses is presented along with an evaluation of research progress to date. Where applicable, I offer speculation regarding mechanisms.

Table 2. Research summary of ginger extracts tested against non-respiratory viruses

Material Used	Virus Studied*	Study Outcome	Reference
Essential oils	HSV1	*in vitro*, reduced plaques in RC-37 cells.	[122]
Essential oils	HSV2	*in vitro*, reduced plaques in RC-37 cells.	[123]
Essential oils	CpHV-1	*in vitro*, reduced viral titer in MDCK cells.	[124]
Aqueous extract of whole ginger	FCV (norovirus model)	*in vitro*, reduced titer CRFK cells.	[125]
6-gingerol	HAV	*in vitro*, reduced head inactivation time and temperature.	[121]
6-gingerol	HCV	*in vitro*, reduced viral titer in PMBC.	[119]
6-gingerol	HPV	*in vivo* (mouse), xenograft tumor growth; *in vitro*, inhibited proliferation of the HPV positive cells; *in silico*, docking to proteosome subunit.	[118]
Essential oils including dodecanal, and n-dodecanol	DV	*in vivo* (mosquito), reduced egg laying	[8]
Aqueous extract of whole ginger	DV3	*in vitro*, inhibit MMP expression, increase TIMP expression in Vero cells	[126]

*HSV1 (Herpes Simplex Virus 1), HSV2 (Herpes Simplex Virus 2), CpHV-1 (Caprine Herpesvirus 1), MDCK (Madin Darby Canine Kidney), FCV (Feline Calicivirus), CRFK (Crandell-Reese feline kidney), HAV (Hepatitis A Virus), HCV (Hepatitis C Virus), PMBC (peripheral blood mononuclear cells), HPV (Human Papillomavirus), DV (Dengue Virus, unspecified), DV3 (Dengue Virus 3), MMP (Matrix metalloproteinase), TIMP (tissue inhibitor of matrix metalloproteinase).

Herpes Simplex Virus

Herpes Simplex Viruses 1 and 2 (HSV-1 and HSV-2) are common human infectious agents producing cold sores and genital herpes [127]. The HSV-1 and HSV-2 virions are enveloped, and each contains a ~152 kbp double stranded DNA genome [128]. The envelope houses several hundred glycoprotein spikes from 11 different viral gene products; 4 of these are essential for entry into cells [129]. Caprine herpesvirus 1 (CapHV-1) is one of several viruses related to human Herpes viruses that infects goats [130]. Viruses like CapHV-1 infect other ruminants including livestock and wild animals [131].

The worldwide infection prevalence with these viruses is astronomical, with estimates of HSV-1 infection reported at 3.7 billion persons under the age of 50 and estimates for HSV-2 infection reported at more than 400 million persons between 17 and 49 [132]. Despite their expansive prevalence, diagnosis can be challenging. Many cases of infection are caused by asymptomatic persons; thus, many remain undiagnosed [133]. In cases where symptoms are evident, diagnosis of herpes viruses is straightforward. Symptomatic HSV can be recognized by orofacial sores (e.g., pharyngitis herpetica, herpes labialis, and herpetic gingivostomatitis) or genital lesions (e.g., genital ulcers and blisters) [129, 132]. In the absence of evident symptoms, diagnosis requires laboratory tests for either serological evidence for glycoproteins G1 and G2 [132], cytologic markers, tissue culture, or PCR [129]. Similar symptomatic lesions [134] and laboratory detection methods are available for detection of CapHV-1 [135, 136].

HSV-1 enters a latent phase by infecting sensory neuron terminals and migrating to cell bodies in the trigeminal ganglion where it can persist indefinitely [137]. HSV-2 employs a similar strategy but resides in sacral ganglia [138]. From this point, both viruses can reinfect innervated mucocutaneous tissues, enter a replicative cycle, and shed infectious virions [139-141], with and without symptoms. Thus, the opportunity for infection to spread to others through salivary or sexual contact is a lifelong risk.

Additional preventative and treatment measures against HSV are needed. These viruses have been difficult to target with vaccination. Live, attenuated HSV strains, though usually more effective at inducing broad, durable immunity, are difficult to maintain as genetically stable strains. Risks for development of latency are also a concern [139]. Despite much effort, no effective vaccines have been developed [142]. Vaccination is feasible for CapHV-1 [143, 144], and protocols continue to be developed [145], though there appears to be minimal interest by pharmaceutical companies. Treatment strategies have similarly been difficult to develop and have been met by viral resistance. Acyclovir is used to treat infections and must be converted to its triphosphate form by HSV thymidine kinase (TK). Mutations in either TK or the viral DNA polymerase are associated with resistance [146, 147]. Thus, a continued search for small molecules that can work as anti-HSV drugs is needed.

Three studies were identified that assessed the presence of anti-HSV activity of ginger. All three studies used ginger essential oils as the source material. Tests of essential oils were found to reduce plaque formation in RC-37 cells by HSV-1 [122] and HSV-2 [123] in a dose-dependent manner. Essential oils were also effective at inactivating CapHV-1 when challenged to infect Madin Darby bovine kidney (MDBK) cells [124]. In all these studies, the virus was pre-treated with the extracts; addition of the extracts to the cells prior to infection or following adsorption was found to be ineffective [122-124]. Collectively, these observations indicate that the target of the activity is the virus, and the compound(s) does not act by competing for a cellular receptor site nor inhibiting aspects of the viral replication cycle once internalized.

Further work will be needed to evaluate the antiviral activities of ginger essential oil. Ginger essential oils were analyzed by Gas Chromatography/Mass Spectrometry (GC/MS) and determined to contain at least 88 detectable compounds. Of these, 5 predominate in the mixture: ar-curcumene (22.1%), zingiberene (11.7%), β-bisabolene (11.2%), β-sesquiphellandrene (10.5%) and cadina-1,4-diene (2.5%). The remainder are present at 1% or less [148]. In each of the reviewed studies, next steps can be to evaluate purified compounds from essential oils against the viral model systems [122-124]. Interestingly, another group has found that essential oils from star anise were an effective inhibitor of HSV-1 when used as a viral pre-treatment [149]. However, these authors identified different chemical species in this extract including trans-anethole, eugenol, β-eudesmol, farnesol, β-caryophyllene, and β-caryophyllene oxide. Given that these lists of primary components show no overlap, it may be that essential oils can cause viral inactivation by a non-specific mechanism. Alternatively, structural motifs shared by subsets of the compounds may mediate binding to a common viral target. Additional studies can help to resolve these uncertainties.

Norovirus

Norovirus, of the family *Caliciviridae*, is a non-enveloped virus with a 7.6 kb, single-stranded, positive sense, RNA genome [150]. The viral protein, VP1, forms an icosahedral capsid of 27-40 nm in size [151]. The genome contains 3 open reading frames (ORF1-3). ORF1 encodes a polyprotein that is processed into non-structural proteins. ORF2 and -3 encode the capsid proteins, VP1 and VP2, respectively [150, 151]. A domain on the VP1 protein, the protruding (P) domain, mediates binding to histo-blood group antigens on the host cell surface [152]. Efforts to identify a protein receptor for human norovirus (HNoV) has not yet been successful [153]. Little is understood about virion internalization into the cell [150, 152].

Norovirus is the major cause of gastroenteritis that is not of bacterial origin [154]. Infection is thought to occur through the fecal-oral route, contaminated food, or water. Viral loads in infected individuals are high, but only a few particles are needed to acquire an infection [152]. Outbreaks commonly occur in areas of high population density where food is served (i.e., hospitals, nursing homes, schools, restaurants, cruise ships). Symptoms of infected persons include nausea, vomiting, diarrhea, and abdominal pain. Infections generally last 2-3 days, however, viral shedding can persist longer [150, 155]. Immunocompromised patients can become chronically infected with durations of infection lasting more than a year [156].

Infection prevention and control strategies are limited. Prevention strategies for health care settings include patient isolation and care policies, hand hygiene protocols, and environmental hygiene protocols [150]. However, these strategies may be less effectively implemented in other settings such as schools arguing for supplemental efforts.

Control strategies implementing various viral inhibitor classes are under active investigation with varying degrees of success to date; how these approaches will bear out in clinical trials remains to be established [155]. Many biological barriers have hampered vaccine development, especially the inability to culture this virus *in vitro*. Much of the *in vitro*-based knowledge has arisen from the use of model viruses such as feline calicivirus

(FCV) [157]. While these obstacles are yet to be overcome, some progress in the use of ginger has been made.

Some progress has been made using ginger as a source of antivirals to target Norovirus. The study by Aboubakr, et al., evaluated the antiviral activity of aqueous extracts of ginger to reduce FCV titers following infection of Crandell-Reese feline kidney (CRFK) cells [125]. Pre-treatment of the cells with the extract was found to be have no effect on viral titer. However, mixing of the virus with the extracts, in advance, or at the time of infection of the cells, was found to reduce viral titer 5 days post-infection. The group further identified R-(-)-1,2-propanediol as the most abundant compound in the ginger extract utilized but did not test the purified compound [125].

Treatment of the virus prior to infection is strongly suggestive of a viral target for the active agents in ginger. Noroviruses are thought to use the histo-blood group antigens (HBGAs) to bind to the cell surface [158]. Previous work has found that tannic acid can block the interactions between the HBGAs and the P domain of the VP1 capsid protein [159]. Thus, it is possible that an extractable compound from ginger could block the viral lifecycle through a similar mechanism. Alternatively, compounds extracted from ginger may alter the structure of the capsid reducing its ability to infect cells. In support of this mechanism, carvacrol from oregano essential oil was found to enlarge the capsid and decrease the infectivity of murine norovirus [160]. Though it should be emphasized that there are other potential targets within the virus, including the viral protease, RNA-dependent RNA polymerase, and other nonstructural proteins with poorly defined functions [161]. Opportunities for future efforts in this area are to evaluate individual compounds from ginger against specific viral targets.

Hepatitis A Virus

Hepatitis A Virus (HAV) is a member of the *Picornaviridae* family. Its genome is a single-strand, positive sense RNA of approximately 7.5 kb [162]. The capsid is an ~30 nm icosahedron and lacks an envelope. The viral polyprotein, P1, is processed into VP0, VP1, and VP3 that assemble to form the capsid [163]. VP0 is cleaved by an RNA-dependent protease activity to form VP2 and VP4 proteins [164]. A putative cellular receptor has been identified, HAVcr-1, however little is understood about the mechanism of viral entry into the host [165, 166].

Hepatitis A is an inflammatory disease of the liver caused by HAV infection [167]. HAV infection commonly occurs through the fecal-oral route, with family members and sexual partners particularly vulnerable [168, 169]. The incubation period is approximately 30 days [167]. Infection with HAV can be recognized by dark urine, fatigue, loss of appetite, and jaundice, among many other symptoms. Laboratory diagnosis can use elevated Alanine aminotransferase (ALT), aspartate aminotransferase (AST) enzymes, bilirubin, and serological detection of circulating antigens [167]. The disease is usually self-limiting [170].

Prevention and treatment strategies of viral hepatitis vary. Because the fecal-oral route is the primary route of transmission for HAV, efforts to minimize viral spread include sanitation, personal hygiene, and increased access to clean water [171]. However, these approaches are limited in many parts of the developing world. Vaccination is available and effective [172], but delivery to those at risk has been challenging. Standard treatment for HAV infection is fluid and nutritional supportive care [173]. Post-infection intravenous immunoglobulin treatment has also been found to be effective [174]. Additional therapies could be used to supplement these efforts.

6-Gingerol, added to viral suspensions at 0.1 milligram/milliliter (mg/ml), was found to reduce the time (D value) needed for heat inactivation of HAV measured in a plaque assay [121]. The D value is the time needed at a specified temperature to reduce the number of infectious agents by a factor of 10 [175]. The effect of 6-gingerol on these values most evident at 60° and 65°C. D values for HAV in phosphate-buffered saline (PBS) at 60°C was 2.63±0.13 minutes (min); addition of 6-gingerol reduced this value to 1.94±0.17 min. The values for HAV at 65°C were 1.8±0.08 min and 1.52±0.12 min in PBS and PBS supplemented with 6-gingerol, respectively [121]. The authors did not attempt to determine the mechanism of 6-gingerol action. It is tempting to speculate that the gingerol may destabilize virus structure acting cooperatively with that promoted by the elevated temperatures. Another possibility is that the elevated temperature may allow access of the 6-gingerol to an inhibitory site on the virus. The inhibitory effect of 6-gingerol was less pronounced at 56°C (D value 9.21±0.24 min and 8.87±0.18 min in PBS and PBS supplemented with 6-gingerol). Further studies are needed to identify the target and mechanism of action of 6-gingerol against HAV.

Hepatitis C Virus

Hepatitis C Virus (HCV) is a member of the *Flaviviridae* family. The genome is a 9.6 kb, single strand, positive sense RNA. The genome is housed in an icosahedral capsid and surrounded by an envelope [176]. Viral glycoproteins E1 and E2 present in the envelope and are needed for fusogenic and receptor-binding activities, respectively [177]. The human scavenger receptor class B type 1 is a putative receptor for HCV through binding by the E2 protein [178]. The low-density lipoprotein (LDL) receptor is another putative receptor; neutralizing antibodies against the LDL receptor were able to block viral entry to host cells [179].

Hepatitis C Virus is primarily spread by contact with the blood from infected individuals; little infection occurs through sexual contact or vertical transmission [180, 181]. Common exposures to infection include use of contaminated needles, medical procedures, and hemodialysis [182]. In addition to some cultural practices that can mediate spread (e.g., circumcision, genital mutilation, ritual scarring, tattooing), biting insects may also facilitate spread in areas where infections rates are high [183]. Many acute infections with HCV are asymptomatic, but the remainder of cases show malaise, loss of appetite, and jaundice [184]. Many patients develop chronic hepatitis despite the absence of symptoms [185]. Laboratory tests include enzyme markers, serological, and detection of the viral RNA [185].

Supportive care and alcohol abstinence are recommended as part of the treatment for HCV. Antiviral treatment with IFN-α and ribavirin has been successful, but high rates of relapse necessitate additional treatment [173]. While many drugs are available for treatment of HCV, the virus exhibits a high mutation rate resulting in mutations that confer resistance to these drugs [176]. Additional prevention and treatment strategies can supplement these efforts.

Anti-viral activity of gingerol against HCV is supported by one study [119]. A small reduction in detectable virus, by RT-PCR, was found in peripheral blood mononuclear cells (PMBC) with various 6-gingerol treatment protocols [119]. For pre-treatment, the cells were exposed to 6-gingerol in the growth medium for 90 minutes and washed with PBS prior to adding the virus [119]. For co-treatment, the 6-gingerol and HCV were added simultaneously and removed after 90 minutes [119]. In the post-treatment protocol, the cells were incubated with the virus, washed, then provided with growth medium supplemented with 6-gingerol [119]. Virus concentration for untreated cells was reported as $1.19 \times 10^{9} \pm 0.001$ copies/ml [119]. The 6-gingerol treated cells were reported to have viral concentrations of $0.97 \times 10^{9} \pm 0.001$ copies/ml (pre-treatment), $0.89 \times 10^{9} \pm 0.001$ copies/ml (co-treatment), and $1.07 \times 10^{9} \pm 0.002$ copies/ml (post treatment). P values were listed as less than 0.0001 [119].

IL-2 expression is increased in chronic infection with HCV [186]. The expression increase may be mediated by direct transcription activation of the IL-2 gene by the HCV core protein [187]. IL-8 is also elevated and may contribute to resistance to Interferon therapy [188]. El Deeb et al., [119] also examined the effects of 6-gingerol on expression of IL-2 and IL-8. Treatment of PMBC with 6-gingerol reduced IL-2 expression to 44.17%, 49.92%, and 20.95% for pre-, co-, and post-treated cells. IL-8 showed lesser reductions to 79.22%, 70.73%, and 70.11% for pre-, co-, and post-treated cells [119]. No efforts to determine the connection between 6-gingerol and expression of IL-2 and IL-8 were reported by the authors [119]. However, other authors have observed reduced interleukin expression in response to ginger extracts *in vitro* and *in vivo* [189, 190]. Modulation of the pro-inflammatory cytokines would be predicted to lessen some of the complications of hepatitis. It is not clear if the reduction in HCV was related to the effects on IL-2 and IL-8 expression. Further work is needed to clarify the target(s) and mechanism of 6-gingerol anti-HCV activity.

Human Papillomavirus

Human Papillomavirus (HPV) is a member of the *papovaviridae* family [191]. The virus is a non-enveloped, icosahedron containing a circular double strand DNA genome [192]. The virus has a remarkable genetic diversity with approximately 200 different types characterized [193, 194]. The capsid is composed of 72 capsomeres that are each assembled from 5 copies of the viral protein, L1 [195]. The L1 protein appears to mediate binding to cell surface heparin sulfate proteoglycans [196], though the protein core may be variable [197]. More recent work suggests that an additional receptor site is critical for infection beyond the initial cell surface binding to heparin sulfate [198].

All HPV types infect squamous epithelial cells [192]. Infection with papillomavirus resolves in most cases without cellular transformation. Transmission can occur through sexual activity or other means. The virus enters the new host through microabrasions in the skin [199]. Clinical symptoms appear in a range of weeks to months following a latency period post-infection [193, 200]. Lesions appear as anogenital warts including cauliflower-like condylomata accuminata on moist surfaces, and keratotic, smooth papular warts on dry surfaces. In addition to the social stigma, the warts may itch, bleed, cause pain/burning, or obstruct urinary output [193, 199, 201]. For infected persons, years or decades may pass before cellular transformation occurs [193, 199, 201]. Transformation is associated with integration of the viral genome into the host cell chromosome and dysregulation of viral gene products, including the viral E6 protein [202]. Though not all HPV strains cause malignant transformation with equal efficiency [193, 200]. The molecular events critical for transformation include degradation of cellular p53 through a viral protein, E6, and a cellular accessory protein, E6AP, that functions as a ubiquitin ligase [203]. In the absence of clinical symptoms, detection of infection can be done with molecular techniques [204].

Current HPV management strategies include cytodestructive, antiviral, immunomodulation, and vaccination. One commonly used cytodestructive drug, derived from the roots of *Berberiacae* (May apple), is Podophyllin. Podophyllin contains podophyllotoxin that has been found to cause necrosis of dermal and epidermal tissues [205, 206]. Antiviral agents are also available including 5-fluorouracil and Cidofovir ((S)-1-(3-hydroxy-2-phosphonylmethoxypropyl)cytosine) that act to disrupt thymidine metabolism and the viral DNA polymerase, respectively [207-209]. Immunological-based therapies include interferon (INF) therapy, Imiquimod (imidazoquinoline) that increases cellular release of IFN-α, -β, -γ, and tumor necrosis factor α (TNFα) [209, 210]. Vaccination has been found to be highly effective though coverage can vary widely for different populations [211].

Promising progress against HPV infection using ginger is supported by one study. As indicated above, one strategy to mitigate HPV infection is through apoptosis of infected cells mediated through p53 [212]. 6-Gingerol was found to inhibit the proliferation of HPV-positive cervical cancer cells. HPV-infected HeLa, CaSki, and SiHa cells were found to have reduced viability in a dose-dependent manner when treated with 6-gingerol using the 3-(4,5-dimethylthiazol-2-yl)-2,5-diphenyltetrazolium bromide (MTT) assay [118]. Further, a key mechanism for survival of infected cells is inhibition of apoptosis through targeted destruction of the p53 protein mediated by the HPV protein E6 [202, 203]. However, 6-gingerol did not appear to influence the expression of the viral E6 protein [118, 213].

Using an *in silico* approach, 6-gingerol was predicted to bind to the 20S beta-5 proteasome subunit where it could potentially inhibit its activity [118, 214]. Inhibition of the proteasome could combat the anti-apoptotic influence of the ubiquitin ligase activity that targets p53 via the E6 protein [118, 203]. Indeed, 6-gingerol was found to block the activity of the proteasome in a dose-dependent manner, blocking degradation of p53 [118]. Thus, through activation of p53, HPV-infected cells may be directed toward the apoptotic pathway, preventing proliferation. Lastly, 6-gingerol was found to inhibit tumor growth of HeLa cells in a xenograft mouse model system when administered at 2.5 and 5.0 mg/kg body weight through a 30-day time course. No loss of body weight was observed indicating that the concentrations of 6-gingerol used were not toxic [118]. Collectively, these results offer a promising start to potential therapeutic practice in patients.

Dengue Virus

Dengue virus (DV) is an enveloped virus with a plus-sense RNA genome and classified in the *Flaviviridae* family. The genome is 10.6 kb in length and codes for 3 structural proteins and 7 nonstructural proteins [215]. The virion has an external icosahedral shell composed of 90 repeating units of E glycoprotein dimers [216]. The next innermost shell is composed of the ectodomain of viral M proteins and the stem region of the E proteins. Within these concentric protein shells is the lipid bilayer surrounding the nucleocapsid and the genome [216]. The E protein contains a hydrophobic domain that is responsible for membrane fusion and a domain that binds to cellular receptors [217, 218]. The E protein is also a major target for neutralizing antibodies. Sequence differences in the E protein give rise to four distinct serotypes. These differences likely mediate binding to distinct cellular receptors [215, 219].

Dengue infection is a tropical, mosquito borne (*Aedes aegypti*), immunopathological disease. Following a bite, the virus is thought to infect dendritic cells near to the wound, then transmission to macrophages and leukocytes, and ultimately enter the blood [220]. An incubation period of 3-14 days is typical following initial infection. For many persons, infection is mild or asymptomatic [215, 221]. For those who show symptoms, the incubation period is followed by Dengue fever, Dengue hemorrhagic fever, or Dengue shock syndrome. When patients recover from an initial infection, they usually have antibodies that can cross react with all 4 serotypes. However, these antibodies only prevent reinfection against the same serotype that caused the infection [218]. Subsequent infection with a different serotype leads to greater risk of developing the hemorrhagic fever.

Mechanistically, it is thought that the non-neutralizing antibodies against the previous infection bind to the virus and promote infection of phagocytes [218, 220].

Dengue fever is usually sudden-onset with headache, retro-orbital pain, nausea and vomiting, anorexia, body ache, weakness, and rash [215, 222]. The hemorrhagic fever is generally considered a worsening of the symptoms of Dengue fever, with increased vascular permeability, hemorrhages of the skin, gums, and gastrointestinal tract. The shock syndrome is caused by hypovolemia and hypotension (< 20 mmHG) [215, 222, 223]. Further to the symptoms of the infection, viremia, and the potential for spreading virus occurs simultaneously. Viral titers can reach 10^5 to 10^6 infectious units per ml during the febrile period; during the hemorrhagic fever and shock syndrome, the titer can be 10 to 100-fold higher [215]. The mosquito can feed from multiple individuals in proximity (e.g., in a household). The virus can be housed in the mosquito salivary gland following feeding from an infected person leading to spread as the insect continues to feed [224]. Thus, it is common to see multiple persons in a household experience onset of symptoms during a 24-36 hour window [222, 224].

Few treatment options are currently available for Dengue virus infection. Supportive measures and fluid therapy are helpful but are most effective when applied within 2-3 days following onset of symptoms [225]. Management efforts have also been directed against the mosquito vector. Insect repellents including DEET (N,N-diethyl-m-toluamide) and other synthetic compounds are also in use. Removal of standing water breeding sites is an additional strategy against the mosquito, though the small volumes needed to support the *Aedes* life cycle can make this strategy impractical on a large area [225, 226]. Mosquito control programs were implemented in different regions in the late 20th century, and though initially successful, were discontinued because they were not considered sustainable [227].

Vaccination development efforts have been evaluated, but significant barriers have prevented success. Animal models, such as mice, are resistant to dengue virus infection, thus cannot be used to verify the efficacy of potential vaccines. The vaccine will need to prevent serologically distinct forms of the virus [220], however the immune response to an infection highlights this challenge. Immunity following an infection with one serotype is thought to be lifelong, but only short-term (2-3 months) against other serotypes [215]. Worse, weakly-bound antibodies can enhance infectivity by enabling virus entry to macrophages through the Fc receptor [218]. Until effective preventative strategies can be deployed, additional treatment options are needed.

Two reports suggest that ginger is a source of phytochemical activities that can be used to fight Dengue fever. Bezerra-Silva et al. [8] found that essential oils isolated from torch ginger (*Etlingera elatior*) deterred oviposition activity against pregnant *A. aegypti* females. Pregnant females were offered a choice of egg-laying in a cup containing water or in a cup containing water supplemented with the oil [8]. The reduction in egg-laying in response to the presence of 100 ppm oil mixture ranged from ~30% to less than 20% compared to controls [8]. Variation in response was observed for different cultivars of the torch ginger (Red > Pink > Porcelain). The oil was found to contain 43 components by gas chromatography including α-pinene, dodecanal, and n-dodecanol as the most abundant [8]. The oviposition deterrent effect could be recapitulated by the purified components dodecanal and n-dodecanol [8]. Further, Bezerra-Silva et al. [8] found that dodecanal and n-dodecanol were able to cause depolarization of the antennae suggesting the compounds could be detected by the mosquito. Docking studies using dodecanal and n-dodecanol (and some similar structures) suggested that they can bind to odorant binding protein 1, that is important for olfaction in *A. aegypti* females [8, 228]. Thus, ginger may serve as a potential source of compounds that interfere with oviposition behavior of some female mosquitos through disruption of normal olfactory responses to environmental clues. This interference could in turn reduce survival of eggs if they are not deposited in appropriate environments to support larval development.

A second approach evaluated the efficacy of ginger to mitigate the pathophysiology of dengue virus infection. In this study, an aqueous extract of ginger was evaluated for its ability to modulate expression of genes important for vascular leakage [126].

In this model system, Vero cells infected with Dengue Virus 3 (DV3), were found to release matrix metalloproteinases (MMP) into conditioned medium as detected by gelatin zymography [126]. The extract of ginger was able to reduce this activity in a dose-dependent manner. Transcription of MMP-2 and -9 was increased by DV3 infection, but this effect was partially reversed by ginger [126]. The reduction of detectable MMP activity by ginger is also partly explained by increasing expression of tissue inhibitors of metalloproteinases (TIMP)-1 and -2, also in a dose-dependent manner [126]. Both MMP-2 and MMP-9 are thought to be important contributors to vascular leakage when overexpressed in response to dengue infection [229, 230].

There is some uncertainty that 6-gingerol is the active agent. The authors determined the quantity of 6-gingerol extracted, but they did not report testing this purified compound in their model system [126]. Other work has found that ginger extracts are able to reduce MMP activity in human vascular endothelial cells [231]. Purified 6-gingerol was found to reduce MMP-2 and -9 in MDA-MB-231 breast cancer cells leading to reduced wound healing migration and motility in a Boyden chamber assay [232]. Similar effects were observed by treating MDA-MB-231 cells with 6-shogaol [233], and by treating HepG2 cells with either 6-gingerol or 6-shogaol [234]. Thus, the effects of ginger observed on DV3-induced MMP and TIMP expression may be due to multiple active compounds acting through potentially different targets [126]. Given that vascular leakage is a contributor to the hemorrhagic effects of DV infection, efforts to mitigate this aspect of the disease may improve patient outcomes. An additional question not yet addressed is whether any component extracted from ginger has the potential to have antiviral activity against DV3 (or other serotypes). With the successes reported elsewhere in this chapter, treatment of the virus prior to infection or the host cells might be used to evaluate if ginger has the capacity to block the viral life cycle at different stages. Collectively, ginger may exert multiple activities that can be used to combat Dengue virus.

Ginger as an Agent against Non-Human Viruses

Further exploration of antiviral activities in ginger was directed toward viruses that infect animals and plant species. This research is summarized in Table 3. The authors of these studies employed a combination of purified 6-gingerol, essential oils, and crude alcoholic extract of ginger.

Table 3. Research summary of ginger extracts tested against non-human viruses

Material Used	Virus Studied*	Study Outcome	Reference
6-gingerol	NDV	*in vivo* (chick), reduced mortality; *in vitro* antioxidant activity.	[120]
Essential oils including Limonene, 1,8-Cineole, and α-Zingiberene	TMV	*in vivo* (plant), viral inactivation, curative, preventative.	[235]
Alcohol extract of whole ginger	FLMaV-1	*in vivo* (plant) reduced severity and presence of symptoms, reduced viral titer	[236]

*NDV (Newcastle Disease Virus), TMV (Tobacco Mosaic Virus), FLMaV-1(Fig Leaf Mottle Associated Virus 1).

Newcastle Disease Virus

Newcastle Disease Virus (NDV) is a pathogenic agent that infects avians, notably chickens, but many bird species appear susceptible [237, 238]. The virus is classified in the family *Paramyxoviridae* and consists of a negative sense RNA surrounded by a capsid and an envelope reaching 200-300 nm in diameter. The genome size varies into three subgroupings of 15,186 nucleotides (nt), 15,192 nt, or 15,198 nt [239]. Two glycoproteins are present in the envelope, hemagglutinin-neuraminidase (HN) and fusion (F) proteins. Within the envelope is a hydrophobic matrix (M) protein. The genome is contained within thousands of copies of the nucleocapsid protein (NP) arranged in a herringbone structure along with several copies of the phosphoprotein (P) and the RNA-directed RNA polymerase (L) [240]. The

HN protein is multifunctional—responsible for receptor binding (to sialic acid-containing receptor sites) and for neuraminidase activity (sialic acid-cleaving) [241]. Interaction between the HN protein and the F protein leads to fusion of the envelope and the cell membrane, leading to infection [242]. Isolates of NDV are classified into groups (i.e., lentogenic, mesogenic, and velogenic) based on the severity of the disease and are associated with sequence variations in the F protein [241, 243].

Management of Newcastle disease occurs through hygiene (i.e., minimizing infection through contamination of feed, equipment, handling, etc.), biosecurity (i.e., prevention of the virus being introduced to a flock), and vaccination [244]. Currently, live-virus vaccination strategies using lentogenic strains are in use and are partially effective. Since all NDV isolates are of the same serotype, vaccination protects against more virulent strains [244]. These treatments can be delivered via drinking water or with atomizer spray; for farmed chickens, this usually occurs at day one following hatching [245]. However, recombinant vaccines are costly and thus pose a barrier to many parts of the world where such expense is prohibitive [244]. In addition, there are some barriers to the complete efficacy of vaccines: Vaccination commonly causes a reduction in egg laying so could potentially decrease harvest or breeding [246]; some vaccinated birds can become infected with more virulent strains and shed small amounts of virus without the appearance of clinical symptoms [248]; vaccine-derived NDV isolates were identified in wild birds on four continents raising the possibility that antigenic drift could increase virulence and hasten infection among other wild birds and commercial stocks [249]; transport and storage to many parts of the developing world lessens the response to the vaccine due to inadequate temperature control [245]. Because of these limitations and challenges, additional strategies are needed to supplement current vaccination, hygiene, and biosecurity efforts.

One study examined the effects of the ginger compound, 6-gingerol, on Newcastle disease. 6-Gingerol was able to block the mesogenic Komarov NDV strain and increase survival *in ovo* in a dose-dependent manner [250, 251]. In the study, embryonated eggs were divided into untreated, 6-gingerol treated, NDV infected, and 3 groups with 6-gingerol treatment and NDV infection that varied by timing (pre-infection, post-infection, and co-infection) [251]. The co-treated groups were further divided into 3 subgroups each that used increasing doses of 6-gingerol; viral infection titer remained constant across all groups [251]. Embryo survival was monitored for 5 consecutive days [251]. Viral titer recovered from the allantoic fluid was measured in a hemagglutination assay [251]. Embryo survival was increased as 6-gingerol dose increased. The NDV titer was at its lowest in the treatment groups with the highest concentration of 6-gingerol [251].

Subbiah et al. [251] went further to characterize the antioxidant effects of 6-gingerol as a potential mechanism to explain their observed antiviral effects. Whole ginger and individual compounds were found to have antioxidant activity in several experimental systems [252-255]. Oxidative stress is known to contribute to the pathology caused by viral infections [256]. Whole ginger lessened hepatic tissue damage, as measured by release of diagnostic enzymes into blood, caused by administration of lead acetate to rats [252]. 6-Shogaol and 10-gingerol were found to reduce lipid peroxidation and to protect rat pheochromocytoma (PC-12) cells from damage by hydrogen peroxide [253]. Purified 6-gingerol was able to scavenge 1,1–Diphenyl–2–picrylhydrazyl (DPPH) and 2'–azinobis–3–ethylbenzothiazoline–6–sulfonic acid (ABTS) radicals [254] *in vitro*. Each of 6-, 8-, and 10-gingerol, as well as 6-shogaol, were able to inhibit N-formyl-methionyl-leucyl-phenylalanine induced production of reactive oxygen species (ROS) in human polymorphonuclear neutrophils [255]. Oxidative stress, accompanying NDV infection, contributed to pathology and tissue damage particularly in the brain and liver. But this effect could be partially mitigated by supplementing treatment with the antioxidant, vitamin E [251]. In evaluating the effects of 6-gingerol, Subbiah et al. [251] determined that this compound exerted antioxidant activities measured in several chemical tests and in erythrocytes. It is suggested that the protective effect of 6-gingerol against NDV infection may, in part, be a consequence of these antioxidant activities [120, 251]. Mitigation of oxidative stress may not be the only mechanism to protect against NDV. Indeed, several studies indicate that phytochemicals can act through immunomodulation [257-259]. Further study is needed to clarify the mechanism of 6-gingerol in this study.

Tobacco Mosaic Virus

Tobacco Mosaic Virus (TMV) is a rod-shaped particle measuring 3000 Angstrom in length and 180 Angstrom in diameter [260]. The 6.4 kb genome is a positive sense RNA that codes for four proteins: two replication-associated proteins (126 and 183 kDa, respectively), the movement protein (MP), and the coat protein (CP) [261, 262].

Transmission of virus from plant to plant occurs through a different mechanism than transmission within a plant. Transmission from plant to plant requires disruption of the cuticle, usually mediated by mechanical injury ("Tobacco Mosaic Virus" n.d.). Infection of adjacent cells with viral replication complexes (VRC) occurs through transport using plasmodesmata and the viral MP [263]. The virus can also spread from the site of infection to more distant cells systemically through the phloem [264]. Infection of plants with TMV causes chlorosis of the leaves and/or vein clearing [265, 266]. Chlorosis of the leaves is associated with depletion of photosystem II complexes and breakdown of the chlorophyll. Malformed chloroplasts can be observed and the reduction in photosynthesis stunts growth [267, 268]. Finally, necrosis is common in plants that have a genotype that can elicit the hypersensitive response and appears to confine the virus to the region of infection [269, 270]. While plants have multiple strategies to defend against viral infection, these mechanisms are imperfect, and viruses continually evolve new countermeasures [271]. The global demand for plant products mandates that innate defense mechanisms are supplemented by human prevention and treatment efforts.

Efforts to manage crop viruses, such as TMV, are vital. One estimate of the economic burden of crop yield losses due to plant viruses is $30 billion USD [272]. In terms of production, approximately 15% of total yield is lost to diseases, of which 30% is caused by plant viruses [273-275]. Efforts to combat TMV have historic roots in the improvement of the yield and quality of tobacco [276]. The crop value of tobacco from the top 10 producing nations is estimated to be close to $8 billion USD [277]; however, TMV is capable of infecting more than 100 other plants including food crops of tomato, cucumber, and pepper [278, 279]. Following infection, removal of the infected crops and monitoring for further infections increases production costs. The virus appears to be able to remain in the soil and survive the winter where it can potentially infect the next crop [267]. TMV can also be transported in irrigation water leading to further spread [280]. Unlike human or animal patients that can be housed and isolated, treatment of infected plants requires *in situ* actions.

Viral infections are difficult to manage in the field. Curative strategies are limited, so much effort is put toward prophylactic control. Chemical treatments, such as the application of plant hormones, can bolster resistance to viruses by pre-activating defensive mechanisms (i.e., systemic acquired resistance) [281]. Compounds such acetylsalicylic acid and benzo-(1,2,3)-thiadiazole-7-carbothiolic acid (BTH) have been found to protect tobacco against TMV [282, 283]. Some drawbacks to this approach are that treated plants expend considerable energy in the form of protein synthesis and metabolic pathways that can lead to stunted growth [284]. Alternatively, cross-protection is used as a plant "vaccination" strategy. Often, when infected with an attenuated virus, the plant gains protection against subsequent challenges [285, 286]. Although, identifying appropriate viruses to serve as the attenuated inoculum has been challenging [281]. Therefore, additional preventative and treatment strategies are needed.

One study was identified that assayed anti-TMV activities in ginger. The authors used *Nicotiana glutinosa* leaves as a host for both *in vitro* and *in vivo* analysis [235]. For *in vitro* study, leaves from plants at growth stage 5-6 were transferred to culture dishes [235]. The leaves were infected using the juice-rubbing method, then cut along the main vein [235]. Following 3 hours of infection, the leaves were immersed in ginger essential oils dissolved in dimethyl sulfoxide (DMSO) [235]. Lu et al. [235] found that ginger essential oils exerted 53.7% TMV inhibition at a concentration of 100 μg/ml. For *in vivo* study, viral inactivation, curative, and protective properties were evaluated separately [235, 287]. Inactivation of TMV was evaluated by pre-mixing the virus suspension with ginger essential oils for 1 hour followed by spreading of the mixture on the leaves [235, 287]. Curative effects were evaluated by spreading the oils on the leaves 5 hours post infection [235, 287]. Protective effects were evaluated by spreading the oils on the leaves 5 hours prior to infection. Following 3-4 days of infection, lesions were counted [235, 287]. The inhibition rates of TMV by ginger essential oils reduced the lesions to ~30% compared to the control [235]. Ginger at the highest concentration was found to have a stronger curative effect (~45%), but a weaker protective effect (~15%) in the virus inactivation study [235]. Other authors have observed similar results using essential oils against TMV [288]. In one study, essential oils of *Satureja montana*, thymol, and carvacrol, were found to reduce the infectivity of TMV to similar values [288]. Additional effort sought to identify active components of the ginger essential oil mixture [288].

In the analysis of essential oils from various sources, the authors determined the individual components using gas chromatography flame ionization detection (GC-FID) and GC-mass spectrometry (GC-MS) [235]. An analysis of the ginger oil identified α-Pinene, Camphene, Myrcene, Limonene, 1,8-Cineole, β-Phellandrene, cis-Piperitol, α-Copaene, Geranyl acetate, β-Elemene, β-Cedrene, β-Farnesene, α-Zingiberene, α-Selinen, β-Bisabolene, γ-Cadinene, and β-Curcumene as the most abundant components of the oil, comprising more than 90% of the total [235]. Of these sourced from ginger, Lu et al. [235] tested Limonene, 1,8-Cineole, and α-Zingiberene in the *in vivo*, curative study. Limonene (~50%), 1,8-Cineole (~45%), and α-Zingiberene (<45%) exerted curative activity when applied to infected leaves at 320 μg/ml [235]. Since their inhibition rates are comparable to the less purified essential oil mixture, it may be that multiple compounds are active and showing cooperative effects [235]. For example, Limonene was reported to represent about 1% of the total peak area for ginger essential oil, but it shows comparable activity to the mixture [235]. This would represent a ~100-fold loss of activity when used as a purified reagent. Future efforts should continue to focus on individual components of the ginger oil, including trials investigating virus inactivation and protection.

Fig Leaf Mottle Associated Virus 1

Fig leaf mottle-associated virus 1 (FLMaV-1) is classified in the *Closteroviridae* family, genus *Closterovirus*, and has a double stranded 19kb RNA genome. The virions are 1800 nm in length and lack an envelope [289]. Virions in this genus typically have a major coat protein (CP) and a divergent CP (CPd) located toward one end [290]. In addition to the genes for CP and CPd, open reading frames for a protease, methyltransferase, helicase, RNA polymerase, and a HSP70-related protein are typical for this genus [289-291].

Figs throughout the world are vulnerable to fig mosaic disease (FMD), caused by multiple different viruses, including FLMaV-1 [292, 293]. Transmission is usually by the eriophyid mite, *Aceria ficus* [290, 294]. Infected fig leaves show chlorotic ring spots and mosaic patterns. On a cellular level, double membrane bodies (DMBs) are evident containing proteins, fibrils, and filamentous materials surrounded by a membrane derived from the endoplasmic reticulum [293, 295]. Often, infected plants have more than one of the viruses present at the time of survey [296-298]. For example, fig trees in Morocco were found to harbor mixed infections of Fig mosaic virus (FMV), FLMaV-1, Fig leaf mottle-associated virus 2 (FLMaV-2), Fig mild mottling-associated virus (FMMaV), Fig latent virus 1 (FLV-1), Fig fleck associated virus (FFkaV), Fig cryptic virus (FCrV), or Fig badnavirus 1 (FBaV-1) in about 50% of the surveyed, infected plants [292]. Diagnosis of individual infecting viruses can be determined by RT-PCR [292, 296, 299-303]. FMD management strategies can be directed toward the eriophyid mite or the viruses, directly.

Economic data on the losses of fig harvest because of FMD are not available. The worldwide fig production in 2018 was 1.14 million tons [304]. The fruit, and various extracts of the tree, are used as phytomedicines to treat more than 40 disorders [305]. A more generalized economic case for crop virus control is presented above in the TMV section. Specific to FLMaV-1, it has been recognized that the severity of infection generally correlates with diminished fruit production [306]. The capacity for FLMaV-1 to infect other crops has not yet been systematically evaluated. Though, since the virus was not isolated until 2006, it suggests a more restricted host range than some other plant viruses [289]. Although FMD had been recognized and described for some time, the contribution made by the various viruses has yet to be fully evaluated [297, 299, 301]. Thus, evaluating the costs associated with any one virus will be problematic.

There does not appear to be a well-documented treatment strategy to cure fig trees of virus infection, so other approaches are used to manage FMD [297, 299, 301]. Infected stocks can be re-cultivated and propagated [306]. The combination of heat treatment and meristem tip culture was able to eradicate FMV from germplasm [306]. But this treatment would not prevent disease once the cultivated plants were exposed to the virus again [306]. An alternative strategy to prevent disease is management of the eriophyid mites. The mites are a pest themselves, in addition to their role as a virus vector [307]. Nontoxic insecticides such as neem oil may be effective [308], but this approach has not yet been evaluated against *Aceria ficus,* specifically. Mites may also be managed by pesticides or biologic controls such as predatory insects [309]. Yet an additional strategy could be to breed figs that are resistant to the viruses. However, this endeavor can take years with no assurance of success [310]. Little evidence available now suggests that any variety of fig harbors resistance alleles [292, 299]. Therefore, additional strategies will be necessary to supplement existing efforts.

Progress using ginger to exert antiviral activity against FLMaV-1 has been reported [236]. A study used an alcoholic extract of ginger root, among other sources including Thuja leaves, Harmal seeds, and Turmeric rhizome, as a source of antiviral phytochemicals [236]. The fig plants were maintained in greenhouse conditions and were not reported to be in contact with *Aceria ficus* mites [311]. Instead, infection challenges occurred through grafting infected buds onto FMD-free potted fig plants [236, 312]. The treatments were delivered to the plants by spray application [236]. These treatments were further divided into pre-infection (treatment performed 7 days prior to grafting) and post-infection groups (treatment performed 3 days following grafting) [236]. Disease severity (DS) was scored by visual inspection and ranked by the presence and severity of the symptoms (e.g., 0, no symptoms; 1, light mottling and vein clearing; 2, mild mosaic and vein banding; 3, severe mosaic and blotch, chlorotic ringspot; and 4, malformation) and converted to a DS score [236, 313]. The ginger was effective when applied as a pre-infection treatment [236]. and dramatically reduced the FLMaV-1 symptoms on the plants. The DS for infected, untreated plants is 100; that for uninfected controls is 0. The ginger-pre-treated, infected plants were evaluated to have a DS score of 2.78. Further, the virus was undetectable in 8 of 9 replicates. In a post-infection treatment experiment, the ginger was found to have no change on the DS score compared to untreated, infected controls (DS = 100). Thus, post-infection treatment had no apparent effect on the disease [236]. Thus, an extractable component of ginger appears able to inhibit infection by FLMaV-1.

Further studies are needed to evaluate the action of ginger against FLMaV-1 infection. The pre-treatment/post-treatment efficacy difference argues that the ginger may stimulate resistance in the host plants [281]. The window of pre-treatment may be needed for expression of gene products and alteration in metabolic pathways needed to resist the action of the virus. The ineffective post-infection treatment may be explained by either an insufficient time for the resistance factors to be expressed or that these factors are ineffective once an infection is established. The extract may be additionally unable to act on the virus when delivered externally by spray application to the grafted plant (assuming the virus is able to pass through plasmodesmata or enter vascular tissues of the uninfected host). The pre-treatment strategy is promising since it may be effective against FLMaV-1 when it is brought to the plant by the mites. Though, it should be cautioned that FMD looks to be caused by multiple viruses and that the efficacy of ginger will need to be evaluated against the other etiological agents [297, 299, 301]. If the ginger is effective against FLMaV-1, but not all the remaining agents, its application in the field to prevent FMD may be limited.

Conclusion and Unanswered Questions

The research summarized here provides promise that ginger joins an expanding list of phytochemical sources that contain antiviral activities. For the most part, much additional work must be completed before bringing such activities into therapeutic use. However, the breadth of action against such very different viruses argues that much may be gained if these activities can be identified and delivered.

Many of the studies focused on one, or a few, individual compound(s). Of these, 6-gingerol stands out as the most investigated. Other studies used less pure aqueous or solvent extracts. A common uncertainty in many of these studies is the identity of the active agent(s). If it is the case that one, or a few, compounds are exerting the effects, then starting with purified samples can permit better defined experiential conditions. Purified agents can also be used to identify target(s) and to serve as a starting point for chemical modifications that may improve their efficacy.

There is also opportunity for multiple sites of action. Some of the studies tested the effects of compounds in the virions and determined that ginger contains agents that may act on the virus directly. Other studies pointed to a role for immunomodulatory effects of ginger compounds. Those studies generally showed that host immunity may be improved in response to ginger compounds. However, it should be noted that there is still much uncertainty as to the mechanisms of immunomodulation by ginger compounds. Identification of the individual compounds and their targets can open future studies to evaluate these mechanisms and to develop treatments.

References

[1] Petrovska, Biljana Bauer. 2012. "Historical Review of Medicinal Plants' Usage." *Pharmacognosy Reviews* 6 (11): 1–5.

[2] Kapoor, R., B. Sharma, and S. S. Kanwar. 2017. "Antiviral Phytochemicals: An Overview." *Biochemie Und Physiologie Der Pflanzen: BPP* 6 (2): 7.

[3] Tang, Weici, and Gerhard Eisenbrand. 1992. "*Zingiber Officinale* (Willd.) Rosc." In *Chinese Drugs of Plant Origin: Chemistry, Pharmacology, and Use in Traditional and Modern Medicine*, edited

by Weici Tang and Gerhard Eisenbrand, 1011–15. Berlin, Heidelberg: Springer Berlin Heidelberg.

[4] Mbaveng, A. T., and V. Kuete. 2017. "Chapter 30 - *Zingiber Officinale*." In *Medicinal Spices and Vegetables from Africa*, edited by Victor Kuete, 627–39. Academic Press.

[5] Ali, Badreldin H., Gerald Blunden, Musbah O. Tanira, and Abderrahim Nemmar. 2008. "Some Phytochemical, Pharmacological and Toxicological Properties of Ginger (*Zingiber Officinale* Roscoe): A Review of Recent Research." *Food and Chemical Toxicology: An International Journal Published for the British Industrial Biological Research Association* 46 (2): 409–20.

[6] Bua-in, Saowaluck, and Yingyong Paisooksantivatana. 2009. "Essential Oil and Antioxidant Activity of Cassumunar Ginger (Zingiberaceae: *Zingiber Montanum* (Koenig) Link Ex Dietr.) Collected from Various Parts of Thailand." *Kasetsart J. (Nat. Sci.)* 43: 467–75.

[7] Klaywong, Konrapob, Gachagorn Khutrakul, Kiattawee Choowongkomon, Chalermpol Lekcharoensuk, Nantawan Petcharat, Porntippa Leckcharoensuk, and Pongrama Ramasoota. 2014. "Screening for Lead Compounds and Herbal Extracts with Potential Anti-Influenza Viral Activity." *The Southeast Asian Journal of Tropical Medicine and Public Health* 45 (1): 62–74.

[8] Bezerra-Silva, Patrícia C., Kamilla A. Dutra, Geanne K. N. Santos, Rayane C. S. Silva, Jorge Iulek, Paulo Milet-Pinheiro, and Daniela M. A. F. Navarro. 2016. "Evaluation of the Activity of the Essential Oil from an Ornamental Flower against *Aedes Aegypti*: Electrophysiology, Molecular Dynamics and Behavioral Assays." *PloS One* 11 (2): e0150008.

[9] Goswami, Dibakar, Mukesh Kumar, Sunil K. Ghosh, and Amit Das. 2020. *Natural Product Compounds in Alpinia Officinarum and Ginger Are Potent SARS-CoV-2 Papain-like Protease Inhibitors.* https://chemrxiv.org/articles/Natural_Product_Compounds_in_Alpinia_officinarum_and_Ginger_are_Potent_SARS-CoV-2_Papain-like_Protease_Inhibitors/12071997.

[10] Ahkam, Ahmad Hafidul, Feri Eko Hermanto, Adzral Alamsyah, Iva Himmatul Aliyyah, and Fatchiyah. 2020. "Virtual Prediction of Antiviral Potential of Ginger (*Zingiber Officinale*) Bioactive Compounds against Spike and MPro of SARS-CoV2 Protein." *Berkala Penelitian Hayati* 25 (2): 52–57.

[11] Rajagopal, Kalirajan, Gowramma Byran, Srikanth Jupudi, and R. Vadivelan. 2020. "Activity of Phytochemical Constituents of Black Pepper, Ginger, and Garlic against Coronavirus (COVID-19): An in Silico Approach." *International Journal of Health & Allied Sciences* 9 (5): 43.

[12] Baatartsogt, Tugsbaatar, Vuong N. Bui, Dai Q. Trinh, Emi Yamaguchi, Dulyatad Gronsang, Rapeewan Thampaisarn, Haruko Ogawa, and Kunitoshi Imai. 2016. "High Antiviral Effects of Hibiscus Tea Extract on the H5 Subtypes of Low and Highly Pathogenic Avian Influenza Viruses." *The Journal of Veterinary Medical Science / the Japanese Society of Veterinary Science* 78 (9): 1405–11.

[13] Rasool, Amir, Muti-Ur-Rehman Khan, Muhammad Asad Ali, Aftab Ahmad Anjum, Ishtiaq Ahmed, Asim Aslam, Ghulam Mustafa, Saima Masood, Muhammad Amjad Ali, and Muhammad Nawaz. 2017. "Anti-Avian Influenza Virus H9N2 Activity of Aqueous Extracts of *Zingiber Officinalis* (Ginger) and *Allium Sativum* (Garlic) in Chick Embryos." *Pakistan Journal of Pharmaceutical Sciences* 30 (4): 1341–44.

[14] Sahoo, Maheswata, Lingaraja Jena, Surya Narayan Rath, and Satish Kumar. 2016. "Identification of Suitable Natural Inhibitor against Influenza A (H1N1) Neuraminidase Protein by Molecular Docking." *Genomics & Informatics* 14 (3): 96–103.

[15] Zhu, Hongmei, Minghua Hu, Dehai Wang, Guowei Xu, Xiquan Yin, Xin Liu, Mingxing Ding, and Li Han. 2020. "Mixed Polysaccharides Derived from Shiitake Mushroom, Poriacocos, Ginger, and Tangerine Peel Enhanced Protective Immune Responses in Mice Induced by Inactivated Influenza Vaccine." *Biomedicine & Pharmacotherapy = Biomedecine & Pharmacotherapie* 126 (June): 110049.

[16] Mansoor, Kenza A., Fadi Qadan, Mathias Schmidt, Nidal A. Qinna, Mujtaba Badr, and Khalid Z. Matalka. 2018. "A Functional Food Mixture 'Protector' Reinforces the Protective Immune Parameters against Viral Flu Infection in Mice." *Nutrients* 10 (6). https://doi.org/10.3390/nu10060743.

[17] Denyer, C. V., P. Jackson, D. M. Loakes, M. R. Ellis, and D. A. Young. 1994. "Isolation of Antirhinoviral Sesquiterpenes from Ginger (*Zingiber Officinale*)." *Journal of Natural Products* 57 (5): 658–62.

[18] Chang, Jung San, Kuo Chih Wang, Chia Feng Yeh, Den En Shieh, and Lien Chai Chiang. 2013. "Fresh Ginger (*Zingiber Officinale*) Has Anti-Viral Activity against Human Respiratory Syncytial Virus in Human Respiratory Tract Cell Lines." *Journal of Ethnopharmacology* 145 (1): 146–51.

[19] Ramphul, Kamleshun, and Stephanie G. Mejias. 2020. "Coronavirus Disease: A Review of a New Threat to Public Health." *Cureus* 12 (3): e7276.

[20] Fehr, Anthony R., Jeremiah Athmer, Rudragouda Channappanavar, Judith M. Phillips, David K. Meyerholz, and Stanley Perlman. 2015. "The nsp3 Macrodomain Promotes Virulence in Mice with Coronavirus-Induced Encephalitis." *Journal of Virology* 89 (3): 1523–36.

[21] Luk, Hayes K. H., Xin Li, Joshua Fung, Susanna K. P. Lau, and Patrick C. Y. Woo. 2019. "Molecular Epidemiology, Evolution and Phylogeny of SARS Coronavirus." *Infection, Genetics and Evolution: Journal of Molecular Epidemiology and Evolutionary Genetics in Infectious Diseases* 71 (July): 21–30.

[22] Almaghaslah, Dalia, Geetha Kandasamy, Mona Almanasef, Rajalakshimi Vasudevan, and Sriram Chandramohan. 2020. "Review on the Coronavirus Disease (COVID-19) Pandemic: Its Outbreak and Current Status." *International Journal of Clinical Practice* 74 (11): e13637.

[23] Li, Guangdi, and Erik De Clercq. 2020. "Therapeutic Options for the 2019 Novel Coronavirus (2019-nCoV)." *Nature Reviews. Drug Discovery* 19 (3): 149–50.

[24] Hoffmann, Markus, Hannah Kleine-Weber, Nadine Krüger, Marcel Müller, Christian Drosten, and Stefan Pöhlmann. 2020. "The Novel Coronavirus 2019 (2019-nCoV) Uses the SARS-Coronavirus Recept or ACE2 and the Cellular Protease TMPRSS2 for Entry into Target Cells." *Cold Spring Harbor Laboratory*. https://doi.org/10.1101/2020.01.31.929042.

[25] Wan, Yushun, Jian Shang, Rachel Graham, Ralph S. Baric, and Fang Li. 2020. "Receptor Recognition by the Novel Coronavirus from Wuhan: An Analysis Based on Decade-Long Structural Studies of SARS Coronavirus." *Journal of Virology* 94 (7). https://doi.org/10.1128/JVI.00127-20.

[26] Hamming, I., W. Timens, M. L. C. Bulthuis, A. T. Lely, G. J. Navis, and H. van Goor. 2004. "Tissue Distribution of ACE2 Protein, the Functional Receptor for SARS Coronavirus. A First Step in Understanding SARS Pathogenesis." *The Journal of Pathology* 203 (2): 631–37.

[27] Sadhukhan, Pritam, M. Talha Ugurlu, and Mohammad O. Hoque. 2020. "Effect of COVID-19 on Lungs: Focusing on Prospective Malignant Phenotypes." *Cancers* 12 (12): 3822.

[28] Jin, Yuefei, Haiyan Yang, Wangquan Ji, Weidong Wu, Shuaiyin Chen, Weiguo Zhang, and Guangcai Duan. 2020. "Virology, Epidemiology, Pathogenesis, and Control of COVID-19." *Viruses* 12 (4). https://doi.org/10.3390/v12040372.

[29] Chaudhuri, Swetaprovo, Saptarshi Basu, Prasenjit Kabi, Vishnu R. Unni, and Abhishek Saha. 2020. "Modeling the Role of Respiratory Droplets in Covid-19 Type Pandemics." *Physics of Fluids* 32 (6): 063309.

[30] Morawska, Lidia, Julian W. Tang, William Bahnfleth, Philomena M. Bluyssen, Atze Boerstra, Giorgio Buonanno, Junji Cao, et al. 2020. "How Can Airborne Transmission of COVID-19 Indoors Be Minimised?" *Environment International* 142 (September): 105832.

[31] Chen, Guang, Di Wu, Wei Guo, Yong Cao, Da Huang, Hongwu Wang, Tao Wang, et al. 2020. "Clinical and Immunological Features of Severe and Moderate Coronavirus Disease 2019." *The Journal of Clinical Investigation* 130 (5): 2620–29.

[32] Chen, Nanshan, Min Zhou, Xuan Dong, Jieming Qu, Fengyun Gong, Yang Han, Yang Qiu, et al. 2020. "Epidemiological and Clinical Characteristics of 99 Cases of 2019 Novel Coronavirus Pneumonia in Wuhan, China: A Descriptive Study." *The Lancet* 395 (10223): 507–13.

[33] Kuipers, Maria T., Tom van der Poll, Marcus J. Schultz, and Catharina W. Wieland. 2011. "Bench-to-Bedside Review: Damage-Associated Molecular Patterns in the Onset of Ventilator-Induced Lung Injury." *Critical Care/the Society of Critical Care Medicine* 15 (6): 235.

[34] Vardhana, Santosha A., and Jedd D. Wolchok. 2020. "The Many Faces of the Anti-COVID Immune Response." *The Journal of Experimental Medicine* 217 (6). https://doi.org/10.1084/jem.20200678.

[35] Diebold, Sandra S., Tsuneyasu Kaisho, Hiroaki Hemmi, Shizuo Akira, and Caetano Reis e Sousa. 2004. "Innate Antiviral Responses by Means of TLR7-Mediated Recognition of Single-Stranded RNA." *Science* 303 (5663): 1529–31.

[36] Mahmudpour, Mehdi, Jamshid Roozbeh, Mohsen Keshavarz, Shokrollah Farrokhi, and Iraj Nabipour. 2020. "COVID-19 Cytokine Storm: The Anger of Inflammation." *Cytokine* 133 (September): 155151.

[37] South, Andrew M., Debra I. Diz, and Mark C. Chappell. 2020. "COVID-19, ACE2, and the Cardiovascular Consequences." *American Journal of Physiology. Heart and Circulatory Physiology* 318 (5): H1084–90.

[38] Lanza, Katharina, Lucas G. Perez, Larissa B. Costa, Thiago M. Cordeiro, Vitria A. Palmeira, Victor T. Ribeiro, and Ana Cristina Simões e Silva. 2020. "Covid-19: The Renin–angiotensin System Imbalance Hypothesis." *Clinical Science* 134 (11): 1259–64.

[39] Conti, P., G. Ronconi, A. Caraffa, C. Gallenga, R. Ross, I. Frydas, and S. Kritas. 2020. "Induction of pro-Inflammatory Cytokines (IL-1 and IL-6) and Lung Inflammation by Coronavirus-19 (COVI-19 or SARS-CoV-2): Anti-Inflammatory Strategies." *Journal of Biological Regulators and Homeostatic Agents* 34 (2): 327–31.

[40] Broers, Annoek E. C., Ron van der Holt, Joost W. J. van Esser, Jan-Willem Gratama, Sonja Henzen-Logmans, Vibeke Kuenen-Boumeester, Bob Löwenberg, and Jan J. Cornelissen. 2000. "Increased Transplant-Related Morbidity and Mortality in CMV-Seropositive Patients despite Highly Effective Prevention of CMV Disease after Allogeneic T-Cell--Depleted Stem Cell Transplantation." *Blood, The Journal of the American Society of Hematology* 95 (7): 2240–45.

[41] Barber, Daniel L., E. John Wherry, David Masopust, Baogong Zhu, James P. Allison, Arlene H. Sharpe, Gordon J. Freeman, and Rafi Ahmed. 2006. "Restoring Function in Exhausted CD8 T Cells during Chronic Viral Infection." *Nature* 439 (7077): 682–87.

[42] Shin, Haina, and E. John Wherry. 2007. "CD8 T Cell Dysfunction during Chronic Viral Infection." *Current Opinion in Immunology* 19 (4): 408–15.

[43] Yu, Xingxia, and Rongrong Yang. 2020. "COVID-19 Transmission through Asymptomatic Carriers Is a Challenge to Containment." *Influenza and Other Respiratory Viruses*. Wiley.

[44] Polack, Fernando P., Stephen J. Thomas, Nicholas Kitchin, Judith Absalon, Alejandra Gurtman, Stephen Lockhart, John L. Perez, et al. 2020. "Safety and Efficacy of the BNT162b2 mRNA Covid-19 Vaccine." *The New England Journal of Medicine*, December. https://doi.org/10.1056/NEJMoa2034577.

[45] Jackson, Lisa A., Evan J. Anderson, Nadine G. Rouphael, Paul C. Roberts, Mamodikoe Makhene, Rhea N. Coler, Michele P. McCullough, et al. 2020. "An mRNA Vaccine against SARS-CoV-2—preliminary Report." *The New England Journal of Medicine*. https://www.nejm.org/doi/full/10.1056/NEJMoa2022483.

[46] Widge, Alicia T., Nadine G. Rouphael, Lisa A. Jackson, Evan J. Anderson, Paul C. Roberts, Mamodikoe Makhene, James D. Chappell, et al. 2020. "Durability of Responses after SARS-CoV-2 mRNA-1273 Vaccination." *The New England Journal of Medicine*, December. https://doi.org/10.1056/NEJMc2032195.

[47] Klemm, Theresa, Gregor Ebert, Dale J. Calleja, Cody C. Allison, Lachlan W. Richardson, Jonathan P. Bernardini, Bernadine Gc Lu, et al. 2020. "Mechanism and Inhibition of the Papain-like Protease, PLpro, of SARS-CoV-2." *The EMBO Journal* 39 (18): e106275.

[48] Han, Yu-San, Gu-Gang Chang, Chiun-Gung Juo, Hong-Jen Lee, Shiou-Hwei Yeh, John Tsu-An Hsu, and Xin Chen. 2005. "Papain-Like Protease 2 (PLP2) from Severe Acute Respiratory Syndrome Coronavirus (SARS-CoV): Expression, Purification, Characterization, and Inhibition." *Biochemistry* 44 (30): 10349–59.

[49] Harcourt, Brian H., Dalia Jukneliene, Amornrat Kanjanahaluethai, John Bechill, Kari M. Severson, Catherine M. Smith, Paul A. Rota, and Susan C. Baker. 2004. "Identification of Severe Acute Respiratory Syndrome Coronavirus Replicase Products and Characterization of Papain-like Protease Activity." *Journal of Virology* 78 (24): 13600–612.

[50] Báez-Santos, Yahira M., Sarah E. St John, and Andrew D. Mesecar. 2015. "The SARS-Coronavirus Papain-like Protease: Structure, Function and Inhibition by Designed Antiviral Compounds." *Antiviral Research* 115 (March): 21–38.

[51] Hegyi, Annette, and John Ziebuhr. 2002. "Conservation of Substrate Specificities among Coronavirus Main Proteases." *The Journal of General Virology* 83 (Pt 3): 595–99.

[52] Jin, Zhenming, Xiaoyu Du, Yechun Xu, Yongqiang Deng, Meiqin Liu, Yao Zhao, Bing Zhang, et al. 2020. "Structure of M pro from SARS-CoV-2 and Discovery of Its Inhibitors." *Nature* 582 (7811): 289–93.

[53] Alves, Vinicius M., Tesia Bobrowski, Cleber C. Melo-Filho, Daniel Korn, Scott Auerbach, Charles Schmitt, Eugene N. Muratov, and Alexander Tropsha. 2020. "QSAR Modeling of SARS-CoV Mpro

Inhibitors Identifies Sufugolix, Cenicriviroc, Proglumetacin, and Other Drugs as Candidates for Repurposing against SARS-CoV-2." *Molecular Informatics*. https://onlinelibrary.wiley.com/doi/abs/10.1002/minf.202000113.

[54] Fearon, D., A. J. Powell, A. Douangamath, C. D. Owen, C. Wild, T. Krojer, P. Lukacik, C. M. Strain-Damerell, M. A. Walsh, and F. von Delft. 2020. "PanDDA Analysis Group Deposition--Crystal Structure of COVID-19 Main Protease in Complex with Z219104216." *Protein Data Base* 10.

[55] Lan, Jun, Jiwan Ge, Jinfang Yu, Sisi Shan, Huan Zhou, Shilong Fan, Qi Zhang, et al. 2020. "Structure of the SARS-CoV-2 Spike Receptor-Binding Domain Bound to the ACE2 Receptor." *Nature* 581 (7807): 215–20.

[56] Jilani, Talha N., Radia T. Jamil, and Abdul H. Siddiqui. 2019. "H1N1 Influenza (Swine Flu)." In *StatPearls*. Treasure Island (FL): StatPearls Publishing.

[57] Peacock, T. Homas P., Joe James, Joshua E. Sealy, and Munir Iqbal. 2019. "A Global Perspective on H9N2 Avian Influenza Virus." *Viruses* 11 (7). https://doi.org/10.3390/v11070620.

[58] Peiris, J. S. Malik, Menno D. de Jong, and Yi Guan. 2007. "Avian Influenza Virus (H5N1): A Threat to Human Health." *Clinical Microbiology Reviews* 20 (2): 243–67.

[59] Bouvier, Nicole M., and Peter Palese. 2008. "The Biology of Influenza Viruses." *Vaccine* 26 Suppl 4 (September): D49–53.

[60] Noda, Takeshi. 2011. "Native Morphology of Influenza Virions." *Frontiers in Microbiology* 2: 269.

[61] Skehel, J. J., and D. C. Wiley. 2000. "Receptor Binding and Membrane Fusion in Virus Entry: The Influenza Hemagglutinin." *Annual Review of Biochemistry* 69: 531–69.

[62] Shtyrya, Y. A., L. V. Mochalova, and N. V. Bovin. 2009. "Influenza Virus Neuraminidase: Structure and Function." *Acta Naturae* 1 (2): 26–32.

[63] Kochs, Georg, Adolfo García-Sastre, and Luis Martínez-Sobrido. 2007. "Multiple Anti-Interferon Actions of the Influenza A Virus NS1 Protein." *Journal of Virology* 81 (13): 7011–21.

[64] Hay, A. J., V. Gregory, A. R. Douglas, and Y. P. Lin. 2001. "The Evolution of Human Influenza Viruses." *Philosophical Transactions of the Royal Society of London. Series B, Biological Sciences* 356 (1416): 1861–70.

[65] Peteranderl, Christin, Susanne Herold, and Carole Schmoldt. 2016. "Human Influenza Virus Infections." *Seminars in Respiratory and Critical Care Medicine* 37 (4): 487–500.

[66] Rust, Michael J., Melike Lakadamyali, Feng Zhang, and Xiaowei Zhuang. 2004. "Assembly of Endocytic Machinery around Individual Influenza Viruses during Viral Entry." *Nature Structural & Molecular Biology* 11 (6): 567–73.

[67] Pinto, Lawrence H., and Robert A. Lamb. 2006. "The M2 Proton Channels of Influenza A and B Viruses." *The Journal of Biological Chemistry* 281 (14): 8997–9000.

[68] Krammer, Florian, Gavin J. D. Smith, Ron A. M. Fouchier, Malik Peiris, Katherine Kedzierska, Peter C. Doherty, Peter Palese, et al. 2018. "Influenza." *Nature Reviews. Disease Primers* 4 (1): 3–3.

[69] Ducatez, M. F., R. G. Webster, and R. J. Webby. 2008. "Animal Influenza Epidemiology." *Vaccine* 26 Suppl 4 (September): D67–69.

[70] Sellers, Subhashini A., Robert S. Hagan, Frederick G. Hayden, and William A. Fischer 2nd. 2017. "The Hidden Burden of Influenza: A Review of the Extra-Pulmonary Complications of Influenza Infection." *Influenza and Other Respiratory Viruses* 11 (5): 372–93.

[71] Kwong, Jeffrey C., Kevin L. Schwartz, Michael A. Campitelli, Hannah Chung, Natasha S. Crowcroft, Timothy Karnauchow, Kevin Katz, et al. 2018. "Acute Myocardial Infarction after Laboratory-Confirmed Influenza Infection." *The New England Journal of Medicine* 378 (4): 345–53.

[72] Gavin, Patrick J., and Richard B. Thomson. 2004. "Review of Rapid Diagnostic Tests for Influenza." *Clinical and Applied Immunology Reviews* 4 (3): 151–72.

[73] Couch, R. B. 2000. “Prevention and Treatment of Influenza.” *The New England Journal of Medicine* 343 (24): 1778–87.

[74] Webster, R. G., W. J. Bean, O. T. Gorman, T. M. Chambers, and Y. Kawaoka. 1992. “Evolution and Ecology of Influenza A Viruses.” *Microbiological Reviews* 56 (1): 152–79.

[75] Neumann, Gabriele, and Yoshihiro Kawaoka. 2019. “Predicting the Next Influenza Pandemics.” *The Journal of Infectious Diseases* 219 (Suppl_1): S14–20.

[76] Neher, Richard A., Trevor Bedford, Rodney S. Daniels, Colin A. Russell, and Boris I. Shraiman. 2016. “Prediction, Dynamics, and Visualization of Antigenic Phenotypes of Seasonal Influenza Viruses.” *Proceedings of the National Academy of Sciences of the United States of America* 113 (12): E1701–9.

[77] Patel, Mitesh S., Kevin G. Volpp, Dylan S. Small, Craig Wynne, Jingsan Zhu, Lin Yang, Steven Honeywell Jr, and Susan C. Day. 2017. “Using Active Choice within the Electronic Health Record to Increase Influenza Vaccination Rates.” *Journal of General Internal Medicine* 32 (7): 790–95.

[78] Han, Julianna, Jasmine Perez, Adam Schafer, Han Cheng, Norton Peet, Lijun Rong, and Balaji Manicassamy. 2018. “Influenza Virus: Small Molecule Therapeutics and Mechanisms of Antiviral Resistance.” *Current Medicinal Chemistry* 25 (38): 5115–27.

[79] Halperin, Scott A., Bruce Smith, Taoufik Mabrouk, Marc Germain, Pierre Trépanier, Thomas Hassell, John Treanor, Richard Gauthier, and Elaine L. Mills. 2002. “Safety and Immunogenicity of a Trivalent, Inactivated, Mammalian Cell Culture-Derived Influenza Vaccine in Healthy Adults, Seniors, and Children.” *Vaccine* 20 (7): 1240–47.

[80] Burmeister, W. P., R. W. Ruigrok, and S. Cusack. 1992. “The 2.2 A Resolution Crystal Structure of Influenza B Neuraminidase and Its Complex with Sialic Acid.” *The EMBO Journal* 11 (1): 49–56.

[81] Harrison, Stephen C. 2008. “Viral Membrane Fusion.” *Nature Structural & Molecular Biology* 15 (7): 690–98.

[82] Chavan, Rahul Dilip, Pramod Shinde, Kaustubh Girkar, Rajendra Madage, and Abhay Chowdhary. 2016. “Assessment of Anti-

Influenza Activity and Hemagglutination Inhibition of Plumbago Indica and Allium Sativum Extracts." *Pharmacognosy Research* 8 (2): 105–11.

[83] Salehi, Bahare, Paolo Zucca, Ilkay Erdogan Orhan, Elena Azzini, Charles Oluwaseun Adetunji, Soheb Anwar Mohammed, Sanjay K. Banerjee, et al. 2019. "Allicin and Health: A Comprehensive Review." *Trends in Food Science & Technology* 86 (April): 502–16.

[84] Schoenknecht, Carola, Gaby Andersen, Ines Schmidts, and Peter Schieberle. 2016. "Quantitation of Gingerols in Human Plasma by Newly Developed Stable Isotope Dilution Assays and Assessment of Their Immunomodulatory Potential." *Journal of Agricultural and Food Chemistry* 64 (11): 2269–79.

[85] Gao, Pei, Lei Fan, Haoyun Du, Bin Xiang, Yulian Li, Minhua Sun, Yinfeng Kang, et al. 2018. "Recombinant Duck Interferon Gamma Inhibits H5N1 Influenza Virus Replication In Vitro and In Vivo." *Journal of Interferon & Cytokine Research: The Official Journal of the International Society for Interferon and Cytokine Research* 38 (7): 290–97.

[86] Sriwilaijaroen, Nongluk, Prapon Wilairat, Hiroaki Hiramatsu, Tadanobu Takahashi, Takashi Suzuki, Morihiro Ito, Yasuhiko Ito, Masato Tashiro, and Yasuo Suzuki. 2009. "Mechanisms of the Action of Povidone-Iodine against Human and Avian Influenza A Viruses: Its Effects on Hemagglutination and Sialidase Activities." *Virology Journal* 6 (August): 124.

[87] To, Kelvin K. W., Cyril C. Y. Yip, and Kwok-Yung Yuen. 2017. "Rhinovirus - From Bench to Bedside." *Journal of the Formosan Medical Association = Taiwan Yi Zhi* 116 (7): 496–504.

[88] Palmenberg, Ann C., and James E. Gern. 2015. "Classification and Evolution of Human Rhinoviruses." *Methods in Molecular Biology* 1221: 1–10.

[89] Hadfield, A. T., W. m. Lee, R. Zhao, M. A. Oliveira, I. Minor, R. R. Rueckert, and M. G. Rossmann. 1997. "The Refined Structure of Human Rhinovirus 16 at 2.15 A Resolution: Implications for the Viral Life Cycle." *Structure* 5 (3): 427–41.

[90] Basnet, Sarmila, Ann C. Palmenberg, and James E. Gern. 2019. "Rhinoviruses and Their Receptors." *Chest* 155 (5): 1018–25.

[91] Fuchs, Renate, and Dieter Blaas. 2010. "Uncoating of Human Rhinoviruses." *Reviews in Medical Virology* 20 (5): 281–97.

[92] Heikkinen, Terho, and Asko Järvinen. 2003. "The Common Cold." *The Lancet* 361 (9351): 51–59.

[93] Makris, Spyridon, and Sebastian Johnston. 2018. "Recent Advances in Understanding Rhinovirus Immunity." *F1000Research* 7 (September). https://doi.org/10.12688/f1000research.15337.1.

[94] Glanville, Nicholas, Gary R. McLean, Bruno Guy, Valerie Lecouturier, Catherine Berry, Yves Girerd, Christophe Gregoire, et al. 2013. "Cross-Serotype Immunity Induced by Immunization with a Conserved Rhinovirus Capsid Protein." *PLoS Pathogens* 9 (9): e1003669.

[95] Khan, Abdul Latif, Hamayun Khan, J. Hussain, M. Adnan, I. Hussain, T. Khan, and A. Rehman. 2008. "Sesquiterpenes: A Potent Antioxidants-A Review." *Pakistan Journal of Scientific and Industrial Research* 51: 343–50.

[96] Chen, Q-F, Z-P Liu, and F-P Wang. 2011. "Natural Sesquiterpenoids as Cytotoxic Anticancer Agents." *Mini Reviews in Medicinal Chemistry* 11 (13): 1153–64.

[97] Rollinger, Judith M., Theodora M. Steindl, Daniela Schuster, Johannes Kirchmair, Kathrin Anrain, Ernst P. Ellmerer, Thierry Langer, Hermann Stuppner, Peter Wutzler, and Michaela Schmidtke. 2008. "Structure-Based Virtual Screening for the Discovery of Natural Inhibitors for Human Rhinovirus Coat Protein." *Journal of Medicinal Chemistry* 51 (4): 842–51.

[98] Bohmwald, Karen, Janyra A. Espinoza, Emma Rey-Jurado, Roberto S. Gómez, Pablo A. González, Susan M. Bueno, Claudia A. Riedel, and Alexis M. Kalergis. 2016. "Human Respiratory Syncytial Virus: Infection and Pathology." *Seminars in Respiratory and Critical Care Medicine* 37 (4): 522–37.

[99] Hacking, D., and J. Hull. 2002. "Respiratory Syncytial Virus—Viral Biology and the Host Response." *The Journal of Infection* 45 (1): 18–24.

[100] Lay, Margarita K., Pablo A. González, Miguel A. León, Pablo F. Céspedes, Susan M. Bueno, Claudia A. Riedel, and Alexis M. Kalergis. 2013. "Advances in Understanding Respiratory Syncytial Virus Infection in Airway Epithelial Cells and Consequential Effects on the Immune Response." *Microbes and Infection / Institut Pasteur* 15 (3): 230–42.

[101] Tayyari, Farnoosh, David Marchant, Theo J. Moraes, Wenming Duan, Peter Mastrangelo, and Richard G. Hegele. 2011. "Identification of Nucleolin as a Cellular Receptor for Human Respiratory Syncytial Virus." *Nature Medicine* 17 (9): 1132–35.

[102] Behera, A. K., H. Matsuse, M. Kumar, X. Kong, R. F. Lockey, and S. S. Mohapatra. 2001. "Blocking Intercellular Adhesion Molecule-1 on Human Epithelial Cells Decreases Respiratory Syncytial Virus Infection." *Biochemical and Biophysical Research Communications* 280 (1): 188–95.

[103] Marr, Nico, and Stuart E. Turvey. 2012. "Role of Human TLR4 in Respiratory Syncytial Virus-Induced NF-κB Activation, Viral Entry and Replication." *Innate Immunity* 18 (6): 856–65.

[104] Teng, M. N., and P. L. Collins. 1998. "Identification of the Respiratory Syncytial Virus Proteins Required for Formation and Passage of Helper-Dependent Infectious Particles." *Journal of Virology* 72 (7): 5707–16.

[105] Lambert, D. M. 1988. "Role of Oligosaccharides in the Structure and Function of Respiratory Syncytial Virus Glycoproteins." *Virology* 164 (2): 458–66.

[106] Asenjo, Ana, Lorena Rodríguez, and Nieves Villanueva. 2005. "Determination of Phosphorylated Residues from Human Respiratory Syncytial Virus P Protein That Are Dynamically Dephosphorylated by Cellular Phosphatases: A Possible Role for Serine 54." *The Journal of General Virology* 86 (4): 1109–20.

[107] Collins, Peter L., and José A. Melero. 2011. "Progress in Understanding and Controlling Respiratory Syncytial Virus: Still Crazy after All These Years." *Virus Research* 162 (1-2): 80–99.

[108] Touch, S. M., and A. R. Spitzer. 1998. "Palivizumab, a Humanized Respiratory Syncytial Virus Monoclonal Antibody, Reduces Hospitalization From Respiratory Syncytial Virus Infection in High-Risk Infants." *Pediatrics* 102 (3): 531–37.

[109] Battles, Michael B., and Jason S. McLellan. 2019. "Respiratory Syncytial Virus Entry and How to Block It." *Nature Reviews. Microbiology* 17 (4): 233–45.

[110] Homaira, Nusrat, William Rawlinson, Thomas L. Snelling, and Adam Jaffe. 2014. "Effectiveness of Palivizumab in Preventing RSV Hospitalization in High Risk Children: A Real-World Perspective." *International Journal of Pediatrics* 2014 (December): 571609.

[111] DeVincenzo, John P., Richard J. Whitley, Richard L. Mackman, Cecilia Scaglioni-Weinlich, Lisa Harrison, Eric Farrell, Stephen McBride, et al. 2014. "Oral GS-5806 Activity in a Respiratory Syncytial Virus Challenge Study." *The New England Journal of Medicine* 371 (8): 711–22.

[112] Stevens, Marita, Sarah Rusch, John DeVincenzo, Young-In Kim, Lisa Harrison, Elizabeth A. Meals, Alison Boyers, et al. 2018. "Antiviral Activity of Oral JNJ-53718678 in Healthy Adult Volunteers Challenged With Respiratory Syncytial Virus: A Placebo-Controlled Study." *The Journal of Infectious Diseases* 218 (5): 748–56.

[113] Beigel, John H., Hannah H. Nam, Peter L. Adams, Amy Krafft, William L. Ince, Samer S. El-Kamary, and Amy C. Sims. 2019. "Advances in Respiratory Virus Therapeutics - A Meeting Report from the 6th Isirv Antiviral Group Conference." *Antiviral Research* 167 (July): 45–67.

[114] Kim, Jae-Sung, Hong Shik Yun, Hong-Duck Um, Jong Kuk Park, Kee-Ho Lee, Chang-Mo Kang, Su-Jae Lee, and Sang-Gu Hwang. 2012. "Identification of Inositol Polyphosphate 4-Phosphatase Type II as a Novel Tumor Resistance Biomarker in Human Laryngeal Cancer HEp-2 Cells." *Cancer Biology & Therapy* 13 (13): 1307–18.

[115] Lieber, Michael, George Todaro, Barry Smith, Andras Szakal, and Walter Nelson-Rees. 1976. "A Continuous Tumor-Cell Line from a Human Lung Carcinoma with Properties of Type II Alveolar Epithelial Cells." *International Journal of Cancer* 17 (1): 62–70.

[116] Jolad, Shivanand D., R. Clark Lantz, Aniko M. Solyom, Guan Jie Chen, Robert B. Bates, and Barbara N. Timmermann. 2004. "Fresh Organically Grown Ginger (*Zingiber Officinale*): Composition and Effects on LPS-Induced PGE2 Production." *Phytochemistry* 65 (13): 1937–54.

[117] Jolad, Shivanand D., R. Clark Lantz, Guan Jie Chen, Robert B. Bates, and Barbara N. Timmermann. 2005. "Commercially Processed Dry Ginger (Zingiber Officinale): Composition and Effects on LPS-Stimulated PGE2 Production." *Phytochemistry* 66 (13): 1614–35.

[118] Rastogi, Namrata, Shivali Duggal, Shailendra Kumar Singh, Konica Porwal, Vikas Kumar Srivastava, Rakesh Maurya, M. L. B. Bhatt, and Durga Prasad Mishra. 2015. "Proteasome Inhibition Mediates p53 Reactivation and Anti-Cancer Activity of 6-Gingerol in Cervical Cancer Cells." *Oncotarget* 6 (41): 43310–25.

[119] El-Deeb, N., H. El-Adawi, M. Sharaf, and H. A. El Enshasy. n.d. *Targeting Pro-Inflammatory Cytokines and Chemokine as Potential Novel Strategy in Adjuvant Development for Anti- HCV Therapy*. http://nopr.niscair.res.in/handle/123456789/44949

[120] Subbaiah, Ganjikunta Venkata, Kesireddy Sathyavelu Reddy, Yagani JayavardhanaRao, Bhasha Shanmugam, Sahukari Ravi, Kondeti Ramudu Shanmugam, and Golla Narasimha. 2018. "6-Gingerol Prevents Free Transition Metal Ion [Fe (Ii)] Induced Free Radicals Mediated Alterations by *In Vitro* and Ndv Growth in Chicken Eggs by *In Ovo*." *Pharmacognosy Magazine* 14 (55): 167.

[121] Patwardhan, Mayuri, Mark T. Morgan, Vermont Dia, and Doris H. D'Souza. 2020. "Heat Sensitization of Hepatitis A Virus and Tulane Virus Using Grape Seed Extract, Gingerol and Curcumin." *Food Microbiology* 90: 103461.

[122] Schnitzler, Paul, Christine Koch, and Jürgen Reichling. 2007. "Susceptibility of Drug-Resistant Clinical Herpes Simplex Virus

Type 1 Strains to Essential Oils of Ginger, Thyme, Hyssop, and Sandalwood." *Antimicrobial Agents and Chemotherapy* 51 (5): 1859–62.

[123] Koch, C., J. Reichling, J. Schneele, and P. Schnitzler. 2008. "Inhibitory Effect of Essential Oils against Herpes Simplex Virus Type 2." *Phytomedicine: International Journal of Phytotherapy and Phytopharmacology* 15 (1-2): 71–78.

[124] Camero, Michele, Gianvito Lanave, Cristiana Catella, Paolo Capozza, Arturo Gentile, Giuseppe Fracchiolla, Domenico Britti, Vito Martella, Canio Buonavoglia, and Maria Tempesta. 2019. "Virucidal Activity of Ginger Essential Oil against Caprine Alphaherpesvirus-1." *Veterinary Microbiology* 230 (March): 150–55.

[125] Aboubakr, Hamada A., Andrew Nauertz, Nhungoc T. Luong, Shivani Agrawal, Sobhy A. A. El-Sohaimy, Mohammed M. Youssef, and Sagar M. Goyal. 2016. "*In Vitro* Antiviral Activity of Clove and Ginger Aqueous Extracts against Feline Calicivirus, a Surrogate for Human Norovirus." *Journal of Food Protection* 79 (6): 1001–12.

[126] Sharma, Binita Koirala, David Charles Klinzing, and John Donnie Ramos. 2015. "Modulatory Activities of *Zingiber Officinale* Roscoe Methanol Extract on the Expression and Activity of MMPs and TIMPs on Dengue Virus Infected Cells." *Asian Pacific Journal of Tropical Disease* 5 (January): S19–26.

[127] Whitley, R. J., and B. Roizman. 2001. "Herpes Simplex Virus Infections." *The Lancet* 357 (9267): 1513–18.

[128] Boehmer, P. E., and I. R. Lehman. 1997. "Herpes Simplex Virus DNA Replication." *Annual Review of Biochemistry* 66: 347–84.

[129] Arduino, P. G., and S. R. Porter. 2008. "Herpes Simplex Virus Type 1 Infection: Overview on Relevant Clinico-pathological Features." *Journal of Oral Pathology & Medicine: Official Publication of the International Association of Oral Pathologists and the American Academy of Oral Pathology*. https://onlinelibrary-wiley-com.ezproxy.philau.edu/doi/abs/10.1111/j.1600-0714.2007.00586.x.

[130] Engels, M., H. Gelderblom, G. Darai, and H. Ludwig. 1983. "Goat Herpesviruses: Biological and Physicochemical Properties." *The Journal of General Virology* 64 (Pt 10) (October): 2237–47.

[131] Ros, C., and S. Belák. 1999. "Studies of Genetic Relationships between Bovine, Caprine, Cervine, and Rangiferine Alphaherpesviruses and Improved Molecular Methods for Virus Detection and Identification." *Journal of Clinical Microbiology* 37 (5): 1247–53.

[132] Rechenchoski, Daniele Zendrini, Ligia Carla Faccin-Galhardi, Rosa Elisa Carvalho Linhares, and Carlos Nozawa. 2017. "Herpesvirus: An Underestimated Virus." *Folia Microbiologica* 62 (2): 151–56.

[133] Pereira, F. A. 1996. "Herpes Simplex: Evolving Concepts." *Journal of the American Academy of Dermatology* 35 (4): 503–20; quiz 521–22.

[134] Tempesta, M., A. Pratelli, G. Normanno, M. Camero, D. Buonavoglia, G. Greco, and C. Buonavoglia. 2000. "Experimental Intravaginal Infection of Goats with Caprine Herpesvirus 1." *Journal of Veterinary Medicine. B, Infectious Diseases and Veterinary Public Health* 47 (3): 197–201.

[135] Elia, Gabriella, Elvira Tarsitano, Michele Camero, Anna Lucia Bellacicco, Domenico Buonavoglia, Marco Campolo, Nicola Decaro, Julien Thiry, and Maria Tempesta. 2008. "Development of a Real-Time PCR for the Detection and Quantitation of Caprine Herpesvirus 1 in Goats." *Journal of Virological Methods* 148 (1-2): 155–60.

[136] Keuser, Véronique, Frédéric Schynts, Bruno Detry, Alfred Collard, Béatrice Robert, Alain Vanderplasschen, Paul-Pierre Pastoret, and Etienne Thiry. 2004. "Improved Antigenic Methods for Differential Diagnosis of Bovine, Caprine, and Cervine Alphaherpesviruses Related to Bovine Herpesvirus 1." *Journal of Clinical Microbiology* 42 (3): 1228–35.

[137] Quinn, J. P., R. G. Dalziel, and A. A. Nash. 2000. "Herpes Virus Latency in Sensory Ganglia—a Comparison with Endogenous Neuronal Gene Expression." *Progress in Neurobiology* 60 (2): 167–79.

[138] Obara, Y., Y. Furuta, T. Takasu, S. Suzuki, H. Suzuki, S. Matsukawa, Y. Fujioka, H. Takahashi, T. Kurata, and K. Nagashima. 1997. "Distribution of Herpes Simplex Virus Types 1 and 2 Genomes in Human Spinal Ganglia Studied by PCR and in Situ Hybridization." *Journal of Medical Virology* 52 (2): 136–42.

[139] Stanberry, L. R., A. L. Cunningham, A. Mindel, L. L. Scott, S. L. Spruance, F. Y. Aoki, and C. J. Lacey. 2000. "Prospects for Control of Herpes Simplex Virus Disease through Immunization." *Clinical Infectious Diseases: An Official Publication of the Infectious Diseases Society of America* 30 (3): 549–66.

[140] Knipe, David M., and Anna Cliffe. 2008. "Chromatin Control of Herpes Simplex Virus Lytic and Latent Infection." *Nature Reviews. Microbiology* 6 (3): 211–21.

[141] Roizman, Bernard, and Richard J. Whitley. 2013. "An Inquiry into the Molecular Basis of HSV Latency and Reactivation." *Annual Review of Microbiology* 67: 355–74.

[142] Alami Chentoufi, Aziz, Elizabeth Kritzer, David M. Yu, Anthony B. Nesburn, and Lbachir BenMohamed. 2012. "Towards a Rational Design of an Asymptomatic Clinical Herpes Vaccine: The Old, the New, and the Unknown." *Clinical & Developmental Immunology* 2012. http://downloads.hindawi.com/journals/cdi/2012/187585.pdf.

[143] Tempesta, M., M. Camero, G. Greco, A. Pratelli, V. Martella, and C. Buonavoglia. 2001. "A Classical Inactivated Vaccine Induces Protection against Caprine Herpesvirus 1 Infection in Goats." *Vaccine* 19 (28-29): 3860–64.

[144] Thiry, Julien, Véronique Keuser, Benoît Muylkens, François Meurens, Sacha Gogev, Alain Vanderplasschen, and Etienne Thiry. 2006. "Ruminant Alphaherpesviruses Related to Bovine Herpesvirus 1." *Veterinary Research* 37 (2): 169–90.

[145] Marinaro, Mariarosaria, Giovanni Rezza, Giuseppe Del Giudice, Valeriana Colao, Elvira Tarsitano, Michele Camero, Michele Losurdo, Canio Buonavoglia, and Maria Tempesta. 2012. "A Caprine Herpesvirus 1 Vaccine Adjuvanted with MF59™ Protects against

Vaginal Infection and Interferes with the Establishment of Latency in Goats." *PloS One* 7 (4): e34913.

[146] Morfin, Florence, and Danielle Thouvenot. 2003. "Herpes Simplex Virus Resistance to Antiviral Drugs." *Journal of Clinical Virology: The Official Publication of the Pan American Society for Clinical Virology* 26 (1): 29–37.

[147] Danve-Szatanek, C., M. Aymard, D. Thouvenot, F. Morfin, G. Agius, I. Bertin, S. Billaudel, et al. 2004. "Surveillance Network for Herpes Simplex Virus Resistance to Antiviral Drugs: 3-Year Follow-Up." *Journal of Clinical Microbiology* 42 (1): 242–49.

[148] Pino, Jorge A., Rolando Marbot, Aristides Rosado, and Aidelys Batista. 2004. "Chemical Composition of the Essential Oil of Zingiber Officinale Roscoe L. from Cuba." *Journal of Essential Oil Research* 16 (3): 186–88.

[149] Astani, Akram, Jürgen Reichling, and Paul Schnitzler. 2011. "Screening for Antiviral Activities of Isolated Compounds from Essential Oils." *Evidence-Based Complementary and Alternative Medicine: eCAM* 2011 (February): 253643.

[150] Robilotti, Elizabeth, Stan Deresinski, and Benjamin A. Pinsky. 2015. "Norovirus." *Clinical Microbiology Reviews* 28 (1): 134–64.

[151] Vinjé, Jan, Mary K. Estes, Pedro Esteves, Kim Y. Green, Kazuhiko Katayama, Nick J. Knowles, Yvan L'Homme, et al. 2019. "ICTV Virus Taxonomy Profile: Caliciviridae." *The Journal of General Virology* 100 (11): 1469–70.

[152] Graaf, Miranda de, Janko van Beek, and Marion P. G. Koopmans. 2016. "Human Norovirus Transmission and Evolution in a Changing World." *Nature Reviews. Microbiology* 14 (7): 421–33.

[153] Graziano, Vincent R., Forrest C. Walker, Elizabeth A. Kennedy, Jin Wei, Khalil Ettayebi, Madison S. Strine, Renata B. Filler, et al. 2020. "CD300lf Is the Primary Physiologic Receptor of Murine Norovirus but Not Human Norovirus." *PLoS Pathogens* 16 (4): e1008242.

[154] Atmar, Robert L., and Mary K. Estes. 2006. "The Epidemiologic and Clinical Importance of Norovirus Infection." *Gastroenterology Clinics of North America* 35 (2): 275–90, viii.

[155] Galasiti Kankanamalage, Anushka C., Pathum M. Weerawarna, Yunjeong Kim, Kyeong-Ok Chang, and William C. Groutas. 2016. "Anti-Norovirus Therapeutics: A Patent Review (2010-2015)." *Expert Opinion on Therapeutic Patents* 26 (3): 297–308.

[156] Siebenga, J. Joukje, Mathias F. C. Beersma, Harry Vennema, Paula van Biezen, Nico J. Hartwig, and Marion Koopmans. 2008. "High Prevalence of Prolonged Norovirus Shedding and Illness among Hospitalized Patients: A Model for in Vivo Molecular Evolution." *The Journal of Infectious Diseases* 198 (7): 994–1001.

[157] Moore, Matthew D., Rebecca M. Goulter, and Lee-Ann Jaykus. 2015. "Human Norovirus as a Foodborne Pathogen: Challenges and Developments." *Annual Review of Food Science and Technology* 6: 411–33.

[158] Ali, Eunüs S., Harinda Rajapaksha, Jillian M. Carr, and Nikolai Petrovsky. 2016. "Norovirus Drug Candidates That Inhibit Viral Capsid Attachment to Human Histo-Blood Group Antigens." *Antiviral Research* 133 (September): 14–22.

[159] Zhang, Xu-Fu, Ying-Chun Dai, Weiming Zhong, Ming Tan, Zhi-Ping Lv, Ying-Chun Zhou, and Xi Jiang. 2012. "Tannic Acid Inhibited Norovirus Binding to HBGA Receptors, a Study of 50 Chinese Medicinal Herbs." *Bioorganic & Medicinal Chemistry* 20 (4): 1616–23.

[160] Gilling, D. H., M. Kitajima, J. R. Torrey, and K. R. Bright. 2014. "Antiviral Efficacy and Mechanisms of Action of Oregano Essential Oil and Its Primary Component Carvacrol against Murine Norovirus." *Journal of Applied Microbiology* 116 (5): 1149–63.

[161] Prasad, Bv Venkataram, Sreejesh Shanker, Zana Muhaxhiri, Lisheng Deng, Jae-Mun Choi, Mary K. Estes, Yongcheng Song, Timothy Palzkill, and Robert L. Atmar. 2016. "Antiviral Targets of Human Noroviruses." *Current Opinion in Virology* 18 (June): 117–25.

[162] Cristina, Juan, and Mauro Costa-Mattioli. 2007. "Genetic Variability and Molecular Evolution of Hepatitis A Virus." *Virus Research* 127 (2): 151–57.

[163] Stuart, David I., Jingshan Ren, Xiangxi Wang, Zihe Rao, and Elizabeth E. Fry. 2019. "Hepatitis A Virus Capsid Structure." *Cold Spring Harbor Perspectives in Medicine* 9 (5). https://doi.org/10.1101/cshperspect.a031807.

[164] Bishop, N. E., and D. A. Anderson. 1993. "RNA-Dependent Cleavage of VP0 Capsid Protein in Provirions of Hepatitis A Virus." *Virology* 197 (2): 616–23.

[165] Feigelstock, D., P. Thompson, P. Mattoo, Y. Zhang, and G. G. Kaplan. 1998. "The Human Homolog of HAVcr-1 Codes for a Hepatitis A Virus Cellular Receptor." *Journal of Virology* 72 (8): 6621–28.

[166] Silberstein, Erica, Li Xing, Willem van de Beek, Jinhua Lu, Holland Cheng, and Gerardo G. Kaplan. 2003. "Alteration of Hepatitis A Virus (HAV) Particles by a Soluble Form of HAV Cellular Receptor 1 Containing the Immunoglobulin- and Mucin-Like Regions." *Journal of Virology* 77 (16): 8765–74.

[167] Koff, R. S. 1992. "Clinical Manifestations and Diagnosis of Hepatitis A Virus Infection." *Vaccine* 10 Suppl 1: S15–17.

[168] Marosevic, Durdica, Anne Belting, Katharina Schönberger, Anja Carl, Jürgen J. Wenzel, and Roland Brey. 2019. "Hepatitis A Outbreak in the General Population due to a MSM-Associated HAV Genotype Linked to a Food Handler, November 2017–February 2018, Germany." *Food and Environmental Virology* 11 (2): 149–56.

[169] Schmid, D., R. Fretz, G. Buchner, C. König, H. Perner, R. Sollak, A. Tratter, et al. 2008. "Foodborne Outbreak of Hepatitis A, November 2007–January 2008, Austria." *European Journal of Clinical Microbiology & Infectious Diseases: Official Publication of the European Society of Clinical Microbiology* 28 (4): 385.

[170] Sagnelli, Evangelista, Nicola Coppola, Cecilia Marrocco, Mirella Onofrio, Ferdinando Scarano, Anna Marotta, Carlo Scolastico, et al. 2003. "HAV Replication in Acute Hepatitis with Typical and Atypical Clinical Course." *Journal of Medical Virology* 71 (1): 1–6.

[171] Franco, Elisabetta, Cristina Meleleo, Laura Serino, Debora Sorbara, and Laura Zaratti. 2012. "Hepatitis A: Epidemiology and Prevention in Developing Countries." *World Journal of Hepatology* 4 (3): 68–73.

[172] Lavanchy, Daniel. 2012. "Viral Hepatitis: Global Goals for Vaccination." *Journal of Clinical Virology: The Official Publication of the Pan American Society for Clinical Virology* 55 (4): 296–302.

[173] Fleming, Jean. 2002. "Current Treatments for Hepatitis." *Journal of Infusion Nursing: The Official Publication of the Infusion Nurses Society* 25 (6): 379–82.

[174] Tai, Chi-Ming, Chun-Jen Liu, and Ming Yao. 2005. "Successful Treatment of Acute Hepatitis A-Associated Hemophagocytic Syndrome by Intravenous Immunoglobulin." *Journal of the Formosan Medical Association = Taiwan Yi Zhi* 104 (7): 507–10.

[175] Kamolsiripichaiporn, Somjai, Supatsak Subharat, Romphruke Udon, Panithan Thongtha, and Suphachai Nuanualsuwan. 2007. "Thermal Inactivation of Foot-and-Mouth Disease Viruses in Suspension." *Applied and Environmental Microbiology* 73 (22): 7177–84.

[176] Rabaan, Ali A., Shamsah H. Al-Ahmed, Ali M. Bazzi, Wadha A. Alfouzan, Shahab A. Alsuliman, Fatimah A. Aldrazi, and Shafiul Haque. 2020. "Overview of Hepatitis C Infection, Molecular Biology, and New Treatment." *Journal of Infection and Public Health* 13 (5): 773–83.

[177] Ashfaq, Usman A., Tariq Javed, Sidra Rehman, Zafar Nawaz, and Sheikh Riazuddin. 2011. "An Overview of HCV Molecular Biology, Replication and Immune Responses." *Virology Journal* 8 (April): 161.

[178] Barth, Heidi, Raffaele Cerino, Mirko Arcuri, Marco Hoffmann, Peter Schürmann, Mohammed I. Adah, Bettina Gissler, et al. 2005. "Scavenger Receptor Class B Type I and Hepatitis C Virus Infection of Primary Tupaia Hepatocytes." *Journal of Virology* 79 (9): 5774–85.

[179] Agnello, V., G. Abel, M. Elfahal, G. B. Knight, and Q. X. Zhang. 1999. "Hepatitis C Virus and Other Flaviviridae Viruses Enter Cells via Low Density Lipoprotein Receptor." *Proceedings of the National*

Academy of Sciences of the United States of America 96 (22): 12766–71.

[180] Shepard, Colin W., Lyn Finelli, and Miriam J. Alter. 2005. "Global Epidemiology of Hepatitis C Virus Infection." *The Lancet Infectious Diseases* 5 (9): 558–67.

[181] Alter, Miriam J. 2011. "HCV Routes of Transmission: What Goes around Comes around." *Seminars in Liver Disease* 31 (4): 340–46.

[182] Brown, Robert S., Jr, and Paul J. Gaglio. 2003. "Scope of Worldwide Hepatitis C Problem." *Liver Transplantation: Official Publication of the American Association for the Study of Liver Diseases and the International Liver Transplantation Society* 9 (11): S10–13.

[183] Pybus, Oliver G., Peter V. Markov, Anna Wu, and Andrew J. Tatem. 2007. "Investigating the Endemic Transmission of the Hepatitis C Virus." *International Journal for Parasitology* 37 (8-9): 839–49.

[184] Dieperink, E., M. Willenbring, and S. B. Ho. 2000. "Neuropsychiatric Symptoms Associated with Hepatitis C and Interferon Alpha: A Review." *The American Journal of Psychiatry* 157 (6): 867–76.

[185] Hoofnagle, J. H. 1997. "Hepatitis C: The Clinical Spectrum of Disease." *Hepatology* 26 (3 Suppl 1): 15S – 20S.

[186] Kasprzak, Aldona, Jolanta Seidel, Agnieszka Adamek, Wiesława Biczysko, Jacek Wysocki, Rafał Spachacz, Jacek Juszczyk, and Maciej Zabel. 2006. "Interleukin-2 (IL-2) Expression in Livers of Patients with Chronic Hepatitis C Virus (HCV) Infection." *Folia Histochemica et Cytobiologica / Polish Academy of Sciences, Polish Histochemical and Cytochemical Society* 44 (2): 103–10.

[187] Bergqvist, A., and C. M. Rice. 2001. "Transcriptional Activation of the Interleukin-2 Promoter by Hepatitis C Virus Core Protein." *Journal of Virology* 75 (2): 772–81.

[188] Polyak, S. J., K. S. Khabar, M. Rezeiq, and D. R. Gretch. 2001. "Elevated Levels of Interleukin-8 in Serum Are Associated with Hepatitis C Virus Infection and Resistance to Interferon Therapy." *Journal of Virology* 75 (13): 6209–11.

[189] Wilasrusmee, Chumpon, Smita Kittur, Josephine Siddiqui, David Bruch, Skuntala Wilasrusmee, and Dilip S. Kittur. 2002. "In Vitro

Immunomodulatory Effects of Ten Commonly Used Herbs on Murine Lymphocytes." *Journal of Alternative and Complementary Medicine* 8 (4): 467–75.

[190] Zhou, Hua-Li, Yang-Mei Deng, and Qiang-Min Xie. 2006. "The Modulatory Effects of the Volatile Oil of Ginger on the Cellular Immune Response in Vitro and in Vivo in Mice." *Journal of Ethnopharmacology* 105 (1-2): 301–5.

[191] Howley PM, Lowy D. R. 2001. "Papillomaviruses and Their Replication." In *Fields Virology*, edited by Howley P. M. Knipe DM, 4th ed., 2:2197–2229. Philadelphia: Lipincott, Williams, and Wilkins.

[192] Brentjens, Mathijs H., Kimberly A. Yeung-Yue, Patricia C. Lee, and Stephen K. Tyring. 2002. "Human Papillomavirus: A Review." *Dermatologic Clinics* 20 (2): 315–31.

[193] Hausen, H. zur, and E. M. de Villiers. 1994. "Human Papillomaviruses." *Annual Review of Microbiology* 48: 427–47.

[194] Chouhy, Diego, Elisa M. Bolatti, Germán R. Pérez, and Adriana A. Giri. 2013. "Analysis of the Genetic Diversity and Phylogenetic Relationships of Putative Human Papillomavirus Types." *The Journal of General Virology* 94 (Pt 11): 2480–88.

[195] Sapp, Martin, and Patricia M. Day. 2009. "Structure, Attachment and Entry of Polyoma- and Papillomaviruses." *Virology* 384 (2): 400–409.

[196] Joyce, Joseph G., Jwu-Sheng Tung, Craig T. Przysiecki, James C. Cook, E. Dale Lehman, Jeffrey A. Sands, Kathrin U. Jansen, and Paul M. Keller. 1999. "The L1 Major Capsid Protein of Human Papillomavirus Type 11 Recombinant Virus-like Particles Interacts with Heparin and Cell-Surface Glycosaminoglycans on Human Keratinocytes." *The Journal of Biological Chemistry* 274 (9): 5810–22.

[197] Shafti-Keramat, Saeed, Alessandra Handisurya, Ernst Kriehuber, Guerrino Meneguzzi, Katharina Slupetzky, and Reinhard Kirnbauer. 2003. "Different Heparan Sulfate Proteoglycans Serve as Cellular Receptors for Human Papillomaviruses." *Journal of Virology* 77 (24): 13125–35.

[198] Day, Patricia M., Douglas R. Lowy, and John T. Schiller. 2008. "Heparan Sulfate-Independent Cell Binding and Infection with Furin-Precleaved Papillomavirus Capsids." *Journal of Virology* 82 (24): 12565–68.

[199] Ljubojevic, Suzana, and Mihael Skerlev. 2014. "HPV-Associated Diseases." *Clinics in Dermatology* 32 (2): 227–34.

[200] Sanclemente, G., and D. K. Gill. 2002. "Human Papillomavirus Molecular Biology and Pathogenesis." *Journal of the European Academy of Dermatology and Venereology: JEADV* 16 (3): 231–40.

[201] Shepherd, Melissa A., and Mary A. Gerend. 2013. "The Blame Game: Cervical Cancer, Knowledge of Its Link to Human Papillomavirus and Stigma." *Psychology & Health* 29 (1): 94–109.

[202] Dürst, M., A. Kleinheinz, M. Hotz, and L. Gissmann. 1985. "The Physical State of Human Papillomavirus Type 16 DNA in Benign and Malignant Genital Tumours." *The Journal of General Virology* 66 (Pt 7) (July): 1515–22.

[203] Martinez-Zapien, Denise, Francesc Xavier Ruiz, Juline Poirson, André Mitschler, Juan Ramirez, Anne Forster, Alexandra Cousido-Siah, et al. 2016. "Structure of the E6/E6AP/p53 Complex Required for HPV-Mediated Degradation of p53." *Nature* 529 (7587): 541–45.

[204] Trottier, Helen, and Eduardo L. Franco. 2006. "The Epidemiology of Genital Human Papillomavirus Infection." *Vaccine* 24 Suppl 1 (March): S1–15.

[205] Krogh, G. von, and H. I. Maibach. 1982. "Cutaneous Cytodestructive Potency of Lignans. I. A Comparative Evaluation of Influence on Epidermal and Dermal DNA Synthesis and on Dermal Microcirculation in the Hairless Mouse." *Archives for Dermatological Research. Archiv Fur Dermatologische Forschung* 274 (1-2): 9–20.

[206] Krogh, G. von, and H. I. Maibach. 1983. "Cutaneous Cytodestructive Potency of Lignans." *Dermatology* 167 (2): 70–77.

[207] Snoeck, R., M. Bossens, D. Parent, B. Delaere, H. Degreef, M. Van Ranst, J. C. Noël, et al. 2001. "Phase II Double-Blind, Placebo-Controlled Study of the Safety and Efficacy of Cidofovir Topical Gel

for the Treatment of Patients with Human Papillomavirus Infection." *Clinical Infectious Diseases: An Official Publication of the Infectious Diseases Society of America* 33 (5): 597–602.

[208] Longley, Daniel B., D. Paul Harkin, and Patrick G. Johnston. 2003. "5-Fluorouracil: Mechanisms of Action and Clinical Strategies." *Nature Reviews. Cancer* 3 (5): 330–38.

[209] Lacey, Charles J. N. 2005. "Therapy for Genital Human Papillomavirus-Related Disease." *Journal of Clinical Virology: The Official Publication of the Pan American Society for Clinical Virology* 32 Suppl 1 (March): S82–90.

[210] Tyring, S. K., I. Arany, M. A. Stanley, M. A. Tomai, R. L. Miller, M. H. Smith, D. J. McDermott, and H. B. Slade. 1998. "A Randomized, Controlled, Molecular Study of *Condylomata Acuminata* Clearance during Treatment with Imiquimod." *The Journal of Infectious Diseases* 178 (2): 551–55.

[211] Garland, Suzanne M., Susanne K. Kjaer, Nubia Muñoz, Stan L. Block, Darron R. Brown, Mark J. DiNubile, Brianna R. Lindsay, et al. 2016. "Impact and Effectiveness of the Quadrivalent Human Papillomavirus Vaccine: A Systematic Review of 10 Years of Real-World Experience." *Clinical Infectious Diseases: An Official Publication of the Infectious Diseases Society of America* 63 (4): 519–27.

[212] Allen, Kristi L., Deidra R. Tschantz, Keytam S. Awad, William P. Lynch, and Angelo L. DeLucia. 2007. "A Plant Lignan, 3′-O-Methyl-Nordihydroguaiaretic Acid, Suppresses Papillomavirus E6 Protein Function, Stabilizes p53 Protein, and Induces Apoptosis in Cervical Tumor Cells." *Molecular Carcinogenesis: Published in Cooperation with the University of Texas MD Anderson Cancer Center* 46 (7): 564–75.

[213] Munagala, Radha, Hina Kausar, Charu Munjal, and Ramesh C. Gupta. 2011. "Withaferin A Induces p53-Dependent Apoptosis by Repression of HPV Oncogenes and Upregulation of Tumor Suppressor Proteins in Human Cervical Cancer Cells." *Carcinogenesis* 32 (11): 1697–1705.

[214] Blackburn, Christopher, Kenneth M. Gigstad, Paul Hales, Khristofer Garcia, Matthew Jones, Frank J. Bruzzese, Cynthia Barrett, et al. 2010. "Characterization of a New Series of Non-Covalent Proteasome Inhibitors with Exquisite Potency and Selectivity for the 20S β5-Subunit." *Biochemical Journal* 430 (3): 461–76.

[215] Whitehead, Stephen S., Joseph E. Blaney, Anna P. Durbin, and Brian R. Murphy. 2007. "Prospects for a Dengue Virus Vaccine." *Nature Reviews. Microbiology* 5 (7): 518–28.

[216] Kuhn, Richard J., Wei Zhang, Michael G. Rossmann, Sergei V. Pletnev, Jeroen Corver, Edith Lenches, Christopher T. Jones, et al. 2002. "Structure of Dengue Virus: Implications for Flavivirus Organization, Maturation, and Fusion." *Cell* 108 (5): 717–25.

[217] Roehrig, John T. 2003. "Antigenic Structure of Flavivirus Proteins." *Advances in Virus Research* 59: 141–75.

[218] Wahala, Wahala M. P. B., and Aravinda M. de Silva. 2011. "The Human Antibody Response to Dengue Virus Infection." *Viruses* 3 (12): 2374–95.

[219] Bielefeldt-Ohmann, H., M. Meyer, D. R. Fitzpatrick, and J. S. Mackenzie. 2001. "Dengue Virus Binding to Human Leukocyte Cell Lines: Receptor Usage Differs between Cell Types and Virus Strains." *Virus Research* 73 (1): 81–89.

[220] Murrell, Sarah, Suh-Chin Wu, and Michael Butler. 2011. "Review of Dengue Virus and the Development of a Vaccine." *Biotechnology Advances* 29 (2): 239–47.

[221] Endy, Timothy P., Supamit Chunsuttiwat, Ananda Nisalak, Daniel H. Libraty, Sharone Green, Alan L. Rothman, David W. Vaughn, and Francis A. Ennis. 2002. "Epidemiology of Inapparent and Symptomatic Acute Dengue Virus Infection: A Prospective Study of Primary School Children in Kamphaeng Phet, Thailand." *American Journal of Epidemiology* 156 (1): 40–51.

[222] Gubler, D. J. 1998. "Dengue and Dengue Hemorrhagic Fever." *Clinical Microbiology Reviews*. https://cmr-asm-org.ezproxy.philau.edu/content/11/3/480.short.

[223] Halstead, S. B. 1970. "Observations Related to Pathogensis of Dengue Hemorrhagic Fever. VI. Hypotheses and Discussion." *The Yale Journal of Biology and Medicine* 42 (5): 350–62.

[224] Halstead, S.B. 2008. "Dengue Virus–mosquito Interactions." *Annual Review of Entomology*. https://www-annualreviews-org.ezproxy.philau.edu/doi/abs/10.1146/annurev.ento.53.103106.093326.

[225] Rajapakse, Senaka, Chaturaka Rodrigo, and Anoja Rajapakse. 2012. "Treatment of Dengue Fever." *Infection and Drug Resistance* 5 (July): 103–12.

[226] Benelli, Giovanni, and Heinz Mehlhorn. 2016. "Declining Malaria, Rising of Dengue and Zika Virus: Insights for Mosquito Vector Control." *Parasitology Research* 115 (5): 1747–54.

[227] Achee, Nicole L., Fred Gould, T. Alex Perkins, Robert C. Reiner Jr, Amy C. Morrison, Scott A. Ritchie, Duane J. Gubler, Remy Teyssou, and Thomas W. Scott. 2015. "A Critical Assessment of Vector Control for Dengue Prevention." *PLoS Neglected Tropical Diseases* 9 (5): e0003655.

[228] Sengul, Meryem S., and Zhijian Tu. 2010. "Expression Analysis and Knockdown of Two Antennal Odorant-Binding Protein Genes in Aedes Aegypti." *Journal of Insect Science* 10: 171.

[229] Luplerdlop, Natthanej, Dorothée Missé, Dorothy Bray, Virginie Deleuze, Jean-Paul Gonzalez, Vijittra Leardkamolkarn, Hans Yssel, and Francisco Veas. 2006. "Dengue-Virus-Infected Dendritic Cells Trigger Vascular Leakage through Metalloproteinase Overproduction." *EMBO Reports* 7 (11): 1176–81.

[230] Luplertlop, Natthanej, and Dorothée Missé. 2008. "MMP Cellular Responses to Dengue Virus Infection-Induced Vascular Leakage." *Japanese Journal of Infectious Diseases* 61 (4): 298–301.

[231] Yanti, Y., N. Steven, A. Wiharja, and S. Fajarianto. 2011. "Anti-Metalloproteinase-9 Activities of Selected Indonesian Zingiberaceae Rhizome Extracts in Lipopolysaccharide-Induced Human Vascular Endothelial Cells In Vitro." *Planta Medica* 77 (12): PJ3.

[232] Lee, Hyun Sook, Eun Young Seo, Nam E. Kang, and Woo Kyung Kim. 2008. "[6]-Gingerol Inhibits Metastasis of MDA-MB-231

Human Breast Cancer Cells." *The Journal of Nutritional Biochemistry* 19 (5): 313–19.

[233] Ling, H., H. Yang, S-H Tan, W-K Chui, and E-H Chew. 2010. "6-Shogaol, an Active Constituent of Ginger, Inhibits Breast Cancer Cell Invasion by Reducing Matrix Metalloproteinase-9 Expression via Blockade of Nuclear Factor-κB Activation." *British Journal of Pharmacology* 161 (8): 1763–77.

[234] Weng, Chia-Jui, Cheng-Feng Wu, Hsiao-Wen Huang, Chi-Tang Ho, and Gow-Chin Yen. 2010. "Anti-Invasion Effects of 6-Shogaol and 6-Gingerol, Two Active Components in Ginger, on Human Hepatocarcinoma Cells." *Molecular Nutrition & Food Research* 54 (11): 1618–27.

[235] Lu, Min, Zhiqiang Han, Yun Xu, and Lei Yao. 2013. "In Vitro and in Vivo Anti-Tobacco Mosaic Virus Activities of Essential Oils and Individual Compounds." *Journal of Microbiology and Biotechnology* 23 (6): 771–78.

[236] Aldhebiani, Amal Y., Esam K. F. Elbeshehy, Areej A. Baeshen, and Toufic Elbeaino. 2017. "Inhibitory Activity of Different Medicinal Extracts from Thuja Leaves, Ginger Roots, Harmal Seeds and Turmeric Rhizomes against Fig Leaf Mottle-Associated Virus 1 (FLMaV-1) Infecting Figs in Mecca Region." *Saudi Journal of Biological Sciences* 24 (4): 936–44.

[237] Diel, Diego G., Patti J. Miller, Paul C. Wolf, Randall M. Mickley, Anthony R. Musante, Daniel C. Emanueli, Kirk J. Shively, Kerri Pedersen, and Claudio L. Afonso. 2012. "Characterization of Newcastle Disease Viruses Isolated from Cormorant and Gull Species in the United States in 2010." *Avian Diseases* 56 (1): 128–33.

[238] Kaleta, Erhard F., and Christine Baldauf. 1988. "Newcastle Disease in Free-Living and Pet Birds." In *Newcastle Disease*, edited by D. J. Alexander, 197–246. Boston, MA: Springer US.

[239] Ganar, Ketan, Moushumee Das, Sugandha Sinha, and Sachin Kumar. 2014. "Newcastle Disease Virus: Current Status and Our Understanding." *Virus Research* 184 (May): 71–81.

[240] Yusoff, K., and W. S. Tan. 2001. "Newcastle Disease Virus: Macromolecules and Opportunities." *Avian Pathology: Journal of the W.V.P.A* 30 (5): 439–55.

[241] Huang, Zhuhui, Aruna Panda, Subbiah Elankumaran, Dhanasekaran Govindarajan, Daniel D. Rockemann, and Siba K. Samal. 2004. "The Hemagglutinin-Neuraminidase Protein of Newcastle Disease Virus Determines Tropism and Virulence." *Journal of Virology* 78 (8): 4176–84.

[242] Morrison, Trudy G. 2003. "Structure and Function of a Paramyxovirus Fusion Protein." *Biochimica et Biophysica Acta* 1614 (1): 73–84.

[243] Seal, B. S., D. J. King, and H. S. Sellers. 2000. "The Avian Response to Newcastle Disease Virus." *Developmental and Comparative Immunology* 24 (2-3): 257–68.

[244] Alexander, D. J. 2000. "Newcastle Disease and Other Avian Paramyxoviruses." *Revue Scientifique et Technique* 19 (2): 443–62.

[245] Kapczynski, Darrell R., Claudio L. Afonso, and Patti J. Miller. 2013. "Immune Responses of Poultry to Newcastle Disease Virus." *Developmental and Comparative Immunology* 41 (3): 447–53.

[246] Gallili, G. E., and D. Ben-Nathan. 1998. "Newcastle Disease Vaccines." *Biotechnology Advances* 16 (2): 343–66.

[247] Senne, D. A., D. J. King, and D. R. Kapczynski. 2004. "Control of Newcastle Disease by Vaccination." *Developments in Biologicals* 119: 165–70.

[248] Guittet, M., H. Le Coq, M. Morin, V. Jestin, and G. Bennejean. 1993. "Distribution of Newcastle Disease Virus after Challenge in Tissues of Vaccinated Broilers." In *Proceedings of the Tenth World Veterinary Poultry Association Congress, Sydney*. Vol. 179.

[249] Ayala, Andrea J., Kiril M. Dimitrov, Cassidy R. Becker, Iryna V. Goraichuk, Clarice W. Arns, Vitaly I. Bolotin, Helena L. Ferreira, et al. 2016. "Presence of Vaccine-Derived Newcastle Disease Viruses in Wild Birds." *PloS One* 11 (9): e0162484.

[250] Reed, L. J., and H. Muench. 1938. "A Simple Method of Estimating Fifty per cent Endpoints 1 2." *American Journal of Epidemiology* 27 (3): 493–97.

[251] Subbaiah, Kadiam C. Venkata, D. Raniprameela, Gopalareddygari Visweswari, Wudayagiri Rajendra, and Valluru Lokanatha. 2011. "Perturbations in the Antioxidant Metabolism during Newcastle Disease Virus (NDV) Infection in Chicken." *Die Naturwissenschaften* 98 (12): 1019–26. [*Natural Sciences*]

[252] Attia, Atef M. M., Fatma A. A. Ibrahim, Ghada M. Nabil, and Samir W. Aziz. 2013. "Antioxidant Effects of Ginger (Zingiber Officinale Roscoe) against Lead Acetate-Induced Hepatotoxicity in Rats." *African Journal of Pharmacy and Pharmacology* 7 (20): 1213–19.

[253] Peng, Fang, Qiaofeng Tao, Xiumei Wu, Hui Dou, Shawn Spencer, Chaoyong Mang, Lu Xu, et al. 2012. "Cytotoxic, Cytoprotective and Antioxidant Effects of Isolated Phenolic Compounds from Fresh Ginger." *Fitoterapia* 83 (3): 568–85.

[254] Yang, J., W. Zhang, L. Du, H. Wu, and J. Guo. 2018. "Comparative Antioxidant Properties of Some Gingerols and Shogaols, and the Relationship of Their Contents with the Antioxidant Potencies of Fresh and Dried Ginger (*Zingiber Officinale* Roscoe)." http://ir.jkuat.ac.ke/handle/123456789/4303.

[255] Dugasani, Swarnalatha, Mallikarjuna Rao Pichika, Vishna Devi Nadarajah, Madhu Katyayani Balijepalli, Satyanarayana Tandra, and Jayaveera Narsimha Korlakunta. 2010. "Comparative Antioxidant and Anti-Inflammatory Effects of [6]-Gingerol, [8]-Gingerol, [10]-Gingerol and [6]-Shogaol." *Journal of Ethnopharmacology* 127 (2): 515–20.

[256] Schwarz, K. B. 1996. "Oxidative Stress during Viral Infection: A Review." *Free Radical Biology & Medicine* 21 (5): 641–49.

[257] Kamboh, Asghar Ali, Muhammad Ammar Khan, Ubedullah Kaka, Elmutaz Atta Awad, Atta Muhammad Memon, Muhammad Saeed, Nazar Ali Korejo, Manatbai Bakhetgul, and Chandar Kumar. 2018. "Effect of Dietary Supplementation of Phytochemicals on Immunity

and Haematology of Growing Broiler Chickens." *Italian Journal of Animal Science* 17 (4): 1038–43.

[258] Rahman, Sajid ur, Sarzamin Khan, Naila Imtiaz, Umar Siddique, Asad Sultan, Fazal Rahim, and Fawad ur Rahman. 2019. "Phytomedicine (*Allium cepa* L.) Effect on Broiler Immunity against Infectious Diseases." *Biomedical Letters* 5 (1): 1–7.

[259] Naveed, Ghania, Syed Ehtisham-Ul-Haque, Iahtasham Khan, Sajjad Ur Rahman, Sidra Anam, Muhammad Usman, Muhammad Zulqarnain Shakir, Ahsan Naveed, Ghazanfar Abbas, and Faisal Rasheed Anjum. 2020. "Enhancement in Humoral Response against Inactivated Newcastle Disease Vaccine in Broiler Chickens Administered Orally with Plant-Derived Soyasaponin." *Poultry Science* 99 (4): 1921–27.

[260] Namba, K., and G. Stubbs. 1986. "Structure of Tobacco Mosaic Virus at 3.6 A Resolution: Implications for Assembly." *Science* 231 (4744): 1401–6.

[261] Meshi, T., M. Ishikawa, F. Motoyoshi, K. Semba, and Y. Okada. 1986. "In Vitro Transcription of Infectious RNAs from Full-Length cDNAs of Tobacco Mosaic Virus." *Proceedings of the National Academy of Sciences of the United States of America* 83 (14): 5043–47.

[262] Liu, Chengke, and Richard S. Nelson. 2013. "The Cell Biology of Tobacco Mosaic Virus Replication and Movement." *Frontiers in Plant Science* 4 (February): 12.

[263] Kawakami, Shigeki, Yuichiro Watanabe, and Roger N. Beachy. 2004. "Tobacco Mosaic Virus Infection Spreads Cell to Cell as Intact Replication Complexes." *Proceedings of the National Academy of Sciences of the United States of America* 101 (16): 6291–96.

[264] Culver, James N. 2002. "Tobacco Mosaic Virus Assembly and Disassembly: Determinants in Pathogenicity and Resistance." *Annual Review of Phytopathology* 40 (February): 287–308.

[265] Nelson, R. S., P. P. Abel, and R. N. Beachy. 1987. "Lesions and Virus Accumulation in Inoculated Transgenic Tobacco Plants Expressing

the Coat Protein Gene of Tobacco Mosaic Virus." *Virology* 158 (1): 126–32.

[266] Banerjee, N., J. Y. Wang, and M. Zaitlin. 1995. "A Single Nuclcotide Change in the Coat Protein Gene of Tobacco Mosaic Virus Is Involved in the Induction of Severe Chlorosis." *Virology* 207 (1): 234–39.

[267] Dawson, W. O. 1999. "Tobacco Mosaic Virus Virulence and Avirulence." *Philosophical Transactions of the Royal Society of London. Series B, Biological Sciences* 354 (1383): 645–51.

[268] Lehto, Kirsi, Mikko Tikkanen, Jean-Baptiste Hiriart, Virpi Paakkarinen, and Eva-Mari Aro. 2003. "Depletion of the Photosystem II Core Complex in Mature Tobacco Leaves Infected by the Flavum Strain of Tobacco Mosaic Virus." *Molecular Plant-Microbe Interactions: MPMI* 16 (12): 1135–44.

[269] Parish, C. L., M. Zaitlin, and A. Siegel. 1965. "A Study of Necrotic Lesion Formation by Tobacco Mosaic Virus." *Virology* 26 (July): 413–18.

[270] Abbink, Truus E. M., Pernilla A. Tjernberg, John F. Bol, and Huub J. M. Linthorst. 1998. "Tobacco Mosaic Virus Helicase Domain Induces Necrosis in N Gene-Carrying Tobacco in the Absence of Virus Replication." *Molecular Plant-Microbe Interactions: MPMI* 11 (12): 1242–46.

[271] Wu, Xiaoyun, Adrian Valli, Juan Antonio García, Xueping Zhou, and Xiaofei Cheng. 2019. "The Tug-of-War between Plants and Viruses: Great Progress and Many Remaining Questions." *Viruses* 11 (3). https://doi.org/10.3390/v11030203.

[272] Subramanya Sastry, K., and Thomas A. Zitter. 2014. *Plant Virus and Viroid Diseases in the Tropics: Volume 2: Epidemiology and Management*. Springer Science & Business Media.

[273] Cerda, Rolando, Jacques Avelino, Christian Gary, Philippe Tixier, Esther Lechevallier, and Clémentine Allinne. 2017. "Primary and Secondary Yield Losses Caused by Pests and Diseases: Assessment and Modeling in Coffee." *PloS One* 12 (1): e0169133.

[274] Islam, Waqar, Madiha Zaynab, Muhammad Qasim, and Zujian Wu. 2017. "Plant-Virus Interactions: Disease Resistance in Focus." *Hosts and Viruses* 4 (1): 5.

[275] Boualem, Adnane, Catherine Dogimont, and Abdelhafid Bendahmane. 2016. "The Battle for Survival between Viruses and Their Host Plants." *Current Opinion in Virology* 17 (April): 32–38.

[276] Scholthof, Karen-Beth G. 2004. "Tobacco Mosaic Virus: A Model System for Plant Biology." *Annual Review of Phytopathology* 42: 13–34.

[277] Goger, Annelies, Penny Bamber, and Gary Gereffi. 2014. "The Tobacco Global Value Chain in Low-Income Countries." *Center on Globalization, Governance and Competitiveness, Duke University*, 1–48.

[278] Peng, Jiyu, Kunlin Song, Hongyan Zhu, Wenwen Kong, Fei Liu, Tingting Shen, and Yong He. 2017. "Fast Detection of Tobacco Mosaic Virus Infected Tobacco Using Laser-Induced Breakdown Spectroscopy." *Scientific Reports* 7 (March): 44551.

[279] Prabahar, Archana, Subashini Swaminathan, Arul Loganathan, and Ramalingam Jegadeesan. 2015. "Identification of Novel Inhibitors for Tobacco Mosaic Virus Infection in Solanaceae Plants." *Advances in Bioinformatics* 2015 (October): 198214.

[280] Chen, Wei, Wenting Liu, Honghong Jiao, Huawei Zhang, Julong Cheng, and Yunfeng Wu. 2014. "Development of a Concentration Method for Detection of Tobacco Mosaic Virus in Irrigation Water." *Virologica Sinica* 29 (3): 155–61.

[281] Gozzo, Franco, and Franco Faoro. 2013. "Systemic Acquired Resistance (50 Years after Discovery): Moving from the Lab to the Field." *Journal of Agricultural and Food Chemistry* 61 (51): 12473–91.

[282] White, R. F. 1979. "Acetylsalicylic Acid (aspirin) Induces Resistance to Tobacco Mosaic Virus in Tobacco." *Virology* 99 (2): 410–12.

[283] Friedrich, Leslie, Kay Lawton, Wilhelm Ruess, Peter Masner, Nicole Specker, Manuela Gut Rella, Beatrice Meier, et al. 1996. "A Benzothiadiazole Derivative Induces Systemic Acquired Resistance

in Tobacco." *The Plant Journal: For Cell and Molecular Biology* 10 (1): 61–70.

[284] Heil, Martin, and Ian T. Baldwin. 2002. "Fitness Costs of Induced Resistance: Emerging Experimental Support for a Slippery Concept." *Trends in Plant Science* 7 (2): 61–67.

[285] Ziebell, Heiko, and John Peter Carr. 2010. "Cross-Protection: A Century of Mystery." *Advances in Virus Research* 76 (March): 211–64.

[286] Nishiguchi, Masamichi, and Kappei Kobayashi. 2011. "Attenuated Plant Viruses: Preventing Virus Diseases and Understanding the Molecular Mechanism." *Journal of General Plant Pathology: JGPP* 77 (4): 221–29.

[287] Chen, Jia, Xiao-Hui Yan, Jia-Hong Dong, Peng Sang, Xin Fang, Ying-Tong Di, Zhong-Kai Zhang, and Xiao-Jiang Hao. 2009. "Tobacco Mosaic Virus (TMV) Inhibitors from Picrasma Quassioides Benn." *Journal of Agricultural and Food Chemistry* 57 (15): 6590–95.

[288] Dunkić, Valerija, Nada Bezić, Elma Vuko, and Dubravka Cukrov. 2010. "Antiphytoviral Activity of *Satureja Montana* L. Ssp. Variegata (Host) P. W. Ball Essential Oil and Phenol Compounds on CMV and TMV." *Molecules* 15 (10): 6713–21.

[289] Elbeaino, T., M. Digiaro, A. De Stradis, and G. P. Martelli. 2006. "Partial Characterisation of a Closterovirus Associated with a Chlorotic Mottling of Fig." *Journal of Plant Pathology: An International Journal of the Italian Phytopathological Society* 88 (2): 187–92.

[290] Martelli, G. P., A. A. Agranovsky, M. Bar-Joseph, D. Boscia, T. Candresse, R. H. A. Coutts, V. V. Dolja, et al. 2002. "The Family Closteroviridae Revised." *Archives of Virology* 147 (10): 2039–44.

[291] Elbeaino, T., M. Digiaro, A. De Stradis, and G. P. Martelli.2007. "Identification of a Second Member of the Family Closteroviridae in Mosaic-Diseased Figs." *Journal of Plant Pathology: An International Journal of the Italian Phytopathological Society* 89 (1): 119–24.

[292] Afechtal, Mohamed. 2020. "Fig Tree Viruses in Morocco." *Moroccan Journal of Agricultural Sciences* 1 (1). https://www.techagro.org/index.php/MJAS/article/view/819.

[293] Martelli, G. P., M. A. Castellano, and R. Lafortezza. 1993. "An Ultrastructural Study of Fig Mosaic." *Phytopathologia Mediterranea* 32 (1): 33–43.

[294] Flock R. A.and Wallace J. M. 1955. "Transmission of Fig Mosaic by Eriophyid Mite Aceria Ficus." *Phytopathology* 45: 52–54.

[295] Appiano, Anna, M. Conti, and N. Zini. 1994. "Cytopathological Study of the Double-Membrane Bodies Occurring in Fig Plants Affected by Fig Mosaic Disease." In *XVI International Symposium on Fruit Tree Virus Diseases 386*, 585–92. actahort.org.

[296] Alkowni, Raed, Michela Chiumenti, A. Minafra, G. P. Martelli, and Others. 2015. "A Survey for Fig-Infecting Viruses in Palestine." *Journal of Plant Pathology: An International Journal of the Italian Phytopathological Society* 97 (2): 383–86.

[297] Martelli, G. P. 2011. "Chapter 52: Fig Mosaic Disease and Associated Pathogens." In *Virus and Virus-Like Diseases of Pome and Stone Fruits*, 281–87. Virology. The American Phytopathological Society.

[298] Elbeaino, Toufic, Michele Digiaro, Abdulkader Alabdullah, Angelo De Stradis, Angelantonio Minafra, Nicole Mielke, Maria Antonietta Castellano, and Giovanni P. Martelli. 2009. "A Multipartite Single-Stranded Negative-Sense RNA Virus Is the Putative Agent of Fig Mosaic Disease." *The Journal of General Virology* 90 (Pt 5): 1281–88.

[299] Aldhebiani, Amal Y., Esam K. F. Elbeshehy, Areej A. Baeshen, and Toufic Elbeaino. 2015. "Four Viruses Infecting Figs in Western Saudi Arabia." *Phytopathologia Mediterranea* 54 (3): 497–503.

[300] Caglar, Behcet Kemal, Hakan Fidan, Mehmet Ertugrul Guldur, and Toufic Elbeaino. 2011. "The Prevalence of Three Viruses Infecting Fig in Southern Turkey." *Journal of Phytopathology* 159 (3): 181–83.

[301] Latinović, Jelena, Sebastjan Radišek, Milija Bajčeta, Jernej Jakše, and Nedeljko Latinović. 2019. "Viruses Associated with Fig Mosaic Disease in Different Fig Varieties in Montenegro." *The Plant*

Pathology Journal/the Korean Society of Plant Pathology 35 (1): 32–40.

[302] Mathioudakis, M. M., V. Stournaras, and T. Elbeaino. 2020. "First Report of Fig Leaf Mottle-Associated Virus 1 Infecting Common Fig Tree in Greece." *Plant Disease*, March, PDIS – 03–20 – 0466 – PDN.

[303] Çağlayan, Kadriye, Çiğdem Ulubaş Serçe, Eminur Barutçu, Kamuran Kaya, Vicente Medina, Mona Gazel, Soner Soylu, and Oğuzhan Çalışkan. 2010. "Comparison by Sequence-Based and Electron Microscopic Analyses of Fig Mosaic Virus Isolates Obtained from Field and Experimentally Inoculated Fig Plants." *Plant Disease* 94 (12): 1448–52.

[304] Anonymous. n.d. *FAOSTAT.* The Food and Agriculture Organization (FAO) of the United Nations. Accessed July 30, 2020. http://www.fao.org/faostat/en/#data/QC.

[305] Badgujar, Shamkant B., Vainav V. Patel, Atmaram H. Bandivdekar, and Raghunath T. Mahajan. 2014. "Traditional Uses, Phytochemistry and Pharmacology of Ficus Carica: A Review." *Pharmaceutical Biology* 52 (11): 1487–1503.

[306] Chiumenti, M., A. Campanale, G. Bottalico, A. Minafra, A. De Stradis, V. Savino, and G. P. Martelli. 2013. "Sanitation Trials for the Production of Virus-Free Fig Stocks." *Journal of Plant Pathology: An International Journal of the Italian Phytopathological Society* 95 (3): 655–58.

[307] Lillo, Enrico de, Alberto Pozzebon, Domenico Valenzano, and Carlo Duso. 2018. "An Intimate Relationship between Eriophyoid Mites and Their Host Plants - A Review." *Frontiers in Plant Science* 9 (December): 1786.

[308] Usharani, K. V., and Dnm Rl. 2019. "Neem as an Organic Plant Protectant in Agriculture." *of Pharmacognosy and Phytochemistry*. http://www.phytojournal.com/archives/2019/vol8issue3/PartBJ/8-2-197-547.pdf.

[309] Abou-Awad, B. A., B. M. El-Sawaf, A. S. Reda, and A. A. Abdel-Khalek. 2000. "Environmental Management and Biological Aspects of the Two Eriophyoid Fig Mites *Aceria Ficus* (Cotte) and

Rhyncaphytoptus Ficifoliae Keifer in Egypt." *Anzeiger Für Schädlingskunde = Journal of Pest Science* 73 (1): 5–12.

[310] Sniezko, Richard A., and Jennifer Koch. 2017. "Breeding Trees Resistant to Insects and Diseases: Putting Theory into Application." *Biological Invasions* 19 (11): 3377–3400.

[311] Antunes, L. E. C., N. N. J. Chalfun, M. Pasqual, L. F. Dutra, and J. M. Cavalcante-Alves. 2001. "Factors Affecting on Rooting of Figs (*Ficus Carica* L.) Cuttings." In *II International Symposium on Fig 605*, 141–46. actahort.org.

[312] Yahyaoui, E., D. Frasheri, M. A. Germanà, S. Burruano, A. M. D'Onghia, and T. Elbeaino. 2015. "Viruses Infecting Different Mediterranean Genotypes of *Ficus Carica* and Their Distribution in Different Plant Organs." In *V International Symposium on Fig 1173*, 273–78. actahort.org.

[313] Yang, Xicai, Liangyi Kang, and P. O. Tien. 1996. "Resistance of Tomato Infected with Cucumber Mosaic Virus Satellite RNA to Potato Spindle Tuber Viroid." *The Annals of Applied Biology* 129 (3): 543–51.

In: Ginger's Antimicrobial ... ISBN: 978-1-68507-117-2
Editor: Diana R. Cundell

Chapter 5

GINGER AND OSTEOARTHRITIS: CURRENT EVIDENCE FOR EFFICACY AND POSSIBLE FUTURE USES FOR EFFECTIVE DELIVERY SYSTEMS

Diana R. Cundell*[*], *PhD and Karren K. Jensen PhD
College of Life Sciences, Jefferson University, Philadelphia, PA, USA
Retired Technical Writer, Stryker Corporation, Kalamazoo, MI, USA

ABSTRACT

Ginger is a traditional medicine used by many cultures as a poultice or compress to alleviate pain and inflammation associated with swollen joints and rheumatic disorders. The primary activity of ginger involves phenolic gingerols, that are unstable and rapidly undergo decomposition to spicy shogaols. Studies have appeared in the literature that reported excellent anti-inflammatory activity for both gingerols and shogaols against isolated cells, as well as in animal models of osteoarthritis. Several meta-analyses of double-blind randomized placebo-controlled clinical trials (DBRPCT) of ginger have also suggested its potential use for human osteoarthritis

[*] Corresponding Author's E-mail: Diana.Cundell@jefferson.edu.

patients. Osteoarthritis is a major cause of significant morbidity worldwide and current pharmaceutical interventions demonstrate both a lack of efficacy combined with significant side effects associated with long-term use. No current strategies exist to halt or reverse the condition. Patients with osteoarthritis and their health providers are therefore seeking newer, safer alternatives to manage this chronic condition. For many, the answer lies in the incorporation of phytomedicines as complementary therapies. To evaluate whether ginger and its bioactive phenols are potential candidates in managing osteoarthritis, this paper will discuss the history of the use of ginger for this condition and evaluate the scientific evidence from *in vitro* studies and animal models to DBRPCT of the condition. Finally, currently available effective delivery systems for gingerols and shogaols will be discussed as well as potential future strategies.

Keywords: herbal medicine, phytochemical, shogaol, gingerol, osteoarthritis

INTRODUCTION

Zingiber officinale Roscoe, commonly referred to as ginger, is used to manage osteoarthritis in the ethnographic medicine practices of China, India (Ayurvedic), Cambodia, the Middle East (Unani) and several African countries [1-3]. Chinese, Ayurvedic and Umani doctrines suggest grinding the plant's rhizomes into a paste, mixing with water or oil [3, 4] and then applying directly to the area affected as a poultice or compress [1-4]. Ingestion of powdered ginger in the form of a tincture or tea is also recommended for alleviation of osteoarthritis in Cambodian [1] and Ayurvedic traditions [2]. Ginger is also used for the alleviation of rheumatic and arthritic conditions in horses and cattle by veterinarians following the Unani system of medicine [5].

Osteoarthritis, has been with us since ancient times with evidence of joint erosion being seen in Egyptian mummies and even 100-million-year-old dinosaur fossils [6]. Thould and Thould [7] suggest that spinal osteoarthritis in Ancient Roman Britain (100 BC) was very common and appeared in approximately two thirds of all individuals under the age of forty. Interestingly at that time, although gout was recognized by healers such as Hippocrates as an independent condition, osteoarthritis and other arthralgias including rheumatoid arthritis were typically grouped together and managed in a similar way [6]. Osteoarthritis only emerged as an independent entity through the work of William Heberden in 1802 [8]. Since then the condition has become recognized as an important, common chronic inflammatory disease that is ultimately associated with significant patient morbidity [9].

As will be discussed in more detail later, osteoarthritic damage involves the loss of articulating cartilage and eventual remodeling of underlying bones in the synovial joints [9]. Osteoarthritis shares many of its underlying pathophysiology with that of other chronic conditions but has specialized mechanisms that corrupt bone-cartilage homeostasis [9]. For example, synovially-released proinflammatory cytokines, such as interleukin-1-beta (IL-1β) and tumor necrosis factor alpha (TNF-α), intensify cartilage damage both directly [10] and via white cell recruitment into the arthritic joint [9]. This inflammatory cascade is amplified through the release of receptor activator of nuclear factor $\kappa\beta$ (RANKL), which increases bone remodeling [11]. RANKL in turn feeds in to the further generation of proinflammatory cytokines [9] as well as upregulating cellular cyclooxygenase-2 (COX-2) expression [12]. This latter effect of RANKL is important as COX-2 upregulation plays a central role in osteoarthritic-cartilage degeneration through generation of prostaglandin E_2 (PGE_2) [12].

Patients with osteoarthritis find themselves faced with questions on long-term pain-management strategies for a progressive underlying cycle of joint erosion and damage that evolves over a period of 15 to 20 years [13]. Pharmaceutical interventions for many patients revolve around the use of non-steroidal anti-inflammatory drugs (NSAIDs), which although accessible and inexpensive, are associated with significant side effects when taken for more than 6 months [13, 14]. Because these agents directly impair homeostatic activation of the cyclooxygenase pathway they in turn disrupt gastrointestinal mucus secretion [13]. As a direct result, every year around two percent of all patients taking these medications go on to develop gastric ulcers and irritation [13]. Hauser [14] also has also suggested that extended usage of NSAIDs increases the likelihood of getting hip or knee replacements by up to 50% [14]. To avoid these complications, it is believed that somewhere between 50 [15] and 90% [16] of patients with osteoarthritis are now turning to alternative, "old fashioned" herbal medicines as they consider them safer and as effective. One such phytomedicine is ginger, with its track record of successful historical use as not only an ingested but a topical anti-inflammatory agent [2]. In contrast, classically designed double-blind randomized placebo-controlled trials (DBRPCT) of the effects of orally-administered ginger on osteoarthritis have, to date, produced conflicting data, even when similar dosages are used [17].

Could ginger's effects represent a placebo effect for osteoarthritis patients? Certainly, the anti-inflammatory effects of its highly bioactive phenolic gingerols and their metabolites the shogaols would argue to the contrary [2, 3]. *In vitro* studies using a variety of cell types have suggested 6-gingerol and or 6-shogaol can inhibit a number of biochemical inflammatory pathways important in osteoarthritis [18-27]. These including cyclooxygenase-2 (COX-2) [18-20], nitric oxide (NO) [21], reactive oxygen species (ROS) [22, 23] and Kelch-like ECH-associated protein 1 (Keap1)–nuclear factor erythroid 2 p45-related factor 2 (Nrf2) generation [24-26] and the wingless-type/ beta catenin pathway (WNT/β catenin) [27]. Animal models have also supported strong antioxidant roles for 6-gingerol and 6-shogaol in terms of their effects on Nrf2 [26, 28] and glutathione synthase (GSH) [29] activity as well as overall joint protection in arthritic models of disease [30-34]. 6-gingerol or gingerol and shogaol-enriched ginger extract was also reported to reduce *in vitro* inflammation in TNF-α-activated human fibroblast-like synoviocytes [32, 35-37], interleukin-1 beta (IL-1β)- [22, 25] or lipopolysaccharide (LPS)-activated [28] cartilage-building chondrocytes and prevented the activation of bone-resorbing osteoclasts [38]. Further, both gingerols and shogaols have been shown to be agonists of the transient receptor potential cation channel subfamily V member 1 (TRPV1) or vanillin (VR1) receptor and therefore block both peripheral and central nervous system pain perception [39].

Given the diversity of *in vitro* anti-inflammatory and pain-blocking capabilities of gingerols and shogaols, this review is therefore timely in that it will evaluate whether either of these phenolic compounds could be used as complementary medicines for osteoarthritis patients. An evaluation of the data coming from isolated cells, animal models of disease and DBRPCT will be accompanied by an exploration of potential safe delivery systems that might be adopted by individuals worldwide that suffer from this debilitating condition. To fully understand how ginger and its components are affecting the altered biochemistry and pathophysiology underpinning OA, it will first be necessary to understand the mechanisms involved.

Osteoarthritis Pathophysiology

Understanding the underlying pathologies that are involved in OA disease is necessary in identifying whether the phenolic components of ginger might have safe, novel or complementary mechanisms of action. OA is a complex disease involving the loss in effective communication (cross-talk) between cells in the synovial membrane, cartilage and underlying (subchondral) bone (Figure 1) [9, 33, 40-55].

Synoviocyte Activation as an Initiating Event

Several pathways of inflammation including those of synoviocyte activation and release of DAMPs, IL-1β, LTB_4 and LTC_4 and TLR-4, RANKL and WNT/β catenin expression by chondrocytes are central to the pathology of OA (Figure 1). As cartilage becomes damaged through various methods in early OA including trauma, naturally through aging or genetically-induced cartilage instability, protein fragments are released that activate macrophages in the synovial membrane (synoviocyte macrophages) [9]. Experimental evidence suggests that during OA the synoviocyte macrophage changes to those able to release DAMP alarmin proteins, chiefly S100A8/A9, which in turn maintain an inflammatory environment in the synovial joint [52].

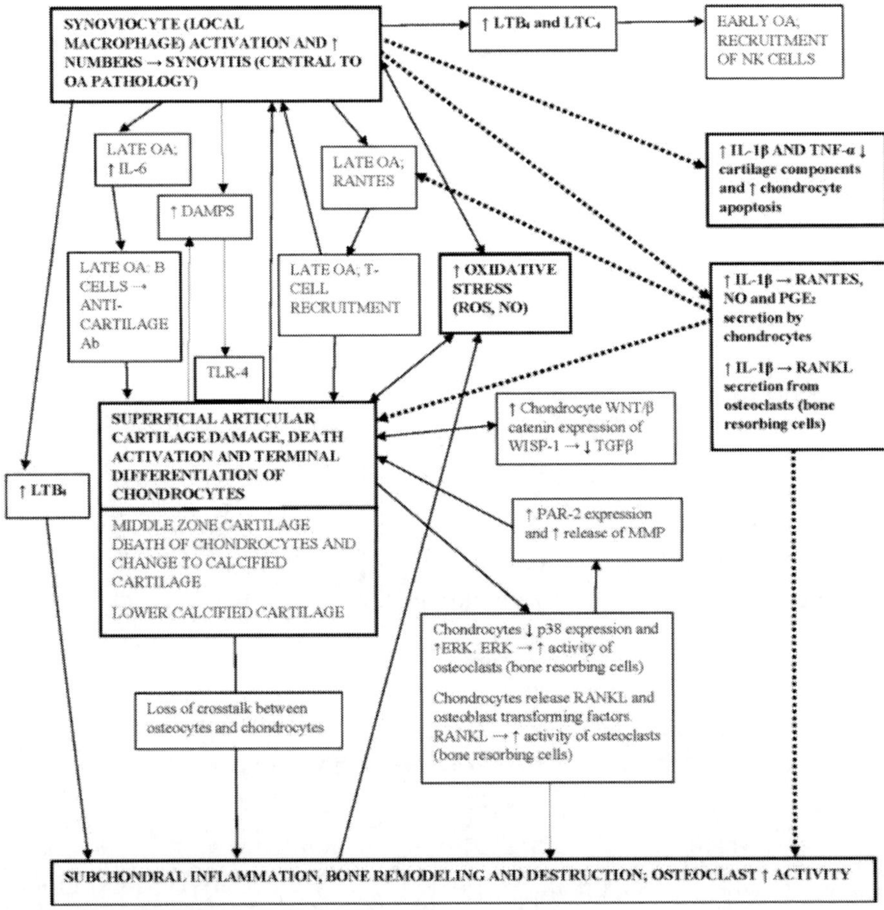

Figure 1. Pathophysiology of OA = major effects of IL-1β in osteoarthritis, heavier lines indicate important pathways. Abbreviations used: Ab (antibodies), COX-2 (cyclooxygenase 2), DAMPS (damage-associated molecular patterns), ERK (extracellular released kinases), IL-1β (interleukin-1 beta), IL-6 (interleukin-6), LTB_4 (leukotriene B_4), LTC_4 (leukotriene C_4), Nrf2 (Kelch-like ECH-associated protein 1 (Keap1)–nuclear factor erythroid 2 p45-related factor 2), NO (nitric oxide), PGE_2 (prostaglandin E_2), RANKL (receptor activator of nuclear factor κβ), RANTES/CCL5 (regulated upon activation, normal T cell expressed and presumably secreted), ROS (reactive oxygen species), TGFβ (transforming growth factor beta), TLR (Toll like receptor), TNF-α (tumor necrosis factor alpha), WNT/β catenin (wingless type/ beta catenin pathway). Legend: Disintegrating cartilage fragments activate synovial cells [40]. Synoviocytes (macrophages) then maintain the inflammatory environment in the joint initially through their release of IL-1β and TNF-α [9, 40, 41]. IL-1β-activated synovial macrophages release inflammatory mediators to recruit immune system cells into the area [42-45]. Early in inflammation LTB_4 and LTC_4 recruit NK cells to the synovium [42]. Later in OA the synovial cell release of RANTES [43, 44] and IL-6 [45] recruit T cells and B cells, respectively. IL-1β directly effects cartilage and bone homogeneity [46-49]. Chondrocytes exposed to IL-1β upregulate RANKL [46], which in turn upregulates secretion of proinflammatory pathways resulting in chemokine RANTES/CCL5 [47], cytokine IL-6 [46] and PGE_2 [48, 49] pathways. Chondrocyte Nrf2 suppression contributes to oxidative stress by upregulating NO [48] and ROS generation [9, 46]. Activated chondrocytes increase their generation of WISP-1 through the WNT/β catenin pathway and depress their generation of TGFβ [9]. Damaged cartilage and activated synoviocytes also release DAMPS, which signals the transition from early to late phase OA [9, 52-55]. Activation of RANKL and ERK pathways in cartilage chondrocytes also stimulates the activities of bone osteoclasts to decrease the integrity of underlying bone [50, 51]. LTB_4 released by activated synovial cells and recruited white cells also directly damages bone [42]. RANKL activation in osteoclasts also occurs directly following IL-1β exposure [33].

Upregulation of TLR-4 expression on chondrocytes occurs following their interaction with these synoviocyte S-100 mobility protein [53, 54]. TLR-4, like all Toll receptors, activates nuclear factor kappa beta (NFκβ); an event central to continued cytokine secretion, arachidonic metabolism and generation of ROS and NO by stimulated cells [55]. Elevated levels of S-100 have been found in the synovial fluid of patients with OA and their levels appear to correlate with disease severity [53].

IL-1β Is Central to Decreased OA Cartilage Integrity

IL-1β has multiple effects on cartilage integrity by promoting matrix reabsorption [41, 48, 49], decreasing cartilage collagen manufacture [9] and increasing chondrocyte death [48, 49]. Indirect damage to the synovial joint occurs when IL-1β interacts with TNF-α to generate the cytokine IL-6, which recruits autoreactive B cells to the synovial joint [9, 45]. Synovial macrophages [43] and chondrocytes [47] exposed to IL-1β stimulation of synovial macrophages [43] and chondrocytes [47] upregulates manufacture of RANTES/CCL5, which recruits damaging T cells into the synovial membrane and cartilage surface [44]. Chondrocytes exposed to IL-1β upregulate expression of RANKL [46]. RANKL activation in chondrocytes creates an inflammatory environment in the articular cartilage through activating pathways that decrease TGFβ expression [9] as well as generate NO, ROS and IL-6 [9, 46].

OA Is an Inflammatory Disease Involving NO and ROS

Normally, cellular elevations in ROS and NO are reduced by the activation of Nrf2 and redox enzymes such as GSH, which in turn switch off inflammation through cross talk with nuclear factor kappa beta (NFκβ) expression [56]. Chondrocytes are particularly sensitive to ROS, and when their levels of these oxidants outstrip those able to be inactivated by scavenging systems like GSH, a cycle of cellular activation, cartilage destruction and cell death results [57]. Activation of nitric oxide synthase (NOS) in both synoviocytes and chondrocytes results in NO and is also associated with continued joint erosion and inflammation characteristic of OA [57]. Chondrocyte RANKL and ERK overexpression in turn increases the reactivity of osteoclast (bone resorbing cells), thus undermining bone integrity by increasing bone resorption [49, 50].

RANKL Activation Results in Mobilization of Arachidonic Acid Mediators

RANKL activation has another major effect on chondrocytes; it upregulates genes that increase arachidonic acid metabolism [9]. Proinflammatory lipid metabolites of arachidonic acid play a major role in OA pathogenesis [48, 49, 51]. Macrophages in the synovial membrane generate LTB_4 and LTC_4 through the lipoxygenase (LOX) pathway which recruit NK cells to the synovium and also directly damage bone [42]. Arachidonic acid, metabolized through the cyclooxygenase COX-2 enzyme pathway to produce PGE_2, also plays a role in cartilage and bone homeostasis by negatively influencing the activity of chondrocytes [48, 49]. As well as participating in cross-talk with NO to increase inflammation, elevated PGE_2 also causes the expression of stromolysin by chondrocytes, which exacerbates cartilage degeneration [48, 49]. Bone homogeneity requires low levels of PGE_2 to be secreted by osteoblasts and during uptick in expression bone is regenerated [50]. This latter effect of PGE_2 may explain why subchondral bone is increased in thickness during OA versus the thinning seen in articular cartilage.

Cartilage Matrix Breakdown Involves the WNT/β Catenin Pathway

WNT/β catenin pathway activation results in the increased expression of induced signaling protein 1 (WISP-1) in the synovial membrane, cartilage and bone [57]. WISP-1 upregulates degrading enzymes such as aggrecans and metalloproteinases (MMP), increasing cartilage matrix breakdown [58]. Osteoblasts divide and mature in the presence of WISP-1, thereby contributing to reactive bone thickening that is characteristic of OA [59]. WISP-1 inhibits the secretion of a TGF-β receptor-regulator protein, termed Smad-2, thus blocking this pathway's signaling [59]. Maintaining TGF-β levels is essential to maintain healthy cartilage and in animal models its removal results in a syndrome resembling OA with synovial inflammation and cartilage destruction [60]. As a result, healthy bone and cartilage demonstrate a low expression of WNT/β catenin [61] and high levels of TGF-β [62], whereas for OA bone this is reversed [62, 63].

Gingerols, Shogaols and Enriched Ginger Extract and OA: *In Vitro* and Animal Studies

Osteoarthritis is a disabling inflammatory process characterized by an interaction between multiple cell types including synoviocyte macrophages, cartilage building chondrocytes and bone building and sculpting osteoblasts and osteoclasts [9]. Management of the progressive damage caused by OA and associated debilitating pain is customarily achieved through the use of pharmaceutical products which carry the risk of unintended consequences due to side-effects of the drug. In contrast, ginger-based treatments are desirable because they are food-based and generally recognized as safe. The challenge in using naturally occurring substances, such as ginger/ginger-based components, is to identify the efficacy of these substances in a quantifiable and evidence-based way. The following classes of experimental studies seek to address this issue using both cellular studies and in vivo systemic treatment protocols.

In Vitro Studies of Ginger and Its Components on OA Cells

To date, eight studies have been performed to directly examine the effects of ginger and its bioactive components on OA cells [22, 25, 28, 31, 32, 36-38]. The findings of these studies and their results are summarized in Table 1.

All eight studies reported positive findings with either pure gingerols [25, 37], shogaols [28, 31], or ginger extract [22, 32, 36, 37]. It is to be noted that two of the ginger extract studies employed the commercially available product EV.EXT77 [36, 37] and one reported it to be as effective as the steroid betamethasone [37]. EV.EXT77 is standardized for its content of gingerols and shogaols but also contains a second inflammatory phytomedicine; *Alpinia galanga* (galangal) [36, 37]. Four studies addressed the effects of ginger and its components on human [22, 25, 28] or murine [31] chondrocytes. Although diverse parameters of OA chondrocyte damage and inflammation were examined in these studies two common themes appeared emerge [22, 25, 28, 31]. The first was a reported improvement in antioxidant status (elevated ROS) [22] in cells exposed to ginger and its extracts, through Nrf2 activation [28]. Abusarah et al. [25], using transfected cells, reported that overexpression of Nrf2 prevented chondrocytes from being damaged by IL-1β. Further, transfected cells with lowered Nrf2 activity were not protected from damage by ginger and its extracts [25]. These findings directly connected ginger with the ability to reverse Nrf2 dysregulation [25].

Further support for ginger affecting Nrf2 activating came from Villavilla et al. [28]. These authors reported that 6-gingerol reversed the effects of IL-1β on cultured human OA chondrocytes with a concomitant increase in the expression of Nrf2 and antioxidant enzymes and decrease in MMP enzymes. Similar cytoprotective effects were also seen in 4-hydroxynonenal (HNE)-damaged chondrocytes pre-treated with 6-gingerol [25] and insulin-transferrin selenium (ITS)-damaged murine chondrocytes [31]. Like IL-1β, HNE has been demonstrated to directly disrupt cartilage and ultimately bone integrity by upregulating MMP and other inflammatory genes [25].

Table 1. Effect of ginger, gingerols and shogaols on isolated OA cells

Study design	Results	Reference
C218 human chondrocyte cells pre-treated with ginger extract (5 or 25 μg/ml) for 24 h then incubated with IL-1β (10 ng/ml) for 24 h. Effects on ROS production, lipid peroxidation and expressions of Bax, Bcl-2, and caspase-3 proteins assessed.	No cytotoxicity for ginger extract at any concentration. Significant ($p<0.05$) ↑gene expression of antioxidant enzymes and reduced IL-1β-induced elevation of ROS, lipid peroxidation, Bax/Bcl-2 ratio, and caspase-3 activity	[22]
Human OA knee cartilage chondrocytes were incubated with IL-1β (1 ng/ml) or HNE (20 μM) in the presence or absence of protandim or 6-gingerol (0-10 μg/ml) for 24 h. Effects on Nrf2 and β-actin expression were assessed.	Protandim and 6-gingerol ↓ OA cartilage degradation via Nrf2 activation. Nrf2 in turn attenuated oxidative stress, catabolic and inflammatory responses through GSTA4-4 activation.	[25]
Human chondrocytes were treated with 6-shaogaol (5 μM) and assayed for cytokine activity after exposure to LPS (1 μg/ml) or IL-1β (1 ng/ml) for 24 h. Assessment of innate immune responses by analysis of TLR-4 signaling, ERK 1/2 activation, NO production and cathepsin K activity. Reduction of cartilage degradation was also determined by measuring MMP2 and MMP9 activity.	6-Shaogaol completely inhibited TLR4-mediated innate immune responses and significantly reduced (p <).05) MMP induction in chondrocytes.	[28]
Murine ATDC chondrocyte line was stimulated with ITS and treated with 6-shogaol (5 μM) for up to 21 days in culture.	6-shogaol significantly MMP-13 expression ($p<0.05$) in the tumor chondrocyte line. Ihh and collagen expression were significantly ($p<0.05$) ↓ results suggesting the chondrocytes were prevented from undergoing terminal differentiation.	[31]
Human synovial cells were isolated from OA patients, treated with ginger extract (1 or 2 mg/ml for 30 minutes) and exposed to IL-1β (10 ng/ml)	Reverse transcriptase analysis of the synoviocytes demonstrated that both ginger extract dosages significantly ($p<0.015$) ↓ expression of both MMP-3 and MMP-13	[32]
Human synovial cells were cultivated for 1h in the presence or absence of a EV.EXT77 ginger extract (100 μg/ml) followed by TNF-α (1 ng/ml) for 1 h and cultured for 24h.	Ginger extract significantly ($p<0.05$) ↓ mRNA expression of the inflammatory chemokines MCP-1 and IP-10	[36]
Human synovial cells were cultivated for 72 h in the presence or absence of TNF-α (1 ng/ml) or in the presence or absence of 1 mg/ml of either betamethasone, ibuprofen or ginger extract (EV.EXT77).	Ginger extract significantly ($p<0.05$) ↓ IL-1β, IL-6 and IL-8 secretion and was as effective an anti-inflammatory as betamethasone	[37]
Co-culture of primary mouse calvarial osteoblasts and bone marrow-derived macrophages was treated with 6-gingerol (0 to 20 μM) for 7 days. Analysis of inflammatory RANKL expression, PGE_2 levels, and COX-2 mRNA expression were made.	6-gingerol inhibited IL-1-induced osteoclast differentiation by ↓ RANKL and PGE_2 levels in osteoblasts.	[38]

Abbreviations used in the table: Bax (Bcl-2 associated X protein), Bcl-2 (B cell lymphoma 2), COX-2 (cyclooxygenase 2), ERK-1/2 (Ras dependent extracellular signal-regulated kinase pathway), h (hours), GSTA4-4 (Glutathione S-Transferase Alpha *4)*, HNE (4-hydroxy-2-nonenal), Ihh (Indian hedgehog), IL (interleukin), IL-1β (interleukin 1-beta), IP-10 (interferon gamma activated protein), ITS (insulin transferrin selenium), LPS (lipopolysaccharide), MMP (matrix metalloproteinase), MCP-1 (macrophage chemotactic factor), mRNA (messenger ribosenucleic acid), NO (nitric oxide), Nrf2 (Nuclear factor erythroid 2-related factor 2), PGE_2 (prostaglandin E2), RANKL (Receptor activator of nuclear factor kappa-B ligand), ROS (reactive oxygen species), TLR-4 (toll-like receptor 4) and TNF-α (tumor necrosis factor alpha).

As previously stated, oxidative stress is one of the major initiating events for OA resulting in chondrocyte damage as well as crosstalk and upregulation of bone resorbing osteoclasts [49, 50, 57].

An additional effect was a decrease in OA chondrocyte apoptosis through mechanisms involving decreased cathepsin B activity [28] and an improved cellular Bcl-2/Bax expression [22]. Interestingly, gingerols and shogaols bear a close structural similarity with extant cathepsin K inhibitors [28] already being tested for use in osteoporosis [63]. Cathepsin K inhibitors are the pharmaceutical holy grail for osteodegenerative diseases as they could prevent bone resorption without effect on cells involved in bone synthesis and sculpting [63]. Unfortunately, all the cathepsin K inhibitors produced have never successfully passed phase III clinical trials [64], but it might be hoped that the natural gingerols and shogaols may be more successful. Gratal et al. [31] also found that 6-shogaol (5 μM), reduced the expression of the Indian hedgehog (Ihh) gene, associated with chondrocyte maturation [65], and collagen X, a product of hypertrophic (terminally differentiating) chondrocytes [66]. These studies all suggest that ginger, gingerol and shogaol are cytoprotective to chondrocytes.

Three studies examined the effects of ginger extracts on cultured human synovial cells [32, 36 37]. Hwang et al. [32], characterized their ginger extract and found it to contain a mixture of primarily 6-shogaol (0.7%) and 6-shogaol (0.24%) with lesser quantities of vanillylacetone (0.11%). These authors reported that the ginger extract significantly ($p<0.05$) decreased the expression of MMP enzymes [32], suggesting an antioxidant effect for the ginger similar to that seen in chondrocytes [28]. Two studies reported it downregulated mRNA expression of various inflammatory cytokines including MCP-1 [36], IP-10 [36] and interleukins IL-1β, Il-6 and IL-8 [37]. The observation by Ribel-Madsen et al. [37] that EV.EXT77 was equivalent to betamethasone and ibuprofen is an interesting one. Both these agents are effective by downregulating NF-κB [9], which would in turn reduce the generation of cytokines by the synoviocyte cells.

Finally, a murine study reported 6-gingerol was able to decrease osteoclast development by impairing PGE_2 and RANKL expression [38]. Although not yet confirmed by other investigators, this latter observation is exciting as RANKL's upregulation in activated osteoblasts plays a central feedback role in osteoarthritic-cartilage degeneration [12].

In Vivo Preclinical (Animal) Studies of Ginger and Its Components on Experimental Arthritis Models

Five studies have been performed to directly examine the effects of ginger and its bioactive components on arthritic models (OA and RA) [30-34] (Table 2).

Each of the five animal studies of OA/RA explored the effects of ginger for a month allowing for at least data comparisons [30-34]. Two studies utilized pure 6-shogaol [31 and 33] and reported that low dosages of > 20 mg/Kg/day were able to significantly ($p<0.05$) reduce inflammation and swelling compared with untreated animals. Two other studies employed ethanol-extracts of *Z. officinale* plant material [30, 34] and reported similar efficacy. Interestingly, ethanolic extraction selectively distills primarily gingerols [67], and although the two rodent studies employed nearly a 10-fold difference in dosages, both reported a similar anti-arthritic efficacy As with many promising naturally occurring pharmacologically significant substances, targeting a single molecule may lead to reduced efficacy and unintended side-effects simply because the naturally occurring system contains multiple factors which work synergistically to achieve the optimum result. This was suggested by the identification of vanillylacetone, 6-gingerol, 6-shogaol, and 1,4-cineol and the primary compounds in the boiling water ginger extract of the study by Hwang et al. [32].

Table 2. Effect of ginger, gingerols and shogaols on animal models of OA

Study design	Results	Reference
Female Lewis rats were injected with *Streptococcus pyogenes* peptidoglycan-polysaccharide polymers to produce an OA/ RA model system. Animals received ethanol-fractionated ginger (26 mg/Kg/day) or crude ginger via IP injection daily for 14 days and thereafter twice daily. Joint and liver histology was assessed on day 28.	Both ginger preparations prevented joint inflammation and destruction. Crude extract was more effective suggesting that other polar compounds enhance the gingerol effects. Gingerols possessed a better safety profile *viz a viz* animal mortality.	[30]
C57BL/6 mice with surgically-induced OA, were given 6-shogaol (15 mg/kg/day) between days 22 and 35 post-induction of OA. Cartilage damage and hypertrophic markers Collagen X and MMP13 were evaluated.	6-shogaol significantly prevented cartilage degradation and synovial inflammation in parallel with reducing the presence of hypertrophic markers.	[31]
Collagen-induced arthritis model (incomplete Freund's adjuvant) of OA/RA was created using DBA/1J mice. Animals were gavaged with water, or ginger extract (boiling water; 100 mg/kg or 200 mg/kg) daily from days 22-35 after arthritis induction.	Ginger extract significantly decreased ($p<0.05$) inflammatory bone destruction in joint tissues at day 36 through inhibition of mRNA expression for the cytokines IFN-γ and IL-17.	[32]
Sprague-Dawley rats were treated with 0.5 mg/ml CFA for 28 days to induce arthritis of the right knee. Animals gavaged with daily oral doses of peanut oil or 6-shogaol (6.2 mg/kg) for 28 days. Histological studies, and synovial leucocyte infiltration was assessed.	6-shogaol treated group showed significantly ↓ ($p<0.05$) knee swelling, serum VCAM-1 and infiltration of leucocytes. Femoral cartilage was preserved in the 6-shogaol group as compared to the control group.	[33]
Albino rats were injected with monosodium iodoacetate in knee joint to induce OA. Ginger (alcohol extract) and curcumin (200 mg/kg and 400 mg/kg, respectively) were orally administered for 28 days. Serum inflammatory parameters and histopathology of joints was assessed at day 28.	Serum levels of COMP, HA, MPO, MDA, and IL-1β were significantly ↓ ($p<0.05$) in rats treated with ginger or curcumin at all doses when compared to control. SOD levels significantly ($p<0.05$) ↑ in treated groups compared to OA groups.	[34]

Abbreviations used in the table: CFA (complete Freund's adjuvant), COMP (cartilage oligomeric matrix protein), HA (hyaluronic acid), IL-1β (interleukin 1 beta), ITS (insulin transferrin selenium), MDA (malondialdehyde), MMP (matrix metalloproteinase), MPO (myeloperoxidase), IP (intraperitoneal), SOD (superoxide dismutase), VCAM-1 (vascular adhesion molecule 1).

IN VITRO AND ANIMAL DATA SUGGEST GINGEROLS AND SHOGAOLS INHIBIT MULTIPLE OA PATHWAYS

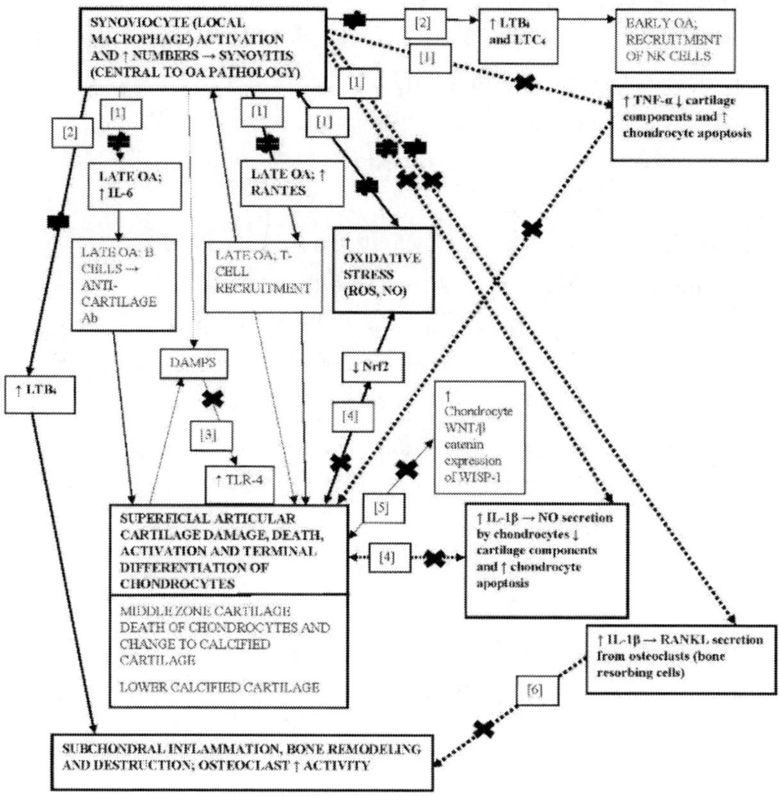

Figure 2. OA pathways inhibited by gingerol, shogaol or enriched ginger extract = major effects of IL-1β in OA = *in vitro* effects of gingerols, shogaols or enriched ginger extract on cells involved in OA = *in vitro* effects of gingerols, shogaols or enriched ginger extract on other human cells. Legend: Only pathways potentially affected by gingerols or shogaols are highlighted in this figure. Heavier lines indicate pathways playing a major role in OA. Six target pathways have been identified for either gingerol and shogaol enriched ginger extract, 6-gingerol, 6 shogaol or 10-shogaol as indicated by numbers [1] through [6]. Pathways [1] and [2] involve synoviocyte mediated effects on cartilage and bone integrity. Three chondrocyte meditated pathways are also affected; DAMPs expression [3], oxidative stress [4] and [4] WNT/β catenin. 6-gingerol inhibits the IL-1β-mediated upregulation of RANKL expression by osteoclasts preventing destabilization of bone integrity [6]. Abbreviations used: Ab (antibodies), COX-2 (cyclooxygenase 2), ERK (extracellular released kinases), IL-1β (interleukin-1 beta), IL-6 (interleukin-6), LTB_4 (leukotriene B_4), LTC_4 (leukotriene C_4), NO (nitric oxide), PGE_2 (prostaglandin E_2), Nrf2 (RANKL (receptor activator of nuclear factor κβ), RANTES/CCL5 (regulated upon activation, normal T cell expressed and presumably secreted), ROS (reactive oxygen species), TGFβ (transforming growth factor beta), TLR-4 (Toll like receptor 4), TNF-α (tumor necrosis factor alpha), WNT/ β catenin (wingless type/ β catenin pathway).

Although OA results from the action of multiple pathways it has become apparent that inhibiting each separately does not eliminate all symptoms [68-70]. For example, although IL-1β is recognized as essential to the pathogenesis of both early and late stage OA all published literature has reported that directly inhibiting IL-1β was ineffective in animal models of OA [68]. Individual recombinant IL-1β has not proven successful in any human trials [68]. Inhibiting PGE_2 levels in the cartilage-bone environment also proved to be a double-edged sword in OA, given that COX-2 inhibitors inhibit bone integrity [69] and also produce a diversion of all arachidonic acid metabolism through the LOX pathway [42]. Attempts to produce a combination COX/LOX inhibitor proved unsuccessful [70]. The only agent developed commercially was Flavocoxid™ and this was later withdrawn following reports of negative liver enzyme effects in some OA patients [70].

In contrast, gingerols and shogaols have been shown, at least *in vitro*, to inhibit several separate OA inflammatory pathways (Figure 2).

References [2, 27, 28, 35, 37, 71-74] were used in preparation of the figure.

OA Synoviocyte Activation and Inflammatory Cell Influx is Reduced or Prevented

Enriched ginger extract [71] and 6-gingerol [73] have effects on a number of OA pathways affecting synoviocyte macrophages [35] or human macrophages [74] including the inhibition of inflammatory cytokines/chemokine TNF-α, IL-1β, RANTES and IL-6 release [35, 71, 72]. Once cytokine production is blocked in these cells they also decrease their secretion of inflammatory ROS and NO [72]. Ginger extract and 10-shogaol can also inhibit the activation of lipoxygenase pathways in U937 human macrophage cells *in vitro* [74]. This decreases lipoxygenase generation of LTB_4 and LTC_4 [74]. Finally, studies by Ribel-Madsen et al. [37] reported that a ginger extract was able to directly inhibit three important inflammatory cytokines in human synoviocytes, namely IL-1β, IL-6 and IL-8. Combined reduction in IL-6, LTB_4 and LTC_4 would in turn prevent the infiltration of NK cells, autoreactive B cells and damaging T cells to the synovial membrane [9].

OA Chondrocyte Apoptosis and Cartilage Turnover Are Reduced or Prevented

Ginger extract and 10-shogaol can also inhibit the activation of both cyclooxygenase and lipoxygenase pathways in U937 human macrophage cells *in vitro* [74]. This decreases COX-2 generation of PGE_2, directly preventing chondrocyte apoptosis [48]. Chondrocyte activation and apoptosis and ROS production induced by IL-1β is down-regulated by gingerol and shogaol-enriched ginger extract *in vitro* [22]. Studies by Gratal et al. [31], also reported that 6-shogaol prevented the terminal differentiation and demise of human chondrocyte cells. TLR-4 expression in chondrocytes stimulated by the bacterial factor lipopolysaccharide (LPS) and the resulting ERK and NO secretion is also decreased by 6-shogaol *in vitro* [28]. Studies by Ahn et al. [75] reported that 6-shogaol was able to directly bind to the TLR-4 receptor *in vitro* and prevent its homodimerization i.e., prevent it from further activating cellular biochemical pathways.

Given that 6-shogaol has been shown to modulate Nrf2 [26, 28] and glutathione synthase (GSH) expression [29], which would combine to decrease ROS and NO generation by these cells [9], part of ginger's efficacy appears to lie in its anti-oxidant effects. Aborehab et al. [34] have also reported that an ethanolic extract of ginger (enriched with gingerols) reduced inflammation in an OA rodent model by increasing superoxide dismutase (SOD) expression 6-Gingerol can upregulate protein USP49 *in vitro* and inhibit the chondrocyte WNT/β catenin signaling pathway [27]. This latter effect would allow a consistent expression of TGF-β [59-61] and a consequent maintenance of cartilage integrity. Finally, one study reported that 6-shogaol treatment was able to reduce serum levels of VCAM-1 [33]. Human studies have found that VCAM-1 expression is predictive of severe OA, since this molecule mediates influx of leukocytes into the synovial joint [9, 76].

OA Reactive Bone Thickening is Reduced or Prevented

In vitro studies reported that 6-gingerol decreased IL-1β-induced RANKL production by osteoclast (bone resorbing cells) *in vitro* and also the increased PGE_2 secretion that resulted upon their activation [38]. Prevention of RANKL activation maintains bone integrity by suppressing osteoclast-induced bone resorption [49, 50]. Lowering PGE_2 secretion promotes effective osteoblast activity and prevents reactive bone thickening [51]. The combined effects of 6-gingerol on these two processes would therefore prevent the reactive bone thickening that is a hallmark of OA disease.

Human Data for Ginger and OA Have Produced Conflicting Data

Human studies are, of course, the most significant indicator that gingerol/shogaol/ginger extract treatments hold a significant promise for OA treatment. Double-blind randomized placebo-controlled trials (DBRPCT) have proven to be the tried and trusted accepted method to ensure observer bias does not affect patient findings in clinical studies [77]. Two large meta-analyses of DBRPCT ginger and its components have appeared in the literature during the past five years that are of note in this respect [17, 78]. Bartels et al. [78] surveyed six major literature studies databases for DBRPCT of the effects of ginger on human OA. They retrieved 123 studies of which seven met their criteria in that they were human studies with full articles and not letters [78]. Two other human studies were discarded as one did not contain a placebo control group and in the second, ginger was not orally administered [78]. Bartels et al. [78] reported that the five studies they analyzed comprised a total of 543 OA patients and their data suggested oral ginger was effective in reducing the pain and stiffness associated with hip and knee arthritis. These authors further stated that oral ginger had a positive safety profile when taking in doses varying between 500 and 1000 mg/ day [78]. Interestingly, two of these human OA studies with positive outcomes employed the EV.EXT77 ginger extract that had been previously investigated on isolated human synovial cells [36, 37].

The second meta-analysis, by Araya-Quintanilla et al. [17] used the same six databases as those of Bartels et al. [78] to identify randomized clinical trials of ginger used either orally or topically for the treatment of human knee OA. Interestingly, although this study was performed five years after that of Bartels et al. [78] they included only seven studies in their original analysis [17]. Araya-Quintanilla et al. [17], eliminated three of the seven initial studies due to "assessing inflammatory aspects", leaving four for their final data. Two studies were common to both meta-analyses and the second meta-analysis also included a DBRPCT by Niempong et al. [79], which did report positive data on knee OA. Araya-Quintanilla et al. [17] were not satisfied that ginger was effective in managing knee OA citing no follow up of patients and no statistical difference in pain or stiffness. Both studies criticized the variability in dosage, source and preparation methodology of the ginger used in the human studies as well as the duration of the study (between 3 and 12 weeks) [17, 78].

None of the DBRPCT utilized purified gingerols or shogaols or preparations standardized for these components, although they were likely to be present in the ginger powders used [36, 37]. In addition, three studies that were not included in the meta-analyses used as they were single blind involved topical applications of ginger to OA affected joints [80-82]. Therkleson [80] used a ginger poultice (hot water extract of ginger powder) applied daily to patients with chronic osteoarthritis. Although this small study of forty patients with mild to moderate osteoarthritis was not repeated, it is to be noted that over the six months that the patients applied the poultice their health satisfaction significantly ($p<0.05$) improved pain, stiffness and overall health satisfaction [80]. Amorndoljai et al. [81, 82] took a slightly different approach, using instead nanoparticle stabilized ginger extract (enriched with gingerols and shogaols). In two separate single-blind, randomized, placebo-controlled trials these authors studied sixty knee osteoarthritis patients who rubbed the nanoparticle-ginger into their knee three times a day for three months. Both studies reported significant ($p< 0.05$) improvement in movement, quality of life and pain [81, 82]. The second study compared the efficacy of the nanoparticle preparation with 0.1% diclofenac gel and reported that the ginger nanoparticles were superior in efficacy ($p<0.05$). All three studies observed these preparations were safe and effective.

Conclusion and Potential Ways Forward for Ginger

Although ginger and its biochemically active constituents the gingerols and shogaols have significant anti-inflammatory activity, as demonstrated using *in vitro*, pre-clinical and some human DBRPCT (Tables 1 and 2, section 4.0) for most of the general population use of this spice is still associated with settling an upset stomach [1, 3]. Many orthopedists are now of the opinion that identification of risk factors and prevention of degenerative changes, in the early phase of osteoarthritis will be key in slowing down or halting the progression of the disease [83].

Gingerols and shogaols simultaneously inhibit at least six different important pathways in OA (Figure 2). In keeping with many anti-inflammatory phytochemical moieties [84], gingerol and shogaol are able to inhibit cytokines including TNF-α, IL-1β, RANTES and IL-6 [36, 41, 42]. Interestingly, several OA pathways inhibited by 6-gingerol, 6-shogaol or 10-shogaol have no currently available pharmaceutical interventions but do have the potential to decrease symptoms as they address the underlying inflammatory mechanisms key to OA symptoms. Of particular interest in this regard are TLR-4 inhibition, Nrf2 regulator and WNT antagonism. Having them combined into one agent, or a pair of related agents like 6-gingerol and 6-shogaol is particularly desirable as it would redirect multiple inflammatory pathways simultaneously [85-87]. In contrast, the NSAID medications used particularly during early to moderate OA, inhibit NFκβ-mediated COX-2 activation [88] and pro-inflammatory cytokine IL-6 and IL-8 release [89]. As was previously stated, inhibition of COX-2 shifts the entire metabolism of arachidonic acid towards the LOX mediators LTB_4 and LTC_4 and is therefore undesirable [42].

TLR-4, Nrf2 and WNT/β Catenin Activities: Three Reasons to Develop 6-Gingerol and 6-Shogoal for OA

The report that 6-shogaol is a specific inhibitor of TLR-4 receptors is one of particular interest [88]. Unlike the other pathways, TLR-expression is both directly connected to the “crossing over” of early to later stage disease and the initiation of inflammatory processes [86]. Prevention of TLR-4 activation of the NFκβ or RANKL pathways would therefore indirectly inhibit the inflammatory pathways seen in OA [56]. Given that oxidative stress is believed by many researchers to be central to the pathophysiology of OA, as it is with most chronic inflammatory diseases [89], the Nrf2 properties of 6-gingerol are also of interest [25]. Nrf2 inhibition has been a “holy grail” for researchers as an answer to managing many chronic inflammatory diseases, including OA, and it is of note that many agents currently in phase II and III clinical trials are plant-derived molecules [56, 90]. This is also the case for research into novel anti-TLR-4 [86] and anti-RANKL molecules [91]. Phytochemicals also feature prominently in the list of WNT/β catenin antagonists being tested as tumoricidal agents as they dampen down the chronic inflammatory processes associated with the condition [92]. If the *in vitro* activities of 6-Gingerol to inhibit the chondrocyte WNT/β catenin signaling pathway are translated to *in vivo* efficacy this could have potential for both OA and tumor interventions [27]. By preventing the early stages of inflammation from progressing into later, aggressive disease, an optimal formulation of gingerols and shogaols has the potential to be of great benefit to many OA sufferers.

Could 6-Gingerol and 6-Shogaol Be Developed into Oral Medicinal AGENTS?

Acceptance of the use of spices and herbal entities by the medical community has encountered two major barriers; a lack of active chemical standardization coupled with poor absorption through the gastrointestinal tract and subsequent lability of the effective phytochemicals [84]. Ginger spice and supplements certainly do vary significantly in their content of gingerols and shogaols, as previously discussed, and may not even contain any bioactive ingredients at all [93-95]. Ginger powder, for example, was reported in three separate studies to contain anywhere from 0.036–13.8 mg/g of gingerols and 0.2-6.62 mg/g of shogaols [93-95]. Analysis of more than twenty commercial ginger supplements, by Marx et al. [94] and Schwertner et al. [95] found that gingerol and shogaol levels ranged from between 0 to 66 mg/kg and 0 to 16 mg/kg, respectively.

Ingested gingerols and shogaols are absorbed from the gastrointestinal tract and appear in the bloodstream as conjugated forms [96, 97]. A study by Zick et al. [96] reported that 6-, 8- and 10-gingerol and 6-shogaol-conjugates appeared in human plasma one hour after ingestion of ginger extract (0.1-2 g). These were fully eliminated two hours following the initial ingestion [88]. As gingerols are phenolic their bioavailability, even in conjugate form, appears poor with maximum plasma concentrations of less than a thousandth of a percent being detected [4]. For example, ingestion of 2 mg of pure 6-gingerol resulted in a maximum plasma concentration of only 0.85 μg/ml [96]. More recent studies by Levita et al. [97], using a higher dosage of ginger (2g/15 ml) have suggested a more rapid human digestive absorption of 10-gingerol and 6-shogaol. In these studies, maximum plasma concentrations were reached after 38 minutes and 43 minutes for 10-gingerol and 6-shogaol, respectively [97]. Further the elimination half-lives for the two components were 336 and 143 minutes, for 10-gingerol and 6-shogaol, respectively [97].

Clearly both studies support the ability of the native bioactive components of ginger being absorbed to some degree following ingestion, but they do raise the question of optimal dosage if the native spice is being studied. Nanoparticles that are able to both successfully release gingerol or shogaol and produce biological effects upon ingestion already exist [98-100]. Demonstrated as safe and non-toxic in animal models of other types of chronic inflammatory disease [98-100], these are now awaiting the results of DBRPCT to confirm their usage in osteoarthritis patients.

Transdermal Delivery for 6-Gingerol and 6-Shogaol Represents an Optimal Safe Use for OA Patients

Developing new oral medications to help manage OA may, however, not what patients with this condition actually want [16]. Studies by Callahan et al. [16] reported that nearly two-thirds of the patients with arthritis they surveyed used rubs (topical applications) and preferred these types of transdermal interventions. Transdermal absorption is an issue for many molecules because of their size and level of lipid solubility or affinity [101]. Early studies by Finnin and Morgan [101], observed that molecules that could penetrate the skin were both highly lipophilic and with a molecular weight of < 500 Daltons. Both gingerols and shogaols fulfill these characteristics making them ideal candidates for transdermal application [102].

Gingerols and shogaols have been reported in several studies to have good transdermal penetration [102-106]. Park et al. [103] reported that topical application of 6-gingerol was able to prevent the phorbol esterase-induced appearance of skin papilloma tumors in mice. Later studies by Minzetti et al. [102] supported these findings and determined that an enriched dry ginger extract of 6-gingerol was able to penetrate both *ex vivo* human and murine epidermal tissue (6.9 and 22.1 μg/cm^2, respectively). Shogaol (10-shogaol) has also been reported to penetrate human skin as well as act as promote the growth of normal human keratinocytes and fibroblasts *in vitro* [104]. Padher [105] produced a cream containing a combination of 6-gingerol (13%) and piperine (10%), which was effective in reducing swelling in a rat paw edema model of arthritis over a one-month period. Using *ex vivo* skin from the animals, Padher reported that approximately

60% of the 6-gingerol was absorbed into the skin from the gingerol-piperine cream [105]. Piperine was used a bioenhancer in this study since it is known to increase the bioavailability of herbal medications by as much as 30% [107]. A similar approach may be needed if native gingerol or shogaols or used topically.

Alternatively, enclosing the phenols in nanoparticles is a strategy that has proven successful in stably delivering other lipid herbal entities into the skin [9]. Viswanathan et al. [106], recently successfully employed just such an approach to incorporate gingerols into lecithin-based vesicles. This group reported rapid and effective passage of the nanoparticles through *ex vivo* goat skin, with an 85% release rate of the stabilized gingerols [106]. This would seem to be a good lead technology for ginger delivery, especially given the preliminary positive data seen in two single blind nanoparticle OA studies [81, 82].

Antinociceptive activities of gingerols and shogaols are able to block pain signals by binding to transient receptor potential cation channel subfamily V member 1 (TRPV1) or vanillin (VR1) receptors [108]. They share this ability as both are structural analogs of capsaicin [108]. Interestingly, most over-the-counter topical pain-relieving creams either contain capsaicin or a second herbal-derived agent, menthol (BenGay™ and Icy Hot™) [16, 109]. Menthol also blocks pain by acting on TRPV1 receptors, albeit via a different mechanism [110]. Both are effective antinociceptive agents, and a recent meta-analysis has even suggested topical capsaicin may be superior to ingested NSAIDS in relieving osteoarthritis pain [110].

Patients with osteoarthritis who are taking aspirin and NSAIDs should avoid ingesting high doses of oral gingerols as these agents can increase clotting times by inhibiting platelet association [111]. Topical application would avoid such interactions and seems to be a good, safe, and relatively inexpensive route to pursue for future gingerol and shogaol management of osteoarthritis. Most pharmaceuticals currently being approved for use by the United States Food and Drug Administration (FDA) are for oral use (62%), injectables and topical medications do constitute 22 and 9% respectively [112]. According to Zhong et al. [112], who recently reviewed this topic, the primary rationale for avoiding the skin as a delivery route is that it provides a "high technical barrier" i.e., are difficult to produce effectively. Conversely, topical medications have fewer limiting factors in terms of safety as they are primarily required only to not produce irritation at the site of injury and to be non-toxic, should they be ingested [112].

Transdermal delivery technologies for pharmaceuticals are relatively recent, with medications of this kind beginning in 1999 [112], and they have become more prevalent over the past decade [113]. By comparison Ayurvedic and traditional Chinese Medicine have used similar, albeit more crude systems for thousands of years so use of this type of strategy is neither new or acceptable for most residents of developing countries [114]. Many new cases of osteoarthritis are predicted to come from residents of developing nations such as India and China, with the condition anticipated to affect over one hundred million people by 2050 [9]. Cost and accessibility are going to be big considerations especially for these populations and, given the established trust in herbal medicines, it is time for scientific technologies to improve on traditional medicine techniques. As the appeal of using natural products increases, these authors would suggest DBRPCT using nanoparticle-stabilized gingerol and or shogaol creams or rubs would provide scientific support for their use and allow the millions of sufferers worldwide a safer pain relief alternative to oral medications, certainly during the early stages of the condition.

FINAL THOUGHTS

As our understanding of OA as a condition with distinct stages, multiple pathways and individual responses has become more apparent, it is clear that treatment strategies must now evolve. Grässer and Muschter in their recent evaluation of OA management state,

> "Recent advances in OA pathology have enlightened key roles of several new pathways, which can be targeted. However, as OA is a highly heterogeneous disease, a single therapeutic targeting a single joint tissue

> may not be effective and no "one size fits all" drug/therapy will ever be developed. Improved patient stratification in combination with advanced DMOADs and cell-based therapies might lead to the development of personalized OA therapeutics." [85].

Phytomedicines with a history of safety and ability to target multiple biochemical pathways simultaneously [84], including ginger, are good prospects for this type of therapy. Whether used as native molecules, incorporated into nanoparticles or as semi-synthetic variants 6-gingerol and 6-shogaol have the potential to be effective in OA management strategies of the future. The family Zingiberaceae has already yielded curcumin from turmeric (*Curcuma longa*) as a now common anti-OA complementary therapy [9] and gingerols and shogaols from ginger have the potential to follow suit once modified into an effective deliverable.

References

[1] Sharifi-Rad, Mehdi, Elena M. Varoni, Bahare Salehi, Javad Sharifi-Rad, Karl R. Matthews, Seyed A. Ayatollahi, Farzad Kobarfard, Salam A. Ibrahim, Dima Mnayer, Zainul A. Zakaria, Majid Sharifi-Rad, Zubaida Yousaf, Marcello Iriti, Adriana Basile, and Daniela Rigano 2017. "Plants of the Genus *Zingiber* as a Source of Bioactive Phytochemicals: From Tradition to Pharmacy". *Molecules (*Basel, Switzerland), 22(12): 2145. Accessed on April 19, 2021. https://doi.org/10.3390/molecules22122145

[2] Therkleson, Tessa 2012. "Chapter 8: Ginger and Osteoarthritis". In *Osteoarthritis - Diagnosis, Treatment and Surgery*. Edited by Qian Chen, IntechOpen. Accessed on April 19, 2021. doi: 10.5772/26274.

[3] Semwal, Ruchi B., Deepak K. Semwal, Sandra Combrinck, and Alvaro M. Viljoen 2015. "Gingerols and shogaols: Important nutraceutical principles from ginger". *Phytochemistry*, 117: 554-468. Accessed on April 19, 2021. http://dx.doi.org/10.1016/j. phytochem.2015.07.012.

[4] Chopra, Arvind, Manjit Saluja, and Girish Tillu 2010. "Ayurveda-modern medicine interface: A critical appraisal of studies of Ayurvedic medicines to treat osteoarthritis and rheumatoid arthritis". *J. Ayurveda Integr. Med.*, 1(3):190-198. Accessed on April 19, 2021. doi:10.4103/0975-9476.72620

[5] Blumenthal, Mark 1999. "Herbal Medicines". *AORN Journal*, 70: 384-384. Accessed on April 19, 2021. doi:10.1016/S0001-2092(06)62318-1

[6] Reginster, Jean-Yves. 2014. "Introduction: historical and current perspectives on osteoarthritis". In: *Atlas of Osteoarthritis*. Springer Healthcare, Tarporley. Accessed on April 19, 2021. https://doi.org/10.1007/978-1-910315-16-3_1

[7] Thould, A.K., and B.T. Thould 1983. "Arthritis in Roman Britain". *Br. Med. J. (Clin. Res. Ed.)*, 287(6409):1909-1911. Accessed on April 19, 2021. doi:10.1136/bmj.287.6409.1909.

[8] Sherk, Henry K. 2004. "Commentaries on the history and cure of diseases". Digitorum Nodi by William Heberden MD. *Clin. Orthop. Relat. Res.*, (427 Suppl): S3-4. Accessed on April 19, 2021. PMID: 15480071.

[9] Cundell, Diana R., and Kathryn Mickle 2018. "Osteoarthritis; potential for herbal medicines as therapies in the management of chronic inflammatory disease". *Current Immunology Reviews*, 14(2): 68-80. Accessed on April 19, 2021. doi:10.2174/157339551 4666180530093702.

[10] Boileau, Christelle, Nathalie Amiable, Johanne Martel-Pelletier, Hassan Fahmi, Nicolas Duval, and Jean-Pierre Pelletier 2007. "Activation of proteinase-activated receptor 2 in human osteoarthritic cartilage upregulates catabolic and proinflammatory pathways capable of inducing cartilage degradation: A basic science study". *Arthritis Res Ther.*, 9: R121:1-R121:10. Accessed on April 19, 2021. doi: 10.1186/ar2329.

[11] Upton, Angus R., Christopher A. Holding, and Anak A.S.S. Dharmapatni, and David R. Haynes 2012. "The expression of RANKL and OPG in the various grades of osteoarthritic cartilage". *Rheumatol.*

Int., 32: 535-540. Accessed on April 19, 2021. doi: 10.1007/s00296-010-1733-6.

[12] Coon, David, Ajay Gulati, Cameron Cowan, and Jianing He J 2007. "The role of cyclooxygenase-2 (COX-2) in inflammatory bone resorption". *J Endod.,* 33(4):432-6. Accessed on April 19, 2021. doi: 10.1016/j.joen.2006.12.001.

[13] Hudson, N., M. Balsitis, S. Everett, and C.J. Hawkey 1993. "Enhanced gastric mucosal leukotriene B4 synthesis in patients taking non-steroidal anti-inflammatory drugs". *Gut*, 34:742-747. Accessed on April 19, 2021. doi: 10.1136/gut.34.6.742.

[14] Hauser, Ross 2010. "The acceleration of articular cartilage degeneration in osteoarthritis by nonsteroidal anti-inflammatory drugs". *Journal of Prolotherapy*, 2(1): 305-322. Accessed on April 19, 2021. https://www.journalofprolotherapy.com/pdfs/issue_05/issue_05_10_nsaids.pdf.

[15] Lapane, K.L., M.R. Sands, S. Yang, T.E. McAlindon, and C.B. Eaton 2012. "Use of complementary and alternative medicine among patients with radiographic-confirmed knee osteoarthritis". *Osteoarthritis Cartilage*, 20(1):22-8. Accessed on April 19, 2021. doi: 10.1016/j.joca.2011.10.005.

[16] Callahan, Leigh F., Elizabeth K. Wiley-Exley, Thelma J. Mielenz, Chiangfu Xiao, Shannon S. Currey, Betsy L. Sleath, Philip D. Sloane, Robert F. DeVellis, Teresa J Brady, and Joseph Sniezek 2009. "Use of complementary and alternative medicine among patients with arthritis". *Prev. Chronic Dis.*, 6(2): A44. Accessed on April 19, 2021. https://www.ncbi.nlm.nih.gov/pmc/articles/PMC2687850/

[17] Araya-Quintanilla, F., H. Gutierrez-Espinoza, M.J. Munoz-Yanez, U. Sanchez-Montoya, and J. Lopez-Jeldes 2020. "Effectiveness of Ginger on Pain and Function in Knee Osteoarthritis: A PRISMA Systematic Review and Meta-Analysis". *Pain Physician*, 23(2): E151-E161. Accessed on April 19, 2021. PMID: 32214292.

[18] Dugasani, Swarnalatha, Mallikarjuna R. Pichika, Vishna D. Nadarajah, Madhu K. Ballijepalli, Satyanaranaya Tandra, and Javaveera N. Korlakunta 2010. "Comparative antioxidant and anti-

inflammatory effects of [6]-gingerol, [8]-gingerol, [10]-gingerol and [6]-shogaol". *Journal of Ethnopharmacology*, 127(2):515-520. Accessed on April 19, 2021. doi: 10.1016/j.jep.2009.10.004.

[19] Lantz, R.C., G.J. Chen, M. Sarihan A.M. Sólyom, S.D. Jolad, and B.N. Timmermann 2007. "The effect of extracts from ginger rhizome on inflammatory mediator production". *Phytomedicine*, 14:123–8. Accessed on April 19, 2021. doi: 10.1016/j.phymed.2006.03.003.

[20] Li, Xiao-Hong, Kristine C.Y. McGrath, Van H. Tran, Yi-Ming Li, Colin C. Duke, Basil D. Roufogalis, and Alison K. Heather 2013. "Attenuation of proinflammatory responses by S-[6]-gingerol via inhibition of ROS/NF-kappa B/COX2 activation of HuH7 cells". *Evidence-Based Complementary and Alternative Medicine,* 2013; 13:146142. Accessed on April 19, 2021. doi: 10.1155/2013/146142.

[21] Pan, Min-Hsiung, Min-Chi Hsieh, Jin-Min Kuo, Ching-Shu Lai, Hou Wu, Shengming Sang, and Chi-Tang Ho 2008. "[6]-Shogaol induces apoptosis in human colorectal carcinoma cells via ROS production, caspase activation, and GADD 153 expression". *Mol. Nutr. Food Res.*, 52:527–37. Accessed on April 19, 2021. doi: 10.1002/mnfr.200700157.

[22] Hosseinzadeh, A., K.B. Juybari, M.J. Fatemi, T. Kamarul, A. Bagheri, N. Tekiyehmaroof, and A.M. Sharifi 2017. "Protective effect of ginger (*Zingiber officinale* Roscoe) extract against oxidative stress and mitochondrial apoptosis induced by interleukin-1 beta in cultured chondrocytes". *Cells Tissues Organs*, 204:241–250. Accessed on April 19, 2021. doi: 10.1159/000479789.

[23] Nonaka, Kohei, Mika Bando, Eijiro Sakamoto, Yuji Inagaki, Koji Naruishi, Hiromichi Yumoto, and Jun-ichi Kido 2019. "6-Shogaol Inhibits Advanced Glycation End-Products-Induced IL-6 and ICAM-1 Expression by Regulating Oxidative Responses in Human Gingival Fibroblasts". *Molecules*, 24(20):3705. Accessed on April 19, 2021. doi:10.3390/molecules24203705

[24] Zhu, Yingdong, Pei Wang, Yantao Zhao, Chun Yang, Anderson Clark, TinChung Leung, Xiaoxin Chen, and Shengmin Sang 2016. "Synthesis, evaluation, and metabolism of novel [6]-shogaol

derivatives as potent Nrf2 activators". *Free Radical Biology and Medicine*, 95: 243-254. Accessed on April 19, 2021. https://doi.org/10.1016/j.freeradbiomed.2016.03.026.

[25] Abusarah, Jamila, Houda Benabdoune, Qin Shi, Bertrand Lussier, Johanne Martel-Pelletier, Michel Malo, Julio C. Fernandes, Fátima P. de Souza, Hassan Fahmi, and Mohamed Benderdour 2017. "Elucidating the Role of Protandim and 6-Gingerol in Protection Against Osteoarthritis". *J. Cell. Biochem.*, 118: 1003-1013. Accessed on April 19, 2021. doi:10.1002/jcb.25659

[26] Chen, Huadong, Junsheng Fu, Hao Chen, Yuhui Hu, Dominique N. Soroka, Justin R. Prigge, Edward E. Schmidt, Feng Yan, Michael B. Major, Xiaoxin Chen, and Shengmin Sang 2014. "Ginger compound [6]-shogaol and its cysteine-conjugated metabolite (M2) activate Nrf2 in colon epithelial cells *in vitro* and *in vivo*. *Chem. Res. Toxicol.*, 27:1575–1585. Accessed on April 19, 2021. doi: 10.1021/tx500211x.

[27] Yang, Lanbo, Zhanchao Wang, Chunyu Zou, Yufei Mi, Hengtao Tang, and Xuejian Wu 2020. "Ubiquitin-specific protease 49 attenuates IL-1β-induced rat primary chondrocyte apoptosis by facilitating Axin deubiquitination and subsequent Wnt/β-catenin signaling cascade inhibition". *Mol. Cell. Biochem.*, 2020; 474: 263–275. Accessed on April 19, 2021. https://doi.org/10.1007/s11010-020-03850-3.

[28] Villalvilla, Amanda, Jame's A. da Silva, Raquel Largo, Oreste Gualillo, Paulo C. Vieira, Gabriel Herrero-Beaumont, and Rodolfo Gómez 2014. "6-Shogaol inhibits chondrocytes' innate immune responses and cathepsin-K activity". *Mol. Nutr. Food Res.*, 58: 256-266. Accessed on April 19, 2021. doi:10.1002/mnfr.201200833.

[29] Saiah, Wassila, Hanane Halzoune, Rabah Djaziri, Khadidja Tabani, Elhadj A. Koceir, and Naomi Omari 2018. "Antioxidant and gastroprotective actions of butanol fraction of *Zingiber officinale* against diclofenac sodium-induced gastric damage in rats". *J. Food Biochem.*, 42: e12456. Accessed on April 19, 2021. doi: 10.1111/jfbc.12456.

[30] Funk, Janet L., Jennifer B. Frye, Janice N. Oyarzo, and Barbara N. Timmermann 2009. "Comparative effects of two gingerol-containing *Zingiber officinale* extracts on experimental rheumatoid arthritis". *J. Nat. Prod.*, 72(3):403-407. Accessed on April 19, 2021. doi:10.1021/np8006183.

[31] Gratal, P., A. Lamuedra, and A. Mediero 2018. "AB0102 The ginger derivative 6-shogaol as a treatment in osteoarthritis. Modulation of chondrocyte hypertrophy and matrix calcification". *Annals of the Rheumatic Diseases,* 77:1246-1247. Accessed on April http://dx.doi.org/10.1136/annrheumdis-2018-eular.4689.

[32] Hwang, Jie H., Hyo W. Jung, Seung Y. Oh, Jong-Seong Kang, Jong-Pil Kim, and Yong-Ki Park 2017. "Effects of *Zingiber officinale* extract on collagen-induced arthritis in mice and IL-1β-induced inflammation in human synovial fibroblasts. *European Journal of Inflammation*, 168-178. Accessed on April 20, 2021. doi:10.1177/1721727X17727997

[33] Levy, Arkene S.A., Oswald Simon, Janet Shelly, and Michael Gardener 2006. "6-Shogaol reduced chronic inflammatory response in the knees of rats treated with complete Freund's adjuvant". *BMC Pharmacol.*, 6:12. Accessed on April 20, 2021. doi:10.1186/1471-2210-6-12.

[34] Aborehab, Nora M., Mahitab H. El Bishbishy, Abeer Refaiy, and Nermien E. Waly. 2017. "A putative Chondroprotective role for IL-1β and MPO in herbal treatment of experimental osteoarthritis." *BMC Complementary and Alternative Medicine* 17(1): 495. Accessed on May 10, 2021. doi:10.1186/s12906-017-2002-y.

[35] Frondoza, Carmelita G., Afshin Sohrabi, Anna Polotsky, Phong V. Phan, David S. Hungerford, and Lars Lindmark 2004. "An in vitro screening assay for inhibitors of proinflammatory mediators in herbal extracts using human synoviocyte cultures". *In Vitro Cell. Dev. Biol. Anim.*, 40(3-4):95-101. Accessed on April 20, 2021. doi: 10.1290/1543-706x(2004)040<0095:aivsaf>2.0.co;2.

[36] Phan, Phong V., Afshin Sohrabi, Anna Polotsky, David S. Hungerford, Lars Lindmark, and Carmelita G. Frondoza CG 2005.

Ginger extract components suppress induction of chemokine expression in human synoviocytes. *The Journal of Alternative and Complementary Medicine*, 11:1, 149-154. Accessed on April 20, 2021. https://doi.org/10.1089/acm.2005.11.149.

[37] Ribel-Madsen, Søren, Else Marie Bartels, Anders Stockmarr, Arne Borgwardt, Claus Cornett, Bente Danneskiold-Sammsøe, and Henning A. Bliddal 2012. "Synoviocyte model for osteoarthritis and rheumatoid arthritis: Response to ibuprofen, betamethasone and ginger extract – a cross-sectional *in vitro* study". *Arthritis*, 2012; Article ID 505842. Accessed on April 20, 2021. https://doi.org/10.1155/2012/505842.

[38] Hwang, Youn-Hwan, Taesoo Kim, Raejong Kim, and Hunil Ha 2018. "The Natural Product 6-Gingerol Inhibits Inflammation-Associated Osteoclast Differentiation via Reduction of Prostaglandin E_2 Levels". *Int. J. Mol. Sci.*, 19(7):2068. Accessed on April 20, 2021. doi:10.3390/ijms19072068.

[39] Fajrin, Fifteen A., Aguna E. Nugroho, Rina Susilowati, and Arief Nurrochmad 2018. "Molecular Docking Analysis of Ginger Active Compound on Transient Receptor Potential Cation Channel Subfamily V Member 1 (TRPV1)". *Indonesian Journal of Chemistry,* 18(1): 179-185. Accessed on April 20, 2021. https://doi.org/10.22146/ijc.28172

[40] Mathiessen, Alexander, and Philip G. Conaghan 2017. "Synovitis in osteoarthritis: current understanding with therapeutic implications". *Arthritis Res. Ther.*, 19(1):18. Accessed on April 20, 2021. doi:10.1186/s13075-017-1229-9.

[41] Lopez-Armada, M.J., B. Carames, M. Lires-Dean, B. Cillero-Pastor, C. Ruiz-Romero, F. Galdo, and F.J. Blanco 2006. "Cytokines, tumor necrosis factor-α and interleukin-1ß, differentially regulate apoptosis in osteoarthritis cultured human chondrocytes". *Osteoarthritis Cartilage*, 14: 660-669. Accessed on April 20, 2021. doi: 10.1016/j.joca.2006.01.005.

[42] Martel-Pelletier, J., R.P. Lajeunesse, and J-P. Pelletieer 2003. "Therapeutic role of dual inhibitors of 5-LOX and COX, selective and

non-selective non-steroidal anti-inflammatory drugs". *Ann. Rheum. Dis.*, 62: 501-509. Accessed on April 20, 2021. doi: 10.1136/ard.62.6.501.

[43] Manferdini, Cristina, Francesca Paolella, Elena Gabusi, Ylenia Silvestri, Laura Gambari, Luca Cattini, Giuseppe Filardo, Sandrine Fleury-Cappellesso, and Gina Lisignoli 2016. "From osteoarthritic synovium to synovial-derived cells characterization: synovial macrophages are key effector cells". *Arthritis Res. Ther.*, 18: 83. Accessed on April 20, 2021. https://doi.org/10.1186/s13075-016-0983-4.

[44] Sakkas, Lazaros I. and Chris D. Platsoucas 2007. "The role of T cells in the pathogenesis of osteoarthritis". *Arthritis & Rheumatism*, 56: 409-424. Accessed on April 20, 2021. doi:10.1002/art.22369.

[45] Haseeb, Abdul, and Tariq M. Haqqi 2013." Immunopathology of Osteoarthritis". *Clinical Immunology*, 146(2): 185-196. Accessed on April 20, 2021. doi: 10.1016/j.clim.2012.12.011.

[46] Tat, Steeve K., Nathalie Amiable, Jean-Pierre Pelletier, Christelle Boileau, Daniel Lajeunesse, Nicolas Duval, and Johanne Martel-Pelletier 2009. "Modulation of OPG, RANK and RANKL by human chondrocytes and their implication during osteoarthritis". *Rheumatology (Oxford)*, 48(12):1482-1490. Accessed on April 20, 2021. doi:10.1093/rheumatology/kep300.

[47] Alaaeddine, Nada, Tsaiwei Olee, Sanshiro Hashimoto, Lilo Creighton-Achermann, and Martin Lotz 2001. "Production of the chemokine RANTES by articular chondrocytes and role in cartilage degradation". *Arthritis Rheum.*, 44: 1633-1643. Accessed on April 20, 2021. doi: 10.1002/1529-0131(200107)44:7<1633::AID-ART286>3.0.CO;2-Z.

[48] Li, Xin, Michael Ellman, Prasuna Muddasani, James H.C. Wang, Gabriella Cs-Szabo, Andre van Wijnen AJ, and Hee-Jeong Im 2009. "PGE_2 and its cognate EP receptors control human adult articular cartilage homeostasis and are linked to the pathophysiology of osteoarthritis". *Arthritis Rheum.*, 60(2): 513-523. Accessed on April 20, 2021. doi: 10.1002/art.24258.

[49] Abramson, S.B. 1999. "The role of COX-2 produced by cartilage in arthritis". *Osteoarthritis Cartilage*, (4):380-1. Accessed on April 20, 2021. doi: 10.1053/joca.1998.0217.

[50] Prasadam, Indira, Thor Friis, Wei Shi, Stijn van Gennip, Ross Crawford R, and Yin Xiao. 2010. "Osteoarthritic cartilage chondrocytes alter subchondral bone osteoblast differentiation via MAPK signaling pathway involving ERK1/2. *Bone*, 46: 226-235. Accessed on April 20, 2021. doi: 10.1016/j.bone.2009.10.014.

[51] Chen, Hao, Bo Hu, Xiao Lv, Shouhan Zhu, Gehua Zhen, Mei Wan, Amit Jain, Bo Gao, Yu Chai, Mi Yang M, Xiao Wang, Ruoxian Deng, Lei Wang, Yong Cao, Shuangfei Ni, Shen Liu, Wen Yuan, Huajiang Chen, Xinzhong Dong, Yun Guan, Huilin Yang, and Xi Cao 2019. "Prostaglandin E2 mediates sensory nerve regulation of bone homeostasis". *Nat. Commun.*, 10: 181. Accessed on April 20, 2021. https://doi.org/10.1038/s41467-018-08097-7.

[52] Cremers, Niels A.J., Martijn van den Bosch, Stephanie van Dalen, Irene Di Ceglie, Giuliana Ascone, Fons van de Loo, Marije Koenders, Peter van der Kraan, Annet Sloetjers, Thomas Vogl, Johannes Roth, Edwin J.W. Geven, Arjen B. Blom, and Peter L.E.M. van Lent 2017. "S100A8/A9 increases the mobilization of pro-inflammatory Ly6C^{high} monocytes to the synovium during experimental osteoarthritis". *Arthritis Res. Ther.*, 19: 217. Accessed on April 20, 2021. https://doi.org/10.1186/s13075-017-1426-6

[53] Van Lent, Peter L.E.M., Arjen B. Blom, Rik F.P. Shelbergen, Annet Slöetjes, Floris P.J.G. Lafeber, Willem F. Lems, Hans Cats, Thomas Vogl, Johannes Roth, and Wim B, van den Berg 2012. "Active involvement of alarmins S100A8 and S100A9 in the regulation of synovial activation and joint destruction during mouse and human osteoarthritis". *Arthritis Rheum.*, 64: 1466-1476. Accessed on April 20, 2021. https://doi.org/10.1002/art.34315.

[54] Crowe, Lindsay A.N., Michael McLean, Susan M. Kitson, Emma G. Melchor, Katharina Patommel, Hai M. Hao, James H. Reilly, William J. Leach, Brian P. Rooney, Simon J. Spencer, Michael Mullen, Max Chambers, George A.C. Murrell, Iain B. McInnes, Moeed Akbar, and

Neal M. Millar 2019. "S100A8 & S100A9: Alarmin mediated inflammation in tendinopathy". *Sci. Rep.*, 9:1463. Accessed on April 20, 2021. https://doi.org/10.1038/s41598-018-37684-3

[55] Choi, Moon-Chang, Jowong Jo, Jonggwan Park, Hee K. Kang, and Yoonkyung Park 2019. "NF-κB Signaling Pathways in Osteoarthritic Cartilage Destruction". *Cells*, 8(7):734. Accessed on April 20, 2021. doi:10.3390/cells8070734.

[56] Ahmed, Syed M.U., Lin Luo, Akhileshwar Namani, Xiuje Wang, and Xiuwen Tang 2016. "Nrf2 signaling pathway: Pivotal roles in inflammation". *Biochmimica et Biophysica Acta*, 1863: 585-597. Accessed on April 20, 2021. https://doi.org/10.1016/j.bbadis.2016.11.005

[57] Zahan, Oana-Maria, Oana Serban, Claudia Gherman, and Daniela Fodor 2020. "The evaluation of oxidative stress in osteoarthritis". *Med. Pharm. Rep.*, 93(1):12-22. Accessed on April 20, 2021. doi:10.15386/mpr-1422.

[58] Blom, Arjen B., Sarah M. Brockbank, Peter L. van Lent, Henk M. van Beuningen, Jeroen Geurts, Nozomi Takahashi, Peter M. van der Kraan, Fons A. van de Loo, B. Wim Schreurs, Kristen Clements, Peter Newham, and Wim B. van den Berg 2009. "Involvement of the WNT signaling pathway in experimental and human osteoarthritis: Prominent role of WNT-induces signaling protein 1". *Arthritis Rheum.*, 60: 501-512. Accessed on April 20, 2021. doi: 10.1002/art.24247.

[59] Inkson, Colette A., Mitsuaki Ono, Sergei A. Kuznetsov, Larry W. Fisher, Pamela G. Robey, and Marion F. Young 2008. "TGF-β1 and WISP-1/CCN-4 can regulate each other's activity to cooperatively control osteoblast function". *J. Cell Biochem.*, 104; 1865-1878. Accessed on April 20, 2021. doi: 10.1002/jcb.21754.

[60] Scharstuhl, Alwin, Elly L. Vitters, Peter M. van der Kraan, and Wim B. van den Berg 2003. "Reduction of osteophyte formation and synovial thickening by adenoviral overexpression of transforming growth factor beta/ bone morphogenetic protein inhibitors during

experimental osteoarthritis". *Arthritis Rheum.*, 48: 3442-3451. Accessed on April 20, 2021. doi: 10.1002/art.11328.

[61] Baron, Roland, and Michaela Kneissel 2013. "WNT signaling in bone homeostasis and disease: From human mutations to treatments". *Nat. Med.*, 19: 179-192. Accessed on April 20, 2021. doi: 10.1038/nm.3074.

[62] Lodewyckx, Liesbet, and Rik J.U. Lories 2009. "WNT signaling in osteoarthritis and osteoporosis: What is the biological significance for the clinician?" *Curr. Rheumatol. Rep.*, 11: 23-30. Accessed on April 20, 2021. doi: 10.1007/s11926-009-0004-6.

[63] Blaney Davidson, Esmerelda N., Elly L. Vitters, Peter L.E.M. van Lent, Fons A. van de Loo, Wim B. van den Berg, and Peter M. van der Kraan 2007. "Elevated extracellular matrix production and degradation upon bone morphogenetic protein-2 (BMP-2) stimulation point toward a role for BMP-2 in cartilage repair and remodeling". *Arthritis Res. Ther.*, 9: R102:1-R102:11. Accessed on April 20, 2021. doi: 10.1186/ar2305.

[64] Rongchen, Dai, Wu Zeting, Chu Hang Yin, Lu Jun, Lyu Aiping, Liu Jin and Zhang Ge. 2020. "Cathepsin K: The Action in and Beyond Bone". *Frontiers in Cell and Developmental Biology*, 8:433. Accessed on April 20, 2021. DOI=10.3389/fcell.2020.00433.

[65] St-Jacques, Benoit, Mathias Hammerschmidt, and Andrew P. McMahon. 1999. "Indian hedgehog signaling regulates proliferation and differentiation of chondrocytes and is essential for bone formation" [published correction appears in Genes Dev 1999 Oct 1;13(19):2617]. *Genes Dev.*, 13(16):2072-2086. Accessed on April 20, 2021. doi:10.1101/gad.13.16.2072.

[66] Kielty, C. M., A.P. Kwan, D.F. Holmes, S.L. Schor, and M.E. Grant.1985. "Type X collagen, a product of hypertrophic chondrocytes". *The Biochemical Journal*, 227(2): 545–554. Accessed on April 20, 2021. https://doi.org/10.1042/bj2270545.

[67] Nguyen, Sinh T., Phuc H. Vo, Thao D. Nguyen, Nghia M. Do, Bao H. Le, Duong T Dinh, Kiet D. Truong, and Phuc D. Pham. "Ethanol extract of Ginger Zingiber *officinale* Roscoe by Soxhlet method

induces apoptosis in human hepatocellular carcinoma cell line." *Biomedical Research and Therapy*, 2019; 6(11): 3433-3442. Accessed on May 21, 2021. https://doi.org/10.15419/bmrat.v6i11.572.

[68] Vincent, Tonia L. 2019. "IL-1 in osteoarthritis: time for a critical review of the literature". *F1000Res.* 2019; 8: F1000 Faculty Rev-934. Accessed on April 20, 2021. doi:10.12688/f1000research.18831.1.

[69] Saxen, Irma 1975. "Associations between oral clefts and drugs taken during pregnancy". *Int. J. Epidemiol.*, 4: 37-44. Accessed on April 20, 2021. doi: 10.1093/ije/4.1.37.

[70] Chalasani, Naga, Raj Vuppalanchi, Victor Navarro, Robert Fontana, Herbert Bonkovsky, Huiman Barnhart, David E. Kleiner, and Jay H. Hoofnagle 2012. "Acute liver injury due to flavocoxid (Limbrel®), a medical food for osteoarthritis: a case series". *Ann. Intern. Med.*, 156(12): 857-860. Accessed on April 20, 2021. https://doi.org/10.7326/0003-4819-156-12-201206190-00006

[71] Tripathi, Sudipta, David Bruch, and Dilip S. Kittur 2008. "Ginger extract inhibits LPS induced macrophage activation and function". *BMC Complement. Altern. Med.*, 8:1. Accessed on April 20, 2021. doi: 10.1186/1472-6882-8-1.

[72] Tripathi, Sudipta, Kristopher G. Maier, David Bruch, and Dilip S. Kittur 2007. "Effect of 6-gingerol on pro-inflammatory cytokine production and costimulatory molecule expression in murine peritoneal macrophages". *J. Surg. Res.*, 138(2):209-13. Accessed on April 20, 2021. doi: 10.1016/j.jss.2006.07.051.

[73] Arango Duque, Guillermo, and Albert Descoteaux 2014. "Macrophage cytokines: involvement in immunity and infectious diseases". *Front. Immunol.*, 5:491. Accessed on April 20, 2021. doi:10.3389/fimmu.2014.00491.

[74] Nievergelt, Andreas, Janine Marazzi, Roland Schoop, Karl-Heinz Altmann, and Jűrg Gertsch 2011. "Ginger Phenylpropanoids Inhibit IL-1β and Prostanoid Secretion and Disrupt Arachidonate-Phospholipid Remodeling by Targeting Phospholipases A_2". *The Journal of Immunology*, 187 (8): 4140-4150. Accessed on April 20, 2021. doi: 10.4049/jimmunol.1100880.

[75] Ahn, Sang-Ihl, Jun-Kyung Lee, and Hyung-Sun Youn H 2009. "Inhibition of homodimerization of toll-like receptor 4 by 6-shogaol". *Mol. Cells* 27: 211–215. Accessed on April 20, 2021. https://doi.org/10.1007/s10059-009-0026-y

[76] Oppl, Bastian, Christian Datz,, Ursula Huber-Schönauer, Emma Husar-Memmer, Wolfgang Brozek, Peter Zenz, Eva Gollob, Christian Wurnig, Alfred Engel, Klaus Klaushofer, Jochen Zwerina, and Johan Bartko. 2019. "Vascular cell adhesion molecule 1 in patients with severe osteoarthritis of the hip: A prospective cross-sectional study". *Wiener Klinische Wochenschrift,* 131(15-16): 369–373. Accessed on May 24, 2021. https://doi.org/10.1007/s00508-019-1497-2.

[77] Kaptchuk, Ted J. 2001. "The double-blind, randomized, placebo-controlled trial: gold standard or golden calf?" *J Clin Epidemiol*, 54(6):541-9. Accessed on May 24, 2021. doi: 10.1016/s0895-4356(00)00347-4.

[78] Bartels, E.M., V.N. Folmer, H. Bliddal, R.D. Altman, C. Juhl, S. Tarp, W. Zhang, and R. Christensen. 2015. "Efficacy and safety of ginger in osteoarthritis patients: a meta-analysis of randomized placebo-controlled trials". *Osteoarthritis and Cartilage*, 123(1):13-21. Accessed on May 28, 2021.

[79] Niempoog, Sunyarn, Kammal K. Pawa, and Chumpot Amatyakul. 2012. "The efficacy of powdered ginger in osteoarthritis of the knee". *J Med Assoc Thai*, 95 Suppl 1: S59-64. Accessed on May 28, 2021. PMID: 23964445.

[80] Therkleson, Tessa 2014. "Topical Ginger Treatment with a compress or patch for osteoarthritis Symptoms". *J. Holist Nurs*., 32(3):173-182. Accessed on April 20, 2021. doi:10.1177/0898010113512182

[81] Amorndoljai, Punyanut, Surasak Taneepanichskul, Suyarn Niempoog, and Ubonthip Nimmannit 2015. "Improving of Knee Osteoarthritic Symptom by the Local Application of Ginger Extract Nanoparticles: A Preliminary Report with Short Term Follow-Up". *J. Med. Assoc. Thai*., 98(9):871-7. Accessed on April 20, 2021. PMID: 26591397.

[82] Amorndoljai, Punyanut, Surasak Taneepanichskul, Suyarn Niempoog, and Ubonthip Nimmannit. 2017. "Comparative of Ginger Extract in Nanostructure Lipid Carrier (NLC) and 1% Diclofenac Gel for Treatment of Knee Osteoarthritis (OA)". *J Med Assoc Thai*, 00(4):447-56. Accessed on April 20, 2021. PMID: 29911849.

[83] Chu, Constance R., Ashley A. Williams, Christian H. Coyle, and Megan E. Bowers 2012. "Early diagnosis to enable early treatment of pre-osteoarthritis". *Arthritis Res. Ther.*, 14(3):212. Accessed on April 20, 2021. doi:10.1186/ar3845.

[84] Cundell, Diana R. 2014. "Herbal phytochemicals as immunomodulators". *Current Immunology Reviews* 10(2): 64-81. Accessed April 20, 2021. http://benthamscience.com/journal/index.php?journalID=cir

[85] Grässel, Susanne, and Dominique Muschter 2020. "Recent advances in the treatment of osteoarthritis". *F1000Res.*,9: F1000 Faculty Rev-325. Accessed on April 20, 2021. doi:10.12688/f1000research.22115.1

[86] Gómez, Rodolfo, Amanda Villalvilla, Raquel Largo, Oreste Gualillo, and Gabriel Herrero-Beaumont 2015. "TLR4 signalling in osteoarthritis—finding targets for candidate DMOADs". *Nat. Rev. Rheumatol.*, 11:159–170. Accessed on April 20, 2021. https://doi.org/10.1038/nrrheum.2014.209

[87] Wang, Yudan, Xinhao Fan, Lei Xing, and Faming Tian 2019. "Wnt signaling: a promising target for osteoarthritis therapy". *Cell Commun. Signal.*, 17: 97. Accessed on April 20, 2021. https://doi.org/10.1186/s12964-019-0411-x

[88] Takada, Yasunari, Anjana Bhardwaj, Pravin Potdar, and Bharat B. Aggarwal 2004. "Nonsteroidal anti-inflammatory agents differ in their ability to suppress NF-kappaB activation, inhibition of expression of cyclooxygenase-2 and cyclin D1, and abrogation of tumor cell proliferation". *Oncogene*, 23(57):9247-58. Accessed on April 20, 2021. doi: 10.1038/sj.onc.1208169.

[89] Lisboa Felipe A., Matthew J. Bradley, Matthew T. Hueman, Seth A. Schobel, Beverly J. Gaucher, Edda L. Styrmisdottir, Benjamin K.

Potter, Jonathan A. Forsberg, and Eric A. Elster 2017. "Nonsteroidal anti-inflammatory drugs may affect cytokine response and benefit healing of combat-related extremity wounds". *Surgery*, 161(4): 1164-1173. Accessed on April 20, 2021. https://doi.org/10.1016/j.surg.2016.10.011.

[90] Sun, Kai, Jiahui Luo, Xingzhi Jing, Jiachao Guo, Xudong Yao, Xiaoxia Hao, Yaping Ye, Shuang Liang, Jiamin Lin, Genchun Wang, and Fengjing Guo 2019. "Astaxanthin protects against osteoarthritis via Nrf2: a guardian of cartilage homeostasis". *Aging (Albany NY)*, 11(22):10513-10531. Accessed on April 20, 2021. doi:10.18632/aging.102474.

[91] Ji, Baochao, Zhendong Zhang, Wentao Guo, Hairong Ma, Boyong Xu, Wenbo Mu, Abdusami Amat, and Li Cao 2018. "Isoliquiritigenin blunts osteoarthritis by inhibition of bone resorption and angiogenesis in subchondral bone". *Sci. Rep.*, 8: 1721. Accessed on April 20, 2021. https://doi.org/10.1038/s41598-018-19162-y.

[92] Clevers, Hans, and Roel Nusse 2012. "Wnt/β-catenin signaling and disease". *Cell*, 149(6):1192-205. Accessed on April 20, 2021. doi: 10.1016/j.cell.2012.05.012.

[93] Park, Ji S., and Mun Y. Jung 2012. "Development of high-performance liquid chromatography-time-of-flight mass spectrometry for the simultaneous characterization and quantitative analysis of gingerol-related compounds in ginger products". *J. Agric. Food Chem.*, 60: 10015-10026. Accessed on April 20, 2021. doi: 10.1021/jf302944p.

[94] Marx, Wolfgang, Elisabeth A. Isenring, and Anna E. Lohning 2017. "Determination of the concentration of major anti-emetic constituents within commercial ginger food products and dietary supplements". *Eur. J. Integ. Med.*, 10:19-24. Accessed on April 20, 2021. 10.1016/j.eujim.2017.02.001.

[95] Schwertner, Harvey A., Deborah C. Rios, and Joshua E. Pascoe 2006. "Variation in concentration and labeling of ginger root supplements". *Obstet. Gynecol.*, 107:1337-1443. Accessed on April 20, 2021. doi: 10.1097/01.AOG.0000217697.33787.8c.

[96] Zick, Suzanna M., Zora Djuric, Mack T. Ruffin, Amie J. Litzinger, Daniel P. Normolle, Sara Alrawi, Meihua R. Feng, and Dean E. Brenner 2017. "Pharmacokinetics of ginger phytochemicals". *Molecules*, 17:1930-1936. Accessed on April 7, 2021. doi: 10.1158/ 1055-9965.EPI-07-2934.

[97] Levita, Jutti, Dina M. Syafitri, Rini D. Supu, Mutakin Mutakin, Sandra Megantara, Maya Febrianti, and Ajeng Diantini 2018. "Pharmacokinetics of 10-gingerol and 6-shogaol in the plasma of healthy subjects treated with red ginger (*Zingiber officinale* var. *Rubrum*) suspension. *Biomedical Reports*, 9: 474-482. Accessed on April 20, 2021. https://doi.org/10.3892/br.2018.1163.

[98] Zhang, Mingzhen, Emilie Viennois, Meena Prasad, Yunchen Zhang, Lixen Wang, Zhen Zhang, Moon K. Han, Bo Xiao, Chanlong Xu, Shanthi Srinivasan, and Didier Merlin 2016. "Edible ginger-derived nanoparticles: A novel therapeutic approach for the prevention and treatment of inflammatory bowel disease and colitis-associated cancer". *Biomaterials*, 101:321-340. Accessed on April 20, 2021. doi:10.1016/j.biomaterials.2016.06.018.

[99] Zhang, Huiyun, Qilong Wang, Congyong Sun, Yuan Zhu, Qiuxuan Yang, Qiuyu Wei, Jiaxin Chen, Wenwen Deng, Michael Adu-Frimpong, Jiangnan Yu, and Ximing Xu 2019. "Enhanced Oral Bioavailability, Anti-Tumor Activity and Hepatoprotective Effect of 6-Shogaol Loaded in a Type of Novel Micelles of Polyethylene Glycol and Linoleic Acid Conjugate". *Pharmaceutics*, 11(3):107. Accessed on April 20, 2021. doi:10.3390/pharmaceutics11030107.

[100] Kalarikkal, Sreeram P., Durga Prasad, Ravi Kasiappan, Sachin R. Chaudhari, and Gopinath M. Sundaraam 2020. "A cost-effective polyethylene glycol-based method for the isolation of functional edible nanoparticles from ginger rhizomes". *Sci. Rep.*, 10: 4456. Accessed on April 20, 2021. https://doi.org/10.1038/s41598-020-61358-8.

[101] Finnin, B.C., and T.M. Morgan 1999. "Transdermal penetration enhancers: applications, limitations, and potential". *J. Pharm. Sci.*, 88(10):955-8. Accessed on April 20, 2021. doi: 10.1021/js990154g.

[102] Minghetti, Paolo, Silvio Sosa, Francesco Cilurzo, Antonella Casiraghi, Elisabetta Alberti, Aurelia Tubaro, Roberto D. Loggia, and Luisa Montanari 2007. "Evaluation of the topical anti-inflammatory activity of ginger dry extracts from solutions and plasters". *Planta Med.*, 73(15):1525-30. Accessed on April 20, 2021. doi: 10.1055/s-2007-993741.

[103] Park, Kwan-Kyun, Kyung-Soo Chun, Jong-Min Lee, Sang-Sup Lee, and Young-Joon Surh Y1998. "Inhibitory effects of [6]-gingerol, a major pungent principle of ginger, on phorbol ester-induced inflammation, epidermal ornithine decarboxylase activity and skin tumor promotion in ICR mice". *Cancer Letters*, 129(2): 139-144. Accessed on April 20, 2021. https://doi.org/10.1016/S0304-3835(98)00081-0.

[104] Chen, Chung-Yi, Kuo-Chen Cheng, Andy Y. Chang, Ying-Ting Lin, You-Cheng Hseu, and Hui-Min Wang 2012. "10-Shogaol, an antioxidant from Zingiber officinale for skin cell proliferation and migration enhancer". *Int. J. Mol. Sci.*, 13(2):1762-1777. Accessed on April 20, 2021. doi:10.3390/ijms13021762.

[105] Padher Shweta 2017. "*In vitro* skin permeation and biological evaluation of gingerol and piperine cream". *Journal of Medicinal Plant Studies*, 5(5): 300-302. Accessed on April 20, 2021. https://www.plantsjournal.com/archives/2017/vol5issue5/PartD/5-5-13-499.pdf

[106] Viswanathan, B, R. Madhan, G. Srinivasan, M. Muralidaran, and K. Selvakumar 2012. "Study on improving bioavailability ratio of anti-inflammatory compound from ginger through nano transdermal delivery". *Asian Journal of Pharmaceutical and Clinical Research*, 5: 241-246.

[107] Kesarwani, Kritika, and Rajiv Gupta 2013. "Bioavailability enhancers of herbal origin: an overview". *Asian Pac. J. Trop. Biomed.*, 3(4):253-266. Accessed on April 20, 2021. doi:10.1016/S2221-1691(13)600 60-X

[108] Dedov, Vadim N., Van H. Tran, Colin C. Duke, Mark Connor, MacDonald J. Christie, Sravan Mandadi, and Basil D. Roufogalis

2002. "Gingerols: a novel class of vanilloid receptor (VR1) agonists". *British Journal of Pharmacology*, 137(6):793-798. Accessed on April 20, 2021. doi: 10.1038/sj.bjp.0704925.

[109] Persson, M.S.M., J. Stocks, D.A. Walsh, M. Doherty, and W. Zhang 2018. "The relative efficacy of topical non-steroidal anti-inflammatory drugs and capsaicin in osteoarthritis: a network meta-analysis of randomised controlled trials". *Osteoarthritis Cartilage*, 26(12):1575-1582. Accessed on April 20, 2021. doi:10.1016/j.joca.2018.08.008

[110] Takaishi, Masayuki, Kunitoshi Uchida, Yoshiro Suzuki, Hiroshi Matsui, Tadashi Shimada, Fumitaka Fujita, and Makoto Tominaga 2016. "Reciprocal effects of capsaicin and menthol on thermosensation through regulated activities of TRPV1 and TRPM8". *J. Physiol. Sci.*, 66(2):143-155. Accessed on April 20, 2021. doi:10.1007/s12576-015-0427-y

[111] Cundell, Diana R., and Anne H. Bower 2015. "Potential for turmeric in preventing chronic inflammatory disease: A review of the clinical evidence". In: Taylor GE Ed, *Tumeric Nutritional Properties, Uses and Potential Benefits*. New York: Nova Science Publishers, pp 51-132.

[112] Zhong, Hao, Ging Chan, Yuanjia Hu, Hao Hu, and Defang Ouyang 2018. "A Comprehensive Map of FDA-Approved Pharmaceutical Products". *Pharmaceutics*, 10(4):263. Accessed on April 20, 2021. doi:10.3390/pharmaceutics10040263.

[113] Alkilani, Ahlam Z., Meliosa T. McCrudden, and Ryan F. Donnelly 2015. "Transdermal Drug Delivery: Innovative Pharmaceutical Developments Based on Disruption of the Barrier Properties of the stratum corneum". *Pharmaceutics*, 7(4):438-470. Accessed on April 20, 2021. doi:10.3390/pharmaceutics7040438.

[114] Benson, Heather A.E., Jeffrey E. Grice, Yousuf Mohammed, Sarika Namjoshi, and Michael S. Roberts 2019. "Topical and Transdermal Drug Delivery: From Simple Potions to Smart Technologies". *Current Drug Delivery,* 16(5):444-460. Accessed on April 20, 2021. doi: 10.2174/1567201816666190201143457.

EDITOR'S CONTACT INFORMATION

Diana R. Cundell, PhD
Professor of Biology,
College of Life Sciences,
Thomas Jefferson University,
Philadelphia, PA, USA
Diana.Cundell@jefferson.edu

INDEX

B

C

D

E

F

I

R

S

W

Z

α

β

γ